# THE S.T.A.B.L.E. Program

## Pre-transport / Post-resuscitation Stabilization Care of Sick Infants
## Guidelines for Neonatal Healthcare Providers – 6th Edition

Learner / Provider Manual

Kristine A. Karlsen

This educational program provides general guidelines for the assessment and stabilization of sick infants in the post-resuscitation / pre-transport stabilization period. These guidelines are based upon evidence-based recommendations in neonatal texts and published literature whenever possible. When necessary, common neonatal stabilization care practices were evaluated and incorporated into this program. Changes in infant care may impact the recommendations contained in this program; such changes should be assessed on a regular basis. While caring for sick infants, healthcare providers may encounter situations, conditions, and illnesses not described in this manual. It is strongly recommended that additional nursing and medical education materials and consultation with neonatal experts are utilized as necessary. Prior to implementing these program guidelines, the content of this manual should be reviewed and approved for use by appropriate policy committees at your institution or facility.

© 2013 Kristine A. Karlsen. All rights reserved
Salt Lake City, S.T.A.B.L.E., Inc.
ISBN: 978-1-937967-02-4

Address communications to:
**Kristine A. Karlsen, PhD, APRN, NNP-BC**
**The S.T.A.B.L.E.® Program**
P.O. Box 980023
Park City, Utah 84098 USA
Phone 1-435-655-8171
Email: stable@stableprogram.org
**www.stableprogram.org**

**Graphic Designer**
Kristin Bernhisel-Osborn, MFA

**PowerPoint Designer**
Mary Puchalski, MS, APN, CNS, NNP-BC

**Medical Illustrators**
John Gibb, MA
Marilou Kundmueller RN, MA

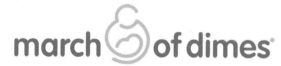

**S.T.A.B.L.E. is endorsed by the March of Dimes**

This book is dedicated to my family – Torbjorn, Annika and Solveig,

whose love and support have sustained me through my long journey with

S.T.A.B.L.E., and to the many incredible and dedicated neonatal healthcare

providers I have had the privilege to meet.

Your expert teaching and guidance does, and will continue to make a difference

in the lives of many babies and their families.

# Content Reviewers

## Specialty Reviewers

**Stephen Baumgart, MD**
Neonatologist,
Department of Neonatology
Professor of Pediatrics
The George Washington University
Medical Center
Children's National Medical Center
Washington, DC
*Temperature module*

**Robert D. Christensen, MD**
Medical Director, Newborn
Intensive Care Unit
McKay Dee Medical Center
Ogden, Utah
Director, Neonatology Research
Intermountain Healthcare
Salt Lake City, Utah
*Lab work module*

**Earl C. (Joe) Downey, MD**
Clinical Professor of Pediatric
Surgery
University of Utah
Salt Lake City, Utah
*Surgery*

**Jennifer L. Grow, MD**
Staff Regional Neonatologist
Associate Professor of Pediatrics at
Northeast Ohio Medical University
Akron Children's Hospital
Akron, Ohio
*Temperature module*

**William W. Hay Jr., MD**
Professor of Pediatrics,
Neonatal Medicine
Associate Director, Colorado Clinical
and Translational Sciences Institute
Scientific Director, Perinatal
Research Center
University of Colorado School of
Medicine
Anschutz Medical Campus
Perinatal Research Center
Aurora, Colorado
*Sugar Module*

**Ross W. McQuivey, MD**
Medical Director, Clinical
Innovations LLC
Murray, Utah
Adjunct Clinical Faculty,
Department of Obstetrics &
Gynecology
Stanford University School of
Medicine
Stanford, California
*Obstetrics*

**Charles Mercier, MD**
Professor of Pediatrics
University of Vermont
Medical Director, Neonatal
Intensive Care
Vermont Children's Hospital
Burlington, Vermont
*Sugar Module*

**Beverley Robin, MD**
Assistant Professor of Pediatrics,
Division of Neonatology
Rush University Medical Center
Chicago, Illinois
*Airway Module*

**Paul J. Rozance, MD**
Associate Professor of Pediatrics,
Neonatal Medicine
University of Colorado School of
Medicine
Anschutz Medical Campus
Perinatal Research Center
Aurora, Colorado
*Sugar Module*

**Michael Varner, MD**
Professor,
Obstetrics and Gynecology
University of Utah
Health Sciences Center
Salt Lake City, Utah
*Obstetrics*

## Physicians

**Joseph Chou, MD, PhD**
Department of Pediatrics, Newborn
Services
Medical Director, Newborn
Intensive Care Unit
MassGeneral Hospital for Children
Boston, Massachusetts

**Alejandro B. Gonzalez, MD, FAAP**
Medical Director, Perinatal
Simulation Program
North Central Baptist Hospital
San Antonio, Texas

**Maggie Meeks, Dip Ed MD
FRCPCH**
Neonatal Paediatrician CDHB
Professional Practice Fellow
University of Otago
Christchurch Women's Hospital
Christchurch, New Zealand

**Prabhu S. Parimi, MD, FAAP**
Professor of Pediatrics
University of Kansas
School of Medicine
Director, Division of Neonatology
Medical Director, Neonatal
Intensive Care Unit
University of Kansas Hospital
Kansas City, Kansas

**Erick Ridout, MD, FAAP**
Medical Director
Neonatal Intensive Unit
Dixie Regional Medical Center
St. George, Utah

**Cynthia Schultz, MD, FAAP**
LCDR MC USN
S.T.A.B.L.E. National Faculty
NICU Medical Director
Naval Hospital Camp Lejeune
Camp Lejeune, North Carolina

**Howard Stein, MD**
Neonatologist,
Director of Neonatal Transport
Toledo Children's Hospital
Clinical Assistant Professor of
Pediatrics
The University of Toledo College of
Medicine
Toledo, Ohio

**John Wareham, MD**
Neonatologist
St. Vincent Women's Hospital
Indianapolis, Indiana

**Mary E. Wearden, MD**
Medical Director NICU
Baptist Health System
San Antonio, Texas

**Bradley A. Yoder, MD**
Medical Director, NICU
University Hospital
Professor of Pediatrics
Division of Neonatology
University of Utah
School of Medicine
Salt Lake City, Utah

## Neonatal Nurses and Nurse Practitioners

**Glenn Barber, RNC-NIC, BSN**
Perinatal Outreach Educator
SSM Cardinal Glennon Children's
Medical Center
St. Louis, Missouri

**Amy Hall, BSN, RN, CCRN, C-NPT**
Senior Flight Nurse
Pediatric/Neonatal Transport Team
Medical City Children's Hospital
Dallas, Texas

**Tracy Karp, MS, NNP-BC**
Chief, Discipline of Advanced
Practice Clinicians
Primary Children's Medical Center
Intermountain Healthcare
Salt Lake City, Utah

**Alta B. Kendall, MN, ARNP,
NNP-BC**
Neonate Intensive Care Unit
Tacoma General Hospital
Tacoma, Washington

**LCDR Jason D. Layton RNC, CNS,
NNP**
NICU Division Officer
Walter Reed National
Military Medical Center
Bethesda, Maryland

**Webra Price-Douglas, PhD, CRNP,
IBCLC**
Coordinator Maryland Regional
Neonatal Transport Program
University of Maryland Medical
Center and Johns Hopkins Hospital
Baltimore, Maryland

**Mary Puchalski, MS, APN, CNS,
NNP-BC**
Director, Neonatal Nurse
Practitioner Services
Rush University Medical Center
Instructor, Rush University
Chicago, Illinois

**Patricia A. Scott, DNP, APN,
NNP-BC, C-NPT**
Advanced Practitioner
Coordinator – Pediatrix Medical
Group of Tennessee
Vanderbilt University
School of Nursing
Coordinator of Neonatal
Transport Services –
Centennial Medical Center
S.T.A.B.L.E. National Faculty
Nashville, Tennessee

## Neonatal Respiratory Therapists

**Kimberly Firestone, BS, RRT**
Neonatal Outreach Educator
Akron Children's Hospital
Akron, Ohio

**John Taylor, BS, RRT**
Manager,
Neonatal Transport and Outreach
Texas Health Presbyterian
Hospital Dallas
Texas Health Presbyterian
Hospital Plano
Dallas, Texas

## Neonatal Pharmacists

**Nhan T. Hoang, Pharm.D.**
Clinical Pharmacist Neonatal
Intensive Care
Intermountain Medical Center
Murray, Utah

**Kara L. Murray, Pharm.D., BCPS**
Manager,
Clinical Therapeutics and Pharmacy
Clinical Services Group, HCA
Nashville, Tennessee

# Table of Contents

## Program Philosophy

All hospitals or birthing centers must be prepared for the resuscitation, stabilization, and transport or transfer of sick and/or preterm infants. This includes hospitals without delivery services because of the occasional unexpected arrival of a newly born sick or preterm infant in the emergency department.

## Program Goals

The S.T.A.B.L.E. Program is designed to provide important information about neonatal stabilization for maternal/infant healthcare providers in all settings – from community hospitals and birth centers, to emergency rooms and more complex hospital environments. A uniform, standardized process of care and comprehensive team approach can improve the infant's overall stability, safety and outcome.[1-3]

**Goal 1:** **Improve patient safety for infants by:**

(a) standardizing processes and approach to care;

(b) encouraging teamwork;

(c) identifying areas where medical errors can and do occur; and,

(d) reducing and eliminating preventable adverse events and errors.

**Goal 2:** **Organize this information using a mnemonic to assist with retention and recall of stabilization activities that are critical for the post-resuscitation / pre-transport care of sick infants.**

## Newborn Transport

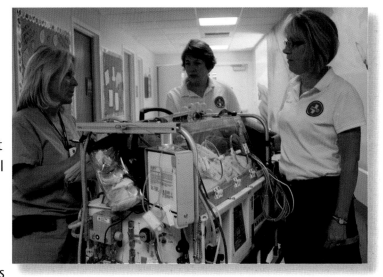

Ideally, mothers with identified high-risk pregnancies should deliver in a level III (subspecialty) perinatal facility so they may have access to care by maternal and infant specialists. However, as many as 30 to 50 percent of infants ultimately requiring neonatal intensive care do not present until the late intrapartum or early neonatal period, thus precluding safe maternal transport prior to delivery.[4] Therefore, it is vitally important that birth hospital providers are prepared to resuscitate and stabilize unexpectedly sick, and/or preterm infants. Adequate preparation of providers includes education and training in resuscitation and stabilization, and immediate access to necessary supplies and equipment.[5] Combined with accurate assessment and appropriate actions, such preparations will contribute to optimizing stabilization efforts prior to arrival of the transport team or prior to transfer of the infant to a neonatal intensive care unit (NICU).

The goal of all neonatal transport teams is to transport a well-stabilized infant. This goal is best achieved when care is provided in a timely, organized, comprehensive manner by all members of the healthcare team.

Because well babies far out-number those who are sick, in some settings healthcare providers may have difficulty remembering what to do for the sick infant. The mnemonic "S.T.A.B.L.E." was created to assist with information recall and to standardize and organize care in the pre-transport / post-resuscitation stabilization period.[6]

 stands for SUGAR and SAFE care

Delivery of safe, quality patient care, including the elimination of preventable errors is a top priority of the S.T.A.B.L.E. Program. Whenever possible, methods to provide safe care are emphasized.

> This symbol ⚠ is used throughout the program to draw attention to safety concerns and precautions so that extra care may be taken.

The Sugar module reviews the importance of establishing IV access when an infant is sick, infants at risk for hypoglycemia, the IV treatment of hypoglycemia, and the initial intravenous (IV) fluid therapy for sick infants. Indications for umbilical catheters and their safe use are included.

 stands for TEMPERATURE

This module reviews special thermal needs of infants including: those at increased risk for hypothermia, ways infants lose body heat, how to reduce heat loss, consequences of hypothermia, and methods for rewarming hypothermic infants. Neuroprotective therapeutic hypothermia for the treatment of hypoxic ischemic encephalopathy (HIE) is also discussed.

 stands for AIRWAY

This module reviews evaluation of respiratory distress, common neonatal respiratory diseases, airway challenges including detection and treatment of a pneumothorax, blood gas interpretation, signs of respiratory failure and when to increase the level of respiratory support, a commonly used method for securing an oral endotracheal tube, useful initial ventilator settings, and basic chest x-ray evaluation.

 stands for BLOOD PRESSURE

This module reviews risk factors for the three major causes of shock in infants: hypovolemic, cardiogenic, and septic shock, and how to assess and treat shock.

 stands for LAB WORK

This module focuses primarily on neonatal infection and includes maternal and neonatal risk factors, signs of infection, interpretation of the complete blood count (CBC) and the initial antibiotic treatment for suspected infection.

 stands for EMOTIONAL SUPPORT

This module reviews the crisis surrounding birth of a sick infant, and how to support families during this emotional and stressful period.

# The ABCs . . . .

When faced with an unexpectedly sick newborn, caregivers often ask: "Where should I start?" In any critical care situation, rapidly assess the infant and attend to immediate resuscitation needs. As we progress through the mnemonic of **S.T.A.B.L.E.**, remember that the ABCs of resuscitation — Airway, Breathing, and Circulation — are first priority. Although the algorithm for cardiac resuscitation care has changed for children and adults,[7] the priority for neonates remains **Airway** first.[8] Therefore, this program mnemonic is based upon:  A B C ➝ S.T.A.B.L.E.

An excellent resource for neonatal resuscitation is the American Heart Association and American Academy of Pediatrics *Textbook of Neonatal Resuscitation*,[9] also known as the Neonatal Resuscitation Program or NRP (www.aap.org). Although a resuscitation course is not a pre-requisite to participating in **S.T.A.B.L.E.**, it is strongly recommended that participants complete the NRP or a similar course prior to studying this program.

**Note:** Throughout this manual, the word "infant" will be used to describe babies from the first through the twenty-eighth day of life.

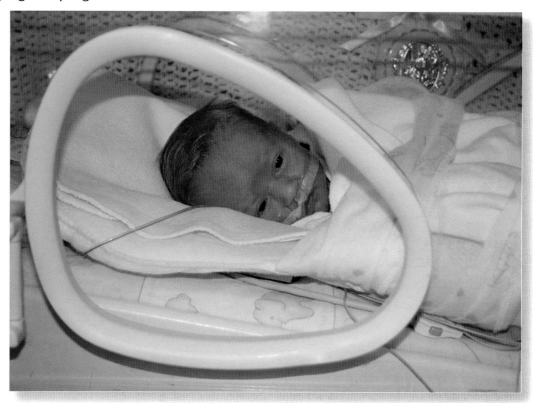

**S**ugar and **S**afe Care

**T**emperature

**A**irway

**B**lood Pressure

**L**ab Work

**E**motional Support

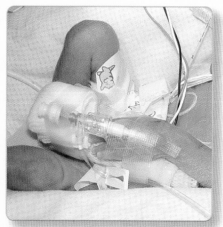

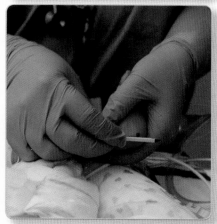

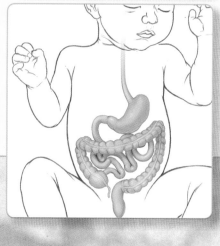

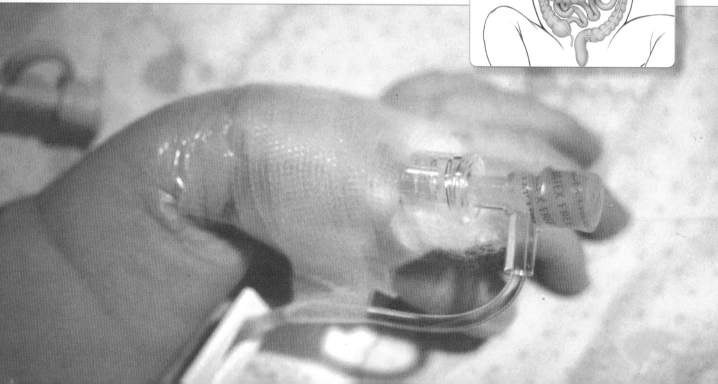

# Sugar and Safe Care – Module Objectives

Upon completion of this module, participants will gain an increased understanding of:

1. Issues of patient safety and error reduction in the delivery of health care to infants.

2. Infants at increased risk for developing hypoglycemia, including preterm and small for gestational age infants, infants of diabetic mothers, and sick, stressed infants.

3. The impact of late-preterm birth on increased morbidity and mortality.

4. Screening recommendations for gestational diabetes.

5. The physiologic basis of aerobic and anaerobic metabolism.

6. The initial intravenous fluid therapy to provide to sick infants.

7. Recommendations for monitoring the blood glucose.

8. Signs of hypoglycemia, IV glucose treatment of hypoglycemia and post-treatment reassessment.

9. Indications for placement of umbilical catheters.

10. The principles for safe use of umbilical catheters.

11. Surgical and medical abdominal conditions that present as bowel obstruction.

## Safe Patient Care

Every year, tens of thousands of infants are transported or transferred to neonatal intensive care units to receive specialized care for a variety of reasons: prematurity, problems related to delivery, infection, cardiac or surgical problems, and complex medical conditions.[10-14] Preparing maternal/child providers for the unexpectedly sick and/or preterm infant includes resuscitation and stabilization education,[15,16] skill acquisition, ensuring proper equipment and supplies are available, and providing an opportunity to practice technical, cognitive, and behavioral aspects of time pressured-emergencies via simulation-based education.[17-20]

The public expects to receive safe quality care every time they interact with healthcare providers and health systems. Simple, standardized care processes use guidelines and protocols to improve effectiveness of patient care and patient safety and to avoid reliance on memory. Vulnerable infants require more technology, medications, treatments, and procedures – all of which increase the potential for making errors. Short- and long-term outcomes may be affected by actions taken in the first minutes, hours and days after birth. Accurate diagnosis, monitoring, and clear, unambiguous communication all contribute to patient safety and improved outcomes. More information about errors, adverse events, and simulation-based training for healthcare teams are discussed in module seven, Quality Improvement.

## Sugar — General Guidelines

### I. If the infant is sick, do not give oral or gavage (enteral) feedings.

When an infant is sick, there are good reasons to withhold breast, bottle, and gavage feedings. Sick infants often have respiratory distress, which places them at increased risk for delayed gastric emptying and aspiration of stomach contents into the lungs.[21] Preterm infants, and/or infants with labored respirations have poor coordination of sucking, swallowing and breathing,[22,23] and some illnesses, including infection, may result in abdominal distension and delayed gastric emptying because of intestinal ileus.[24,25] If feedings are given under any of these circumstances, there is an increased risk that the infant will aspirate stomach contents into the lungs.

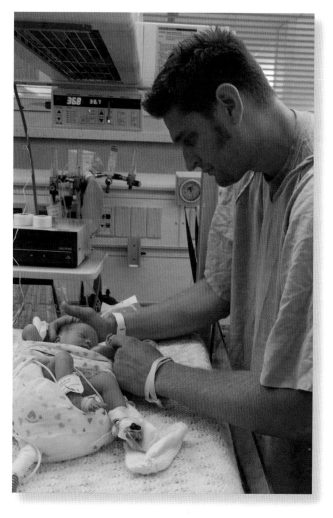

If the fetus or newborn experienced severely low blood oxygen levels (hypoxemia) or low blood pressure (hypotension) prior to, during, or after birth, intestinal blood flow may be reduced, making the intestine susceptible to ischemic injury.[26,27] Therefore, it is important to withhold enteral feedings and allow the bowel enough time to recover from any injury that may have occurred.

Finally, if the infant has a bowel obstruction he is at high risk for aspirating stomach contents. Feedings should be withheld and gastric decompression should be provided while awaiting transport or transfer to the neonatal intensive care unit.

Causes of bowel obstruction include:[28,29]

- Atresia anywhere in the intestinal tract: esophageal, duodenal, jejunal, ileal, or anal (see Figure 1.1 and Appendix 1.1);
- Malrotation with volvulus (see Figure 1.2);
- Functional causes, such as Hirschsprung's disease, meconium plug, or meconium ileus.

If the maternal history includes **polyhydramnios**, the infant should be observed closely for signs of bowel obstruction.[28] Excessive urine output in utero secondary to abnormalities in the genitourinary tract may also lead to polyhydramnios.[30,31] If the infant is coughing or choking with feedings, or he has excessive drooling, then **esophageal atresia (EA) and/or tracheoesophageal fistula (TEF)** should be suspected.[29] See Appendix 3.2 in the Airway module for additional information on EA/TEF.

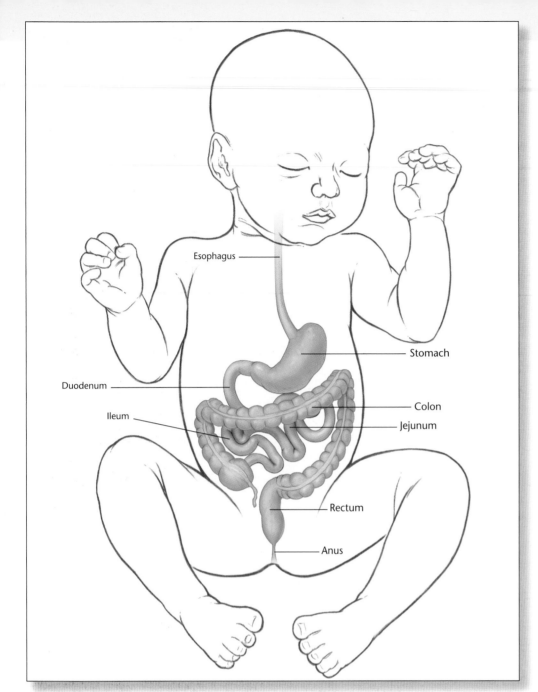

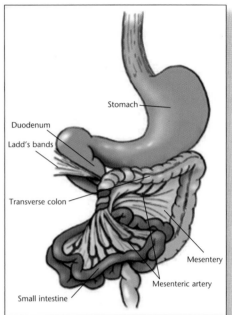

**Figure 1.1 Anatomical locations where bowel obstruction may occur.**

**Figure 1.2. Malrotation with midgut volvulus.** Rotation and twisting of the freely mobile bowel cuts off mesenteric artery blood supply to the intestine. Immediate surgery is necessary to untwist the bowel and restore blood flow.

## Malrotation with midgut volvulus[28-29]

Early in fetal life, between the 6th and 12th week of gestation, the developing, elongating intestine rotates and returns to the abdominal cavity. Upon entry into the abdomen, the duodenal-jejunal region becomes fixed by the ligament of Treitz which is located in the upper left part of the abdomen. The cecum then proceeds to return to the abdominal cavity and rotates counterclockwise until it is positioned correctly in the right lower quadrant, where it becomes fixed to the posterior abdominal wall.

This process of rotation and fixation is designed to prevent the intestine from being able to twist or become obstructed. At times however, upon entering the abdomen, the bowel fails to properly rotate. This condition is called **malrotation**. Bands of tissue that normally attach the colon to the posterior abdominal wall instead extend from the cecum to the region of the duodenum. Some infants with malrotation will present with duodenal obstruction. When the diagnostic work-up is performed, malrotation is discovered. Surgery is then required to cut the obstructing bands (also called Ladd's Procedure after a pediatric surgery pioneer) and to widen the mesentery so that **volvulus** (twisting of the bowel) will be prevented. Midgut volvulus occurs because the gut is not fixed or secured. Instead of a stable, secure "tacked down" small intestine, the small intestine is left mobile and freely able to twist. When twisting occurs, the mesenteric artery blood supply to the intestine is cut off. This life-threatening condition can occur at any age, however it most commonly occurs in the first few weeks of life. Figure 1.2 is an illustration of strangulated bowel secondary to midgut volvulus.

⚠ **One of the cardinal signs of bowel obstruction is bilious (green colored) emesis.**[29] Bilious emesis is worrisome and should be reported immediately to the medical staff provider. Physical examination of the infant and a diagnostic workup, which may include blood tests, an abdominal x-ray and radiographic studies, should be initiated quickly. Preferably, radiographic diagnostic studies are performed at a hospital with pediatric surgical services and by radiologists experienced in pediatric evaluation, as well as radiology staff that are prepared to monitor the infant and protect him from aspiration during the procedure. If unsure about the correct work-up, consult the tertiary neonatal intensive care physician for assistance.

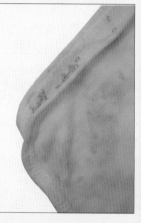
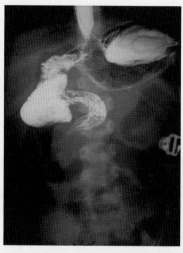

*Upper gastrointestinal study in an infant with midgut volvulus*

## II. Provide glucose via intravenous (IV) fluids.

Supporting the energy needs of sick infants with IV fluids containing glucose is an important component of stabilization. Glucose is one of the body's primary fuels. Unlike the liver, skeletal muscle or cardiac muscle, the brain cannot store adequate amounts of glucose in the form of glycogen and requires a steady supply of glucose to function normally.[32-35]

As soon as it is evident that the infant is sick, glucose-containing solutions should be given intravenously. It is important to also remain alert to the infant who has been identified as high risk for feeding intolerance or hypoglycemia, as these infants may also need an IV glucose infusion while feedings are being established.

For infants, the best peripheral IV insertion sites are in the hand, foot, or scalp veins. Figure 1.3 and the Clinical Tip: *pointers from intensive care nursery nurses on starting IVs in infants,* provides useful information for starting and securing IVs.

### IV Access

At times it may be difficult to insert an IV, especially if the infant is in shock or if caregivers have had little opportunity to practice this skill. If having difficulty inserting a peripheral IV, remember the **umbilical vein** can be used for delivering IV fluid and medications. The umbilical vein can usually be cannulated for up to one week after birth. Low-lying umbilical venous catheters are acceptable for urgent to emergent need for glucose infusion.[36] If unable to establish intravenous access, then the **intraosseous route** may be used.[37]

**Figure 1.3. Setting up for and securing a peripheral IV.**

## Insertion of a Peripheral IV

**For most infants, appropriate sizes are:**

24 gauge IV catheter or 23 or 25 gauge butterfly needle (with ¾ inch needle length).

> ⚠️ To reduce the risk of a needle stick injury and exposure to bloodborne pathogens, use a needle or catheter system with a safety device. When finished with the procedure, promptly and properly dispose the shielded stylet or needles in a regulation sharps container and wash hands or apply an antibacterial cleansing solution to hands.

## Preparation for Insertion of a Peripheral IV

- Wash and dry hands or apply an antiseptic solution to hands before beginning.
- Assemble all of the equipment that will be necessary for the procedure.
- Prepare the tape and clear surgical dressing so that it is ready to use when the IV is inserted.
- Apply gloves.
- Clean the skin with antiseptic solution around the insertion site and allow the solution to dry.
- Optional: a non-latex material tourniquet may be placed on the extremity above the area where you will insert the needle (take care to not cut off the blood supply).

> ⚠️ Observe evidence-based guidelines for hand hygiene before and after patient contact![38]

### Step 1

A (cold light) transillumination light or a bright pen light held beneath the hand or foot helps the veins become visible. Insert the needle or catheter into the vein and ensure there is good blood return. Hypotensive infants may have very slow blood return, so be patient. Remove the tourniquet (if one was used) when blood return is noted. If using a catheter, follow the manufacturer's recommendation for advancing the catheter and for discarding or securing the needle stylet.

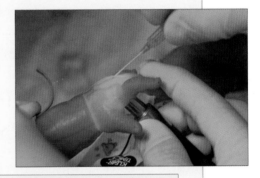

> ⚠️ Take care to check that any light source used does not transmit heat, which could burn the skin.

### Step 2

If using a catheter, secure it by placing a small piece of sterile transparent semipermeable membrane dressing over the catheter from the hub down to below the insertion site. If this dressing is not available, then secure the hub with a piece of ½ inch tape.

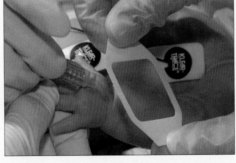
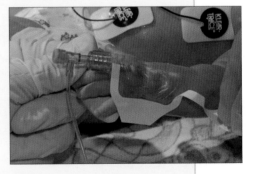

Avoid covering the needle insertion site with tape as this will obscure observation of the site for infiltration or redness. If using a butterfly needle, place the tape such that it also covers the butterfly wings.

### Step 3

While taping, periodically ensure patency by flushing the IV with a small amount of sterile normal saline (NS).

## Step 4

Place a ½ inch piece of tape over the hub. Avoid placing tape over the insertion site of the needle or catheter so that the site can be monitored during infusion of fluids or medications. The sterile transparent semipermeable membrane dressing will allow for optimal observation, yet hold the needle/catheter securely.

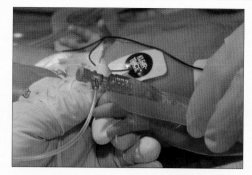
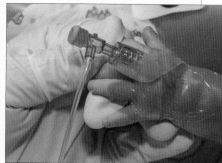
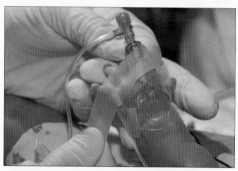
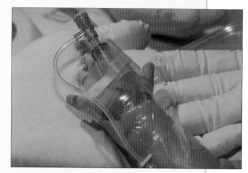

## Step 5

At times it may be necessary to use a padded "board" to prevent flexion of the arm or leg. Try to secure the area in the most anatomically correct position. To help prevent accidental dislodgment of the IV, secure the tubing with a ½ inch piece of tape such that the tape does not touch the hub or wings of the IV needle. Double back tape or cushion the tape with a gauze pad to prevent unnecessary contact with the skin.

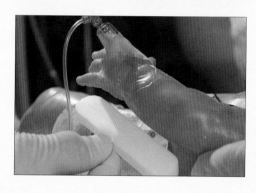
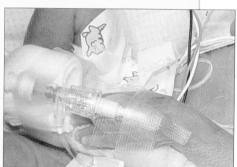
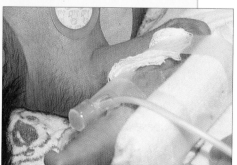

## Monitoring

Observe the IV site closely for swelling or redness which may indicate infiltration. If these signs are observed then it is safest to remove the IV and insert a new one in another area. Document hourly the appearance of the IV and the amount of fluid that was infused in the past hour. Protect the IV from dislodgment whenever the infant is moved.

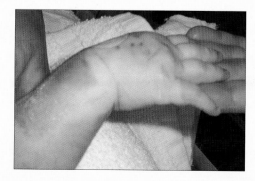
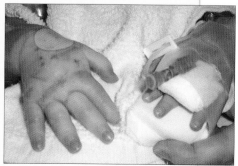

## Clinical Tip

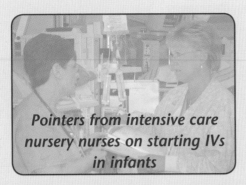

*Pointers from intensive care nursery nurses on starting IVs in infants*

1. Use two people to start the IV. One should bundle and comfort the infant while the other prepares the materials and places the IV.

2. This is a painful procedure. If the infant is able to suck on a pacifier, this may reduce discomfort during the procedure. When possible, a few drops of sucrose placed on the tongue should be provided for pain and comfort.

3. When placing an IV in the scalp, swab the skin with alcohol immediately before piercing the vein. This will help to briefly dilate the vein. Because the alcohol dries quickly, the infant should not feel a sting.

4. Palpate for arterial pulsation prior to placing an IV in scalp veins. If a pulse is felt, the vessel is likely an artery and should not be used. If the skin blanches once the IV is inserted, the IV is in an artery and should be removed. Apply pressure to the site for at least several minutes to be sure all bleeding has stopped.

5. Move slowly and be patient. Blood return may be very slow in infants who are hypotensive or otherwise compromised. Once you see the flashback of blood, slowly advance the IV catheter off the stylet into the vein.

6. Use any protective devices provided with your IV equipment to protect against accidental needle sticks and immediately discard needles in a proper disposal container.

7. When using a butterfly needle, enter the skin approximately ¼ inch away from where you plan on entering the vein. This will improve stability of the IV needle once it is placed. Once you have a blood return, don't try to cannulate the vein further because the butterfly needle may go through the vein.

## III. Some infants are at increased risk for low blood sugar (glucose) or "hypoglycemia."

Preterm infants (less than 37 weeks gestation), small for gestational age (SGA) infants, large for gestational age (LGA) infants, infants of diabetic mothers (IDM), and stressed, sick infants are at increased risk for becoming hypoglycemic.[39,40] In addition, some medications given to pregnant women increase the risk for neonatal hypoglycemia. These medications and their effect on glucose metabolism are described in Table 1.1.

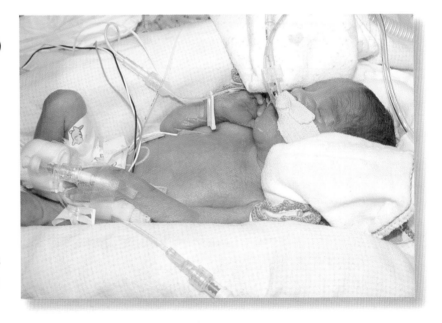

| Medication[a] | Used for treatment of: | Effect on neonate's glucose metabolism |
|---|---|---|
| **Beta-sympathomimetics**[32,41-43]<br>Terbutaline | Preterm labor | Maternal hyperglycemia leads to fetal pancreatic beta cell stimulation and increased fetal insulin secretion.<br><br>Drug crosses the placenta and breaks down glycogen in the fetus. |
| **Sulfonylureas**[44-48]<br>Chlorpropamide [b]<br>Glyburide [c]<br>Glipizide | Type 2 diabetes | Maternal hyperglycemia leads to fetal pancreatic beta cell stimulation and increased insulin secretion.<br><br>Drug crosses the placenta and promotes insulin secretion directly. |
| **Beta blockers**[49,50]<br>Labetalol<br>Propranolol<br>Metoprolol<br>Pindolol<br>Atenolol | Hypertension<br>Migraine headaches<br><br>Propranolol is also used for thyrotoxicosis | **Blocks** fetal $\beta_2$ adrenergic receptors (adrenocepters) preventing their stimulation of hepatic glycogen breakdown (glycogenolysis) and pancreatic release of glucagon.<br><br>Drug persists in the neonate after birth and prevents glycogenolysis. |
| **Thiazide diuretics**[51]<br>Chlorothiazide<br>Hydrochlorothiazide<br>Chlorthalidone | Hypertension<br>Edema | Maternal hyperglycemia leads to fetal pancreatic beta cell stimulation and increased insulin secretion. |
| **Tricyclic antidepressants**[52,53]<br>Amitriptyline<br>Nortriptyline<br>Imipramine<br>Desipramine | Depression | Maternal hyperglycemia leads to fetal pancreatic beta cell stimulation and increased insulin secretion. |
| Maternal IV dextrose [d] administration during labor[54] | Labor hydration | Glucose crosses the placenta and causes increased fetal insulin secretion. |

**Table 1.1.** Maternal medications and effect on the neonate's glucose metabolism.[55,56]

Notes:

a Not all medications are listed for each class described.

b First generation sulfonylurea implicated as possible teratogen.

c Increasing evidence that glyburide achieves similar glycemic control as insulin therapy and risk for hypoglycemia and macrosomia in neonate is not increased.[45,47]

d Appropriate IV fluid administration during labor varies based on maternal indication and includes NS, $D_5W$, $D_5NS$, $D_5LR$.

# Preparation for Extrauterine Life and Factors that Affect Glucose Stability after Birth

In preparation for extrauterine life, the fetus stores glucose in the form of glycogen. The fetus has limited ability to convert glycogen to glucose, and so relies primarily on placental transfer of glucose and amino acids to meet energy demands.[32,57] When the cord is cut, the infant no longer receives glucose from the mother. Enzymes activate the breakdown of glycogen back into glucose molecules which are released into the blood stream. This process makes glucose available to meet the infant's energy needs after birth.[58]

## Three Main Factors that Impact Blood Glucose after Birth

Three main factors that negatively affect an infant's ability to maintain normal blood glucose after birth include:

- Inadequate glycogen stores and decreased glucose production.
- Hyperinsulinemia, which suppresses glucose production and increases glucose utilization.
- Increased glucose utilization.

### Inadequate Glycogen Stores and Decreased Glucose Production: *High Risk Groups*

#### Preterm infants

Glycogen is stored in the liver, heart, lung and skeletal muscle.[56] Although glycogen stores increase slowly during the first and second trimesters, the majority of glycogen is stored during the latter part of the third trimester.[32] At term, glycogen accounts for approximately 5 to 8 percent of the liver and muscle weight, and 4 percent of the cardiac muscle weight.[59] Infants born preterm may have inadequate amounts of stored glycogen and available glycogen stores may be depleted rapidly after birth, thus placing these infants at increased risk for hypoglycemia.[58]

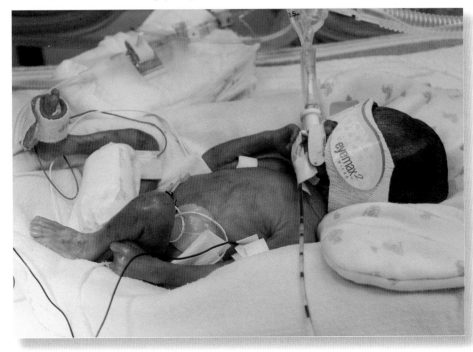

## Inadequate Glycogen Stores and Decreased Glucose Production: *High Risk Groups*
(continued)

### Late preterm infants

Infants born between 34-0/7 and 36-6/7 weeks are classified as "late preterm".[60] In the United States, approximately 71% of all preterm births are infants born in the late preterm age group.[61] Regardless of their weight, infants born before 37 weeks are metabolically and physiologically immature. The earlier the gestation, the more pronounced this becomes. Late preterm infants are at increased risk for clinical complications including hypoglycemia, feeding problems - including delayed or problematic breastfeeding, temperature instability, respiratory distress, apnea, hyperbilirubinemia, and higher hospital readmission rates.[60,62-65]

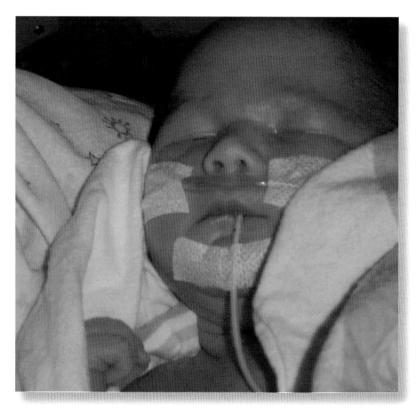

There are a variety of medical reasons why an infant may deliver or be delivered before term gestation is reached, including maternal indications such as placental abruption or previa, spontaneous labor, hypertension, cardiac disease or other maternal diseases that jeopardize maternal health; or fetal indications such as fetal heart abnormalities, oligohydramnios, intrauterine growth restriction, or other indications that place the fetus in jeopardy.[66] However, it is important to recognize that late preterm infants have a three-fold higher mortality rate when compared with term infants,[61] and there is evidence that neurodevelopmental outcomes are negatively impacted when infants are born late preterm.[67,68]

 When an infant is born in the late preterm gestation period, provide appropriate vigilance and surveillance monitoring! **Anticipate problems** that may occur, **recognize problems** when they do occur, and **act on problems** quickly to restore stability. **Reassess** the infant at regular intervals, as changes may occur that were not evident during earlier assessments.

## Inadequate Glycogen Stores and Decreased Glucose Production: *High Risk Groups* (continued)

### Small for gestational age infants (SGA) with symmetric and asymmetric growth patterns

SGA infants are usually defined as those with a birth weight below the 10th percentile for their gestational age.[69] Other definitions of SGA include when the birthweight is more than 2 standard deviations (SD) below the mean for gestational age,[70] or when the birthweight is below the 3rd or 5th percentile.[71] When compared with appropriately grown (AGA) preterm and term infants, SGA infants have higher complication rates, including death.[56,72,73] Growth in utero is influenced by genetics, the ability of the placenta to deliver oxygen and nutrients, and intrauterine growth factors and hormones.[69] Causes of insufficient growth of the fetus include the following:

### Fetal factors[71,76]

1 day old, 35 weeks gestation, 1850 grams

- ◇ Chromosomal abnormalities
- ◇ Genetic abnormalities
- ◇ Syndromes
- ◇ Metabolic disorders
- ◇ Intrauterine viral infection, especially early in gestation (cytomegalovirus, rubella, toxoplasmosis, syphilis, varicella, malaria)
- ◇ Multiple gestation

### Maternal factors[71,74-77]

- ◇ Nutritional status before and during pregnancy
- ◇ Chronic illness: hypertension, diabetes with underlying vascular disease, cyanotic congenital heart disease, renal disease, anemia, chronic pulmonary illness (asthma, cystic fibrosis)
- ◇ Uterine factors: uteroplacental vascular insufficiency, anatomy, size, multiple gestation, short interpregnancy interval (less than six months)
- ◇ Impaired placental function and ability to deliver oxygen and nutrients: preeclampsia, hypertension, diabetes
- ◇ Ingestion of drugs of abuse and toxins: nicotine, heroin, methadone, cocaine, morphine, methamphetamine, alcohol, toluene (glue and paint sniffing)
- ◇ Prescription medications used for chemotherapy (methotrexate, aminopterin, busulfan), seizure control (diphenylhydantoin, trimethadione), hypertension (propranolol), anticoagulant therapy (warfarin)
- ◇ Genetic and familial factors for small infant size
- ◇ Note: some infants may be "constitutionally small" but otherwise healthy
- ◇ Chronic psychosocial stress

Inadequate Glycogen Stores and Decreased Glucose Production: *High Risk Groups*
(continued)

**A chronically stressed fetus** may use most, if not all, of the placentally transferred glucose for growth and survival. This limits the ability to make or store glycogen for use after birth. The risk for hypoglycemia in term infants who have intrauterine growth restriction (IUGR) is estimated at 25 percent. Preterm infants with IUGR are at even higher risk.[78]

## Clinical Tip

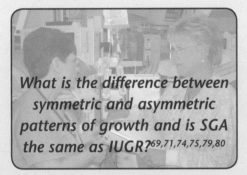

*What is the difference between symmetric and asymmetric patterns of growth and is SGA the same as IUGR?*[69,71,74,75,79,80]

**Symmetric growth restriction** (or symmetric SGA) infants have a lower weight, length, and head circumference for their gestational age. When these parameters are plotted on a graph, each will usually be at or below the 10th percentile. Symmetric SGA growth often results from intrauterine viral infection in early gestation, longstanding maternal disease with placental growth restriction present throughout most of pregnancy, or from chromosomal or genetic causes.

**Intrauterine growth restriction** (IUGR) is a term used to describe infants who have altered fetal growth, especially in the third trimester when lipid accumulation is greatest and growth is rapid. However, IUGR can at times be detected on a second trimester ultrasound.

The term "IUGR" is often used interchangeably with "SGA", however, they are not the same thing. Infants with IUGR have **asymmetric growth restriction**. Their weight will be low for their gestational age, followed by some impact on length, but with relatively less restriction in brain growth and head circumference (often referred to as "head sparing"). IUGR infants may appear "wasted," long and thin. This asymmetric pattern of growth usually results from maternal medical conditions or poor placental function that disrupts oxygen and nutrient delivery to the fetus during the last trimester of pregnancy. While the cause of growth restriction may not be easily apparent, assessment of the above factors (genetics, infection, maternal medical conditions, and placental function) must be considered as they may impact future pregnancies.

It is important to perform an accurate gestational age assessment before plotting the weight, head circumference, and length on the growth chart. If the gestational age assessment is incorrect, then the assessment of the infant's size may be inaccurate. See Appendices 1.2 and 1.3 for female and male growth charts.[81]

## Hyperinsulinemia*: *High Risk Groups*

### Infant of a diabetic mother (IDM)

The only source of glucose available to a fetus is that transferred across the placenta from the maternal circulation. This transfer occurs by combined mechanisms of facilitated diffusion and active transport. The blood glucose concentration in the fetus is typically only 70 to 80 percent of that in the mother's blood, because some maternal glucose is utilized in the placenta and therefore is not available to the fetal circulation.[32] If the maternal blood glucose concentration is abnormally elevated, the fetal blood glucose level will also be abnormally elevated. In contrast to glucose, insulin does not cross the placenta, thus when a fetus has elevated blood glucose levels, fetal insulin production increases. When the fetus is delivered and the umbilical cord is cut, glucose supply is abruptly stopped, yet the infant's insulin level can remain elevated.[40] Compared to non-IDM infants, the expected nadir (low point) of the blood glucose value is reached more quickly for IDM infants, often within one hour after birth.[82] It may take several

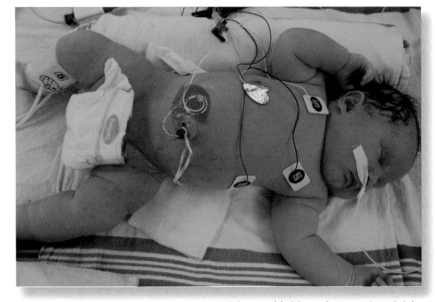

*6 hours old, 39 weeks gestation, 5.1 kg*

days, or longer, for the neonate's insulin level to down-regulate appropriately. During this time, in addition to regular enteral feedings, IV dextrose may be required in order to maintain the newborn's blood sugar at a safe concentration.[83,84]

### Large for gestational age (LGA) infants

LGA infants are defined as those with a birth weight greater than the 90th percentile for their gestational age.[79,85] Infants may be LGA because of ethnic[69] or genetic factors,[86] or in the case of male infants, because of a higher percentage of lean body mass.[87] However, infants may also be LGA because of effects of elevated maternal glucose levels during pregnancy and the consequent fetal hyperinsulinemia.[85] Since insulin is a major growth hormone in the fetus, too much insulin may cause the fetus to deposit more body fat than would otherwise occur; thus the infant grows larger than appropriate for gestational age.[87]

When an infant is born LGA, the underlying cause should be investigated. This includes the possibility that the mother was not recognized as being diabetic or that she developed gestational diabetes mellitus (GDM). Risk factors for developing GDM include maternal obesity, past history of GDM, glycosuria, past history of delivering a LGA infant, a maternal family history of type II diabetes, ethnicity, and a diagnosis of polycystic ovarian syndrome.[45,88-91]

## Hyperinsulinemia*: *High Risk Groups*   (continued)

*If an infant is LGA and hyperinsulinemic, the blood glucose may fall rapidly when the umbilical cord is cut.*

### Early evaluation for hypoglycemia is recommended as follows:

1. Evaluate the blood glucose concentration within 1 to 2 hours after birth and then every 1 to 3 hours based on the glucose values identified, the interventions provided, and the health status of the infant (e.g., able to feed the infant versus the infant requires IV therapy, and vital sign stability). Ideally, the blood glucose should be evaluated prior to a feeding if the infant is stable enough to tolerate feedings.

2. When the blood glucose demonstrates a pattern of stability and remains consistently in the normal range of 50 to 110 mg/dL (2.8 to 6.1 mmol/L),[97] glucose monitoring can be slowed and eventually stopped. It is not uncommon for the infant of a diabetic mother to require glucose testing for 24 to 72 hours after birth, and in some cases even longer.

*\*Other causes of hyperinsulinemia (usually accompanied by persistent severe hypoglycemia) can result from chromosomal, genetic or other conditions including inborn errors of metabolism and endocrine disorders such as hypopituitarism and hypothyroidism. These rare, but severe causes of persistent and difficult to treat hypoglycemia are beyond the scope of this program and will not be further discussed in this module.[40,56,58]*

 Infants with persistent, severe hypoglycemia should be referred quickly to subspecialty neonatology and endocrinology care.

## Clinical Tip

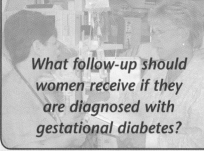

*What follow-up should women receive if they are diagnosed with gestational diabetes?*

Women who are diagnosed with GDM should receive follow-up testing and evaluation 6 to 12 weeks postpartum as they have a seven-fold increased risk for developing type 2 diabetes mellitus; half of these cases develop within the 10 years following pregnancy.[89,92] These women should also be counseled regarding their increased risk for GDM in subsequent pregnancies, as well as other healthcare consequences for themselves and their offspring.[45] Consequences for the offspring include future diabetes, childhood obesity, cardiovascular disease, and hypertension.[87,93-96] Screening the mother for the development of prediabetes or diabetes should occur at least every 3 years.[90]

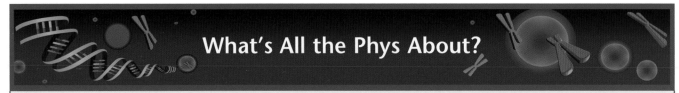

## What's All the Phys About?

### What is hemoglobin A1c (HbA1c) and how is this test used to evaluate maternal glucose levels during pregnancy?

In adults, hemoglobin A is the most abundant variety of hemoglobin in the red blood cell (RBC).[98] When the plasma glucose is higher than normal, the excessive quantity of glucose enters the RBC. In the RBC, the glucose attaches to hemoglobin A and this glycosylated hemoglobin A is quantified as hemoglobin A1c.[99] A normal hemoglobin A1c in those without diabetes is approximately 5%, meaning 5% of the hemoglobin is "glycosylated".

The hemoglobin A1c estimates the average blood glucose level over the previous three month period (the average lifespan of the RBC is 120 days). In this way, the hemoglobin A1c test has become a reliable and valuable indicator of blood glucose control.

### Key Points:

- If the blood glucose concentration is elevated, more hemoglobin A1c will be formed (the percent of hemoglobin A1c will increase).

- Formation of hemoglobin A1c is an irreversible process which means, until the RBCs die and new hemoglobin is formed, (which is on average a period of 120 days[98]), hemoglobin A1c reflects overall glucose control.[99]

- Individuals with a hemoglobin A1c range of 5.7 to 6.4% are at high risk for future diabetes and are considered pre-diabetic. Counseling about strategies to prevent diabetes is strongly recommended for these individuals.[90]

- The threshold for diagnosing overt diabetes is when the hemoglobin A1c is greater than, or equal to 6.5%.[88]

- Assessment of hemoglobin A1c is of limited value in the presence of certain conditions: rapid RBC turnover (hemolytic anemia, some hemoglobinopathies, and sickle-cell disease), kidney disease, and when a patient has received a blood transfusion. In these cases, glucose testing (fasting and following administration of a glucose load) should be used to assess for diabetes.[88]

# Clinical Tip

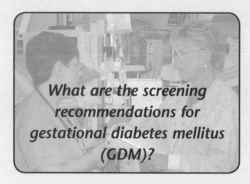

*What are the screening recommendations for gestational diabetes mellitus (GDM)?*

If the mother has risk factors for diabetes, she should be screened at her first prenatal visit for undiagnosed type 2 diabetes. This testing may include a hemoglobin A1c evaluation.

**There are currently two screening recommendations for diagnosing GDM.**

The first is from the International Association of Diabetes and Pregnancy Study Groups (IADPSG) Consensus Panel,[100] which is endorsed by the American Diabetes Association (ADA),[90] and the second is from the American College of Obstetricians and Gynecologists (ACOG).[93] ACOG has not yet endorsed the recommendations from the IADPSG and the ADA and are awaiting the National Institutes of Health consensus development conference on Diagnosing Gestational Diabetes, which is planned for October 2012, to investigate whether their current recommendations should be changed. ACOG raises concerns regarding the increased number of women who would be identified as gestational diabetic using the new IADPSG criteria and the lack of evidence that the identification and treatment of these women would result in improved maternal and neonatal outcomes, as well as concerns about the significantly increased health care costs and potential for increased obstetric interventions as a result of a GDM diagnosis.[93]

**The IADPSG[100] Consensus Panel and the ADA,[90] recommends the following:**

- At the first prenatal visit, screen for risk factors for undiagnosed type 2 diabetes and perform any diagnostic screening that is indicated, which may include a fasting plasma glucose, hemoglobin A1c, or random plasma glucose.[90,100]

- For those who have not been diagnosed with diabetes, between 24 and 28 weeks gestation, screen for diabetes with a 75 gram, 2-hour oral glucose tolerance test (75-g OGTT). Perform the test in the morning after an overnight fast of 8 hours.[90,100]

- The diagnosis of GDM is made if results are above any of the following plasma glucose values:[90,100]

  ✧ Fasting ≥ 92 mg/dL (5.1 mmol/L).
  ✧ 1 hour ≥ 180 mg/dL (10 mmol/L).
  ✧ 2 hours ≥ 153 mg/dL (8.5 mmol/L).

- The diagnosis of overt (not GDM) diabetes in pregnancy is made if any of the following are present:[100]

  ✧ Fasting ≥ 126 mg/dL (7 mmol/L).
  ✧ Hemoglobin A1c is ≥ 6.5%.
  ✧ If a random plasma glucose is ≥ 200 mg/dL (11.1 mmol/L), then confirmatory testing should be performed by obtaining a fasting plasma glucose or hemoglobin A1c.

**The ACOG recommends the following:93**

- Screen all pregnant women for GDM. Screening methods include patient history, clinical risk factors, or a 50 gram, 1-hour glucose loading test (50-g OGTT) at 24 to 28 weeks gestation.

- If a 100 gram 3-hour oral glucose tolerance test is indicated, (50-g OGTT screen > 140 mg/dL [7.8 mmol/L], or other strong clinical suspicion), the diagnosis of GDM is made when two or more elevated plasma or serum glucose levels are obtained.

  ✧ Fasting ≥ 95 mg/dL (5.3 mmol/L).
  ✧ 1 hour ≥ 180 mg/dL (10 mmol/L).
  ✧ 2 hours ≥ 155 mg/dL (8.6 mmol/L).
  ✧ 3 hours ≥ 140 mg/dL (7.8 mmol/L).

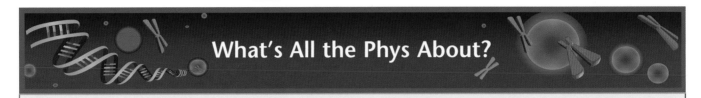

## What's All the Phys About?

### What is the relationship between hyperinsulinemia and macrosomia?[32,34,69,70,79,94,101-104]

Insulin works in synergy with growth hormone and is very important for fetal growth. When the fetus has higher than normal levels of insulin, such as when the maternal blood glucose level is excessive, then glycogen, fat, and protein synthesis are accelerated. This leads to overgrowth of the fetus, which is called *macrosomia* (birthweight greater than 4000 grams).

Macrosomic infants are at increased risk for birth complications including shoulder dystocia, brachial plexus injury, arm and clavicle fractures, organ injury and perinatal asphyxia.

Infants of diabetic mothers have a higher mortality rate and are at increased risk for cardiac and other malformations, preterm birth, respiratory distress syndrome, polycythemia, hyperviscosity, renal vein thrombosis, hyperbilirubinemia, hypoglycemia, hypocalcemia, and hypomagnesemia.

## Increased Utilization of Glucose: *High Risk Groups*

All sick infants including preterm and small for gestational age infants as well as those with infection, shock, respiratory and cardiac disease, hypothermia, or hypoxia

Under aerobic conditions, when oxygen content in the blood is sufficient to satisfy tissue needs, glucose is metabolized into energy. Stressed, sick infants have higher energy needs than well newborns and may rapidly deplete their glycogen stores. Hypoxic infants (infants with oxygen delivery to the tissues less than what is needed by the cells to function normally), may need to rely on anaerobic glycolysis for energy production. Anaerobic glycolysis is very inefficient: large quantities of glucose are consumed for a very low yield of energy.[27,56] For short periods of time – often only minutes – this type of

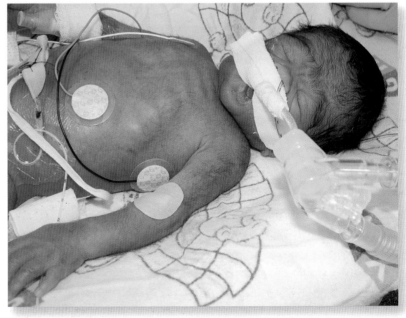

*Preterm infant with sepsis and hypotension*

metabolism can provide enough energy to sustain cellular function.[105] Figures 1.4 and 1.5 illustrate energy production under aerobic and anaerobic conditions.

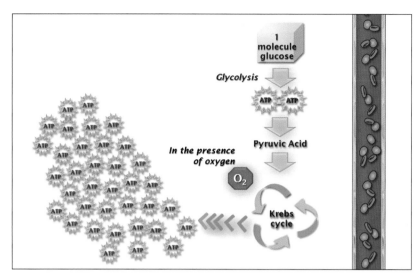

**Figure 1.4. Model of aerobic metabolism.** Under aerobic conditions, adequate amounts of oxygen are present inside cells to allow for the complete metabolism of glucose into adenosine triphosphate (ATP). For every molecule of glucose that is completely metabolized, 38 molecules of ATP are produced: 2 molecules from glycolysis of glucose to pyruvic acid and 36 molecules from metabolism of pyruvic acid to ATP via the Krebs cycle.[105,106]

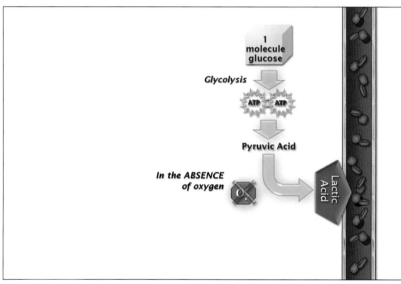

**Figure 1.5. Model of anaerobic metabolism.** Under anaerobic conditions (when oxygen content in the cells is low), incomplete metabolism of glucose occurs: only two molecules of ATP are produced for every molecule of glucose that is metabolized to pyruvic acid. Pyruvic acid is further metabolized into lactic acid. Evidence of anaerobic glycolysis may be seen as an elevated lactate level, and on a blood gas, as a low pH, low bicarbonate value, and worsening base deficit value.[105,106]

# REVIEW

## Infants at increased risk for hypoglycemia:

✧ Preterm infants (< 37 weeks).

✧ Small for gestational age (SGA) infants.

✧ Infants of diabetic mothers (IDM).

✧ Large for gestational age (LGA) infants.

✧ Stressed, sick infants, especially those with a history of perinatal stress, respiratory distress, hypoxia, shock, hypothermia, sepsis, and cardiac disease.

✧ Infants exposed to certain maternal medications (see Table 1.1).

## Glucose Monitoring

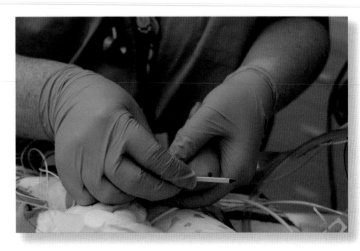

Carbohydrates, as simple sugars, are the major source of metabolic fuel for the newborn. Glucose is the principal simple sugar: as glucose is transported to organs and tissues in the blood, it is also the principal 'blood sugar'. The gold standard for monitoring the level of blood sugar is the plasma glucose value. However, measuring a plasma glucose value requires a sample of whole blood be obtained and processed by the laboratory. More commonly, a whole blood glucose screening test is performed at the bedside and is used as an estimate of the plasma sugar level.[39]

### Bedside Monitoring of Blood Glucose

When an infant is sick or displays signs or symptoms consistent with hypoglycemia (see Table 1.2), evaluate the blood sugar by the method most rapidly available. For an asymptomatic infant who has risk factors for hypoglycemia, perform bedside evaluation of the blood sugar by whatever method your nursery has selected (for example, SureStep®, i-STAT®, OneTouch®, ACCU-CHEK®, Nova StatStrip™ etc.).

## Clinical Tip

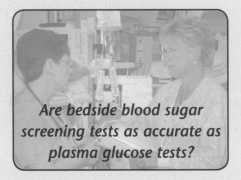

*Are bedside blood sugar screening tests as accurate as plasma glucose tests?*

It is important to recognize that a whole blood glucose test may be 10 to 18 percent lower than a measured plasma glucose value.[39] In addition, when the infant's blood sugar is low, the bedside (whole blood glucose) screening test may be less accurate and result in over or under-treatment of the infant. Therefore, if the bedside test is low, it is often helpful to confirm the blood sugar value with plasma glucose analysis. **However, do not delay treatment while awaiting confirmatory laboratory test results.**

⚠ To improve accuracy of results, notify the laboratory that a whole blood sample has been sent for plasma glucose measurement. Testing should be performed immediately upon receipt of the sample.

# Signs and Symptoms of Hypoglycemia

Some infants may have a low blood sugar and not exhibit any signs. Therefore, if the infant is sick or there are risk factors for hypoglycemia, it is important to continue monitoring the blood sugar by bedside screening. Table 1.2 describes the common signs and symptoms that may be observed when the blood sugar is low.[56,107] Remember that these signs may also be observed because of other medical problems.[40,107]

**Table 1.2.** Signs and symptoms of hypoglycemia.

| General findings | Neurologic signs | Cardiorespiratory signs |
|---|---|---|
| Abnormal cry: weak, high-pitched | Tremors | Tachypnea |
| Poor feeding: poor suck, coordination | Jitteriness | Apnea |
| Hypothermia | Irritability | Cyanosis |
| Diaphoresis | Hypotonia | |
| | Lethargy | |
| | Seizures | |

Adapted with permission from S. Karger AG, Basel, publisher, from Rozance & Hay (2006).[107]

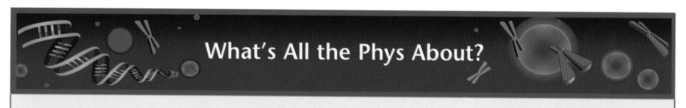

## What's All the Phys About?

**At the same low blood glucose value, why do some infants have clinical signs and other infants do not?**

This observation has complicated the discussion regarding what glucose value should be used to trigger treatment with IV dextrose. A lack of clinical signs as outlined in Table 1.2 during periods when the blood sugar is low may mean that other energy substrates, such as lactate or ketone bodies are providing adequate fuel for the brain.[32,39] However, evidence is lacking regarding the impact, if any, of asymptomatic hypoglycemia on neurodevelopmental outcomes.[108,109] In addition, it is important to realize that the signs commonly attributed to hypoglycemia are somewhat non-specific and may be present because of other clinical problems including infection, brain injury, drug withdrawal, metabolic derangements, or respiratory distress.[40,109,110] Until more definitive research is available that evaluates these complicated issues, the S.T.A.B.L.E. Program recommends a margin of safety be maintained in sick infants by ensuring the blood sugar is in a normoglycemic range.

## Recommended Target Blood Sugar for Infants Who Require Neonatal Intensive Care

The S.T.A.B.L.E. Program defines hypoglycemia as "glucose delivery or availability which is inadequate to meet glucose demand". The exact blood glucose value which defines hypoglycemia remains controversial.[108,111] Furthermore, glucose values tolerated by individual infants may vary because of their individual diagnoses and medical problems. If an infant has a low blood or plasma glucose value, this does not imply that permanent neurologic damage will occur; however, it does mean that action should be taken to restore the blood sugar to a euglycemic, or normal blood glucose concentration.[56,83]

There is controversy regarding what glucose value constitutes hypoglycemia. Furthermore, there is lack of definitive evidence regarding at which glucose values and under what conditions neurologic damage occurs. **Therefore, to provide a safe and reasonable target for treatment, the S.T.A.B.L.E. Program recommends the following:**

For sick infants who cannot be enterally fed, a glucose value (whether by bedside or laboratory method of analysis) of 50 mg/dL (2.8 mmol/L)[40,58] is the value below which the S.T.A.B.L.E. Program recommends corrective intravenous therapy and on-going monitoring until the glucose is stabilized between 50 and 110 mg/dL (2.8 and 6.1 mmol/L).

The goal of therapy is to maintain the blood sugar between 50 and 110 mg/dL (2.8 and 6.1 mmol/L).[83,97] Individual evaluation of the infant's age and cause of hypoglycemia must be considered in all cases. This recommendation is consistent with most current recommendations and published literature.

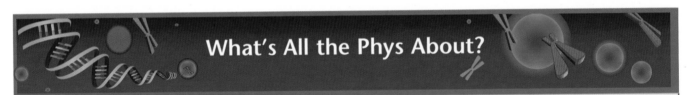

### What's All the Phys About?

#### Are there alternative sources of fuel?

When infants are healthy, glucose is provided by carbohydrate intake in the form of breast milk or formula. When infants are sick and cannot feed, carbohydrates are supplied in the form of IV dextrose. When the blood sugar drops as a result of fasting or other factors such as increased glucose utilization, inadequate glycogen storage, or hyperinsulinemia, the term infant will compensate for the low blood sugar by using other substrates such as lactate or ketone bodies as alternative fuels for brain energy.[32,57,107,112,113] Preterm and SGA or intrauterine growth restricted (IUGR) infants are at a disadvantage however, because they lack the adipose (fat) tissue required for ketone production, or they are unable to mobilize free fatty acids from adipose tissue.[40,57] In addition, preterm infants may not have matured enough to have the enzymes required for the breakdown of glycogen into glucose molecules, a process called glycogenolysis.[32,57]

# Initial IV Fluid and Rate

Establish intravenous (IV) access and administer a 10% dextrose solution ($D_{10}W$), without electrolytes, at a rate of 80 mL per kilogram per day (80 mL/kg/day). This provides a glucose infusion rate of 5.5 mg/kg/minute, which is similar to the liver glucose production rate in healthy term newborns — 4 to 6 mg/kg/minute.[32,57,97]

**Figure 1.6. Initial IV fluid management for the sick infant.**

$D_{10}W$ without electrolytes*

80 mL per kilogram per 24 hours (80 mL/kg/day)

Infuse via an infusion pump

*If the infant is older than 24 hours, it may be necessary to add electrolytes to the IV solution.[114]*

In the absence of conditions related to hyperinsulinemia, for infants with limited or no glycogen stores (for example, preterm and small for gestational age infants), or those without significantly increased glucose utilization, a glucose infusion rate of 5.5 mg/kg/minute (80 mL/kg/day of $D_{10}W$), should adequately maintain the blood sugar above 50 mg/dL (2.8 mmol/L). Figures 1.6 and 1.7 summarize the initial IV fluid to provide for sick infants and how to calculate the hourly infusion rate. Table 1.3 shows the glucose infusion rate that is provided with varying fluid infusion rates and varying dextrose concentrations. Treatment of a blood glucose less than 50 mg/dL (2.8 mmol/L) is outlined in Table 1.4.

| Dextrose concentration | Infusion volume mL/kg per 24 hours (mL/kg/day) | Glucose infusion rate mg/kg delivered per minute (mg/kg/min) |
|---|---|---|
| $D_{10}W$ | 60 | 4.2 |
| $D_{10}W$ | 80 (usual starting rate) | 5.5 (usual starting dose) |
| $D_{10}W$ | 100 | 6.9 |
| $D_{12.5}W$ | 60 | 5.2 |
| $D_{12.5}W$ | 80 | 6.9 |
| $D_{12.5}W$ | 100 | 8.7 |
| $D_{15}W$ | 60 | 6.3 |
| $D_{15}W$ | 80 | 8.3 |
| $D_{15}W$ | 100 | 10.4 |

**Table 1.3.** Effect of varying dextrose concentrations and infusion rates on the rate of glucose that is delivered in mg/kg/minute.

**Figure 1.7. Calculating the hourly fluid delivery rate to provide 80 mL/kg/day.**

## Desired infusion rate: 80 mL/kg/day

**Step 1.** Multiply the body weight in kilograms by 80 (mL): kg x 80

**Step 2.** To find the hourly rate, divide this number by 24 (hours):
(kg x 80) ÷ 24 = fluid rate in mL per hour to infuse the IV fluid

**Example: Body weight 1800 grams (1.8 kg)**

**Step 1.** 1.8 x 80 = 144 (mL)

**Step 2.** 144 (mL) divided by 24 (hours) = 6 (mL per hour)

**Step 3.** Round up to the nearest whole number

**Step 4.** Infuse the fluid via an infusion pump at 6 mL per hour

Note: a pounds/ounces to grams conversion chart may be found on the inside back cover of this manual.

**Figure 1.8. How to calculate a $D_{10}W$ bolus.**

## Desired dose: 2 mL/kg $D_{10}W$ bolus
## This dose equals 200 mg of glucose per kg

**Step 1.** Multiply the body weight in kilograms by 2

**Step 2.** Infuse this volume of $D_{10}W$ intravenously at a rate of 1 mL per minute

**Example: Body weight 1800 grams (1.8 kg)**

1.8 (kg) x 2 (mL) = 3.6 (mL)

Give 3.6 mL of $D_{10}W$ IV over four minutes (rate of 1 mL per minute)

## Clinical Tip

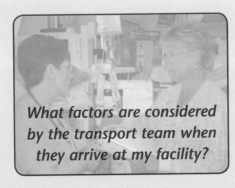

*What factors are considered by the transport team when they arrive at my facility?*

When the transport team arrives, they assess the infant's history, diagnosis, current condition, and therapies that have been provided. They use this information to decide what is best to continue the stabilization process. This includes whether they need to make changes, including to the IV fluid and/or rate and the need for additional IVs. Do not be alarmed or discouraged by any changes made by this team as they are expected to make necessary adjustments as they continue the stabilization process that you started.

**Table 1.4.** S.T.A.B.L.E. Program guideline for sick infants who require IV treatment when the plasma or bedside blood glucose test is less than or equal to 50 mg/dL (2.8 mmol/L).

If the bedside blood glucose test is less than 50 mg/dL (2.8 mmol/L), proceed with the following treatment. Confirm low glucose values with a laboratory plasma glucose, **but do not delay treatment while awaiting results!**

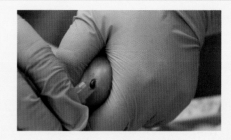

This information about IV treatment of a blood glucose less than 50 mg/dL (2.8 mmol/L) by either a bedside screening test or plasma analysis **pertains to a sick infant who cannot receive oral or gavage feedings**. Infants with a low blood sugar who are otherwise healthy can usually tolerate oral feedings unless the blood sugar value is very low, in which case the infant will require IV therapy. For additional guidance regarding the infant who can tolerate enteral feedings, the S.T.A.B.L.E. Program recommends the algorithm in reference McGowan 2011, in Figure 15-5, p. 368: Decision tree for management of neonate with acute hypoglycemia.[56]

**Step 1.** Begin an intravenous infusion of $D_{10}W$ at 80 mL/kg/day.

**Step 2.** Administer a bolus of 2 mL/kg of $D_{10}W$ at a rate of 1 mL per minute. This dose equals 200 mg per kg of glucose.[39,115] Figure 1.8 shows how to calculate the bolus.

⚠ To prevent hyperglycemia and rebound hypoglycemia, use $D_{10}W$; do not give 25% ($D_{25}W$) or 50% ($D_{50}W$) glucose boluses.

**Step 3.** Recheck the bedside blood glucose test within 15 to 30 minutes after the completion of any glucose bolus or increase in IV rate.

**Step 4.** If the blood glucose is again less than 50 mg/dL (2.8 mmol/L), repeat the bolus of 2 mL/kg of $D_{10}W$ and increase the IV to 100 mL per kg per day. Figure 1.9 shows how to calculate a higher infusion rate.

**Step 5.** If the blood glucose is not 50 mg/dL (2.8 mmol/L) or greater after two glucose boluses, then repeat the glucose bolus and increase the amount of delivered glucose.

*Two options for increasing the amount of delivered glucose are:*
    a. Increase the IV infusion to 120 mLs per kg per day (see Figure 1.9), or,

    b. Increase the IV dextrose concentration to $D_{12.5}W$. Appendix 1.4 explains how to make higher (or lower) dextrose concentrations for IV infusion.

**Note:** If the infant is hypoglycemic because of hyperinsulinemia, it may be necessary to increase the dextrose concentration of the infused fluid to provide a glucose infusion rate of 12 to 15 mg/kg/minute (or more). This means the dextrose concentration will exceed a 12.5% solution. Solutions containing greater than $D_{12.5}W$ should be infused via a central venous line (umbilical venous catheter, percutaneously inserted central catheter, or surgically inserted central catheter).

**Step 6.** Continue to evaluate the blood glucose (bedside or laboratory test) every 30 to 60 minutes until 50 mg/dL (2.8 mmol/L) or greater on at least two consecutive evaluations. Follow the trend in blood glucose and use clinical judgment to decide when blood glucose testing can be safely decreased.

**Step 7.** If the blood glucose remains persistently low after these steps, the attending physician or transport control physician should be called immediately for additional advice.

## Clinical Tip

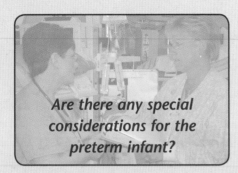

*Are there any special considerations for the preterm infant?*

**Fluid requirements:** Preterm infants may require a higher volume of fluid than term infants because of increased water losses through their thinner, less developed skin. Various factors increase water loss, including skin immaturity, providing care under a radiant warmer, and use of phototherapy lights.[114,116]

**HYPERglycemia:** Preterm infants, especially those less than 32 weeks gestation and those who are SGA, may become hyperglycemic (blood glucose greater than 125 mg/dL or 6.9 mmol/L) when they receive an infusion of 80 mL/kg/day of $D_{10}W$. This occurs because of their immature endocrine system. If the blood glucose is persistently elevated, consult with the neonatal intensive care physician for guidance regarding fluid management. Preterm infants may need less glucose delivery (a lower IV dextrose concentration) and more fluid delivery (a higher fluid infusion rate) because of glucose intolerance and increased insensible water loss[40,56] See Appendix 1.4 for a dextrose preparation chart.

**Figure 1.9. How to calculate a higher IV infusion rate.**

### Desired infusion rate: 100 mL/kg/day

**Step 1.** Multiply the body weight in kilograms by 100

**Step 2.** Divide this number by 24 (hours) to calculate the hourly infusion rate

(Weight in kg multiplied by 100), divide by 24 = the hourly infusion rate

**Example:** Body weight 4.2 kg

**Step 1.** 4.2 (kg) X 100 = 420 (mL)

**Step 2.** 420 (mL) divided by 24 (hours) = 17.5 mL/hour, round up to 18 mL/hour

**Step 3.** Infuse the IV fluid at 18 mL/hour on an infusion pump

### Desired infusion rate: 120 mL/kg/day

**Step 1.** Multiply the body weight in kilograms by 120

**Step 2.** Divide this number by 24 (hours) to calculate the hourly infusion rate

(Weight in kg multiplied by 120), divide by 24 = the hourly infusion rate

**Example:** Body weight 4.2 kg

**Step 1.** 4.2 (kg) X 120 = 504 (mL)

**Step 2.** 504 (mL) divided by 24 (hours) = 21 mL/hour

**Step 3.** Infuse the IV fluid at 21 mL/hour on an infusion pump

# SUMMARY

## General Recommendation for the Initial Fluid and Glucose Management of Sick Infants

1. Make infant NPO. Do not offer enteral feedings, which includes oral, gavage or tube feedings.

2. Begin $D_{10}W$ IV fluid (without electrolytes) at 80 mL per kg per day, via a peripheral vein or umbilical vein. If the infant is older than 24 hours, then electrolytes are usually added to the IV fluid.

3. Monitor the blood glucose at an appropriate interval and maintain between 50 and 110 mg/dL (2.8 to 6.1 mmol/L).

4. If fluids are given via an umbilical venous or artery catheter, add 0.5 to 1 unit heparin per mL of IV fluid.

5. If the glucose is less than 50 mg/dL (2.8 mmol/L), give a 2 mL/kg bolus of $D_{10}W$ and continue the IV infusion of $D_{10}W$ at 80 mL per kg per day.

6. Evaluate the blood glucose within 15 to 30 minutes:

   • Of completion of any glucose bolus.

   • After starting an IV infusion.

   • In any infant with an initially or subsequently low blood glucose.

   Use clinical judgment based upon the infant's condition and risk factors for hypoglycemia to determine how often the blood glucose should be evaluated once a pattern of stability has been established.

7. The highest concentration of dextrose that is infused by peripheral IV is $D_{12.5}W$. If a dextrose concentration greater than $D_{12.5}W$ is required, the fluid should be infused through a central venous line. Another indication for central venous line infusion may include when electrolytes or calcium are added to $D_{12.5}W$.[117] When total parenteral nutrition is provided, check with your pharmacist to determine whether the fluid can be infused peripherally or if central line infusion is necessary.

8. If the blood glucose is above 125 mg/dL (6.9 mmol/L) and not decreasing, this may be secondary to glucose intolerance (as may be seen with preterm infants), or as a stress response. Consult with the referral center for guidance as needed.

# Umbilical Catheters

## Indications for Umbilical Catheterization

In the pre-transport and post-resuscitation stabilization period, it may be necessary to insert an umbilical vein catheter (UVC), an umbilical artery catheter (UAC), or a peripheral arterial line.

### A UVC should be selected if:[118-120]

- Rapid IV access is required and, given the infant's condition, the UVC is the best option for administering emergency fluids and medications.

- Based on the infant's health status and condition, there is ongoing difficulty establishing a peripheral IV within a reasonable period of time or attempts.

- More than one intravenous line is required.

- It is necessary to administer glucose concentrations exceeding 12.5% dextrose.

- To perform an exchange transfusion.

### A UAC or peripheral arterial line should be selected if:[121,122]

- Continuous arterial blood pressure monitoring is required.

- Frequent arterial blood gas evaluation is necessary.

Table 1.5 summarizes indications for placement of umbilical venous and arterial catheters, catheter size, infusion solutions, heparin dose, medication administration and contraindications for use. Table 1.6 contains information about the correct UVC tip location and complications related to malposition, and Table 1.7 explains how to calculate the dose of heparin to add to central line fluids.

⚠ In a life-threatening emergency, (e.g. severe shock or pre-cardiac arrest state), if not able to rapidly establish reliable venous access via peripheral IV or umbilical venous catheter, consider placing an 18-gauge intraosseous needle into the medial aspect of the tibial bone just below the tibial tuberosity.[37,123] When an intraosseous needle or intraosseous needle placement device is not available, then an 18- or 20-gauge short spinal needle (with stylet) may be used.[123] Medications, blood products, and fluids can be administered via the intraosseous route.[123]

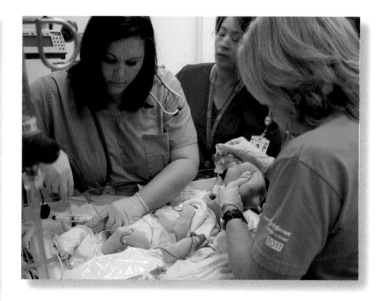

**Table 1.5.** UAC and UVC: Indications for placement, catheter size, infusion solutions, heparin dose, medication administration and contraindications.

## Umbilical Vein Catheter (UVC)

| Indications for placement UVC[118-120] | Catheter size[a] UVC[125] | Infusion solutions UVC[126] | Heparin dose (Units per mL IV fluid) UVC[127] | Medication administration UVC[126,128] | Contraindications UVC[118] |
|---|---|---|---|---|---|
| 1. To provide emergency fluids and medications during resuscitation<br><br>2. Unable to start a peripheral IV in a reasonable time or number of attempts<br><br>3. To provide a glucose concentration greater than D$_{12.5}$W<br><br>4. When additional IV access is required for fluids or medications<br><br>5. When an exchange transfusion is necessary | < 1.5 kg: 3.5 French<br><br>>1.5 kg: 5 French<br><br>Consider using a double-lumen catheter so that medications and fluids may be administered simultaneously | 5 to 20% dextrose solution (D$_5$W to D$_{20}$W) is appropriate if the tip is in good position | 0.5 to 1 unit per mL of IV fluid | If the catheter tip is properly positioned at the IVC / RA junction, then all medications, including vasopressors (dopamine, dobutamine, epinephrine), may be given in the UVC | Omphalitis<br><br>Peritonitis<br><br>Omphalocele<br><br>Necrotizing enterocolitis |

**Clinical Tip:** A spongy, "bouncing back" feeling of resistance during placement usually indicates the catheter tip is malpositioned in the liver or portal venous system.

[a]Some neonatal texts recommend a 3.5 Fr UAC when the infant weighs less than 1.25 kg.[122,124,134]

**Table 1.5.** UAC and UVC: Indications for placement, catheter size, infusion solutions, heparin dose, medication administration and contraindications.   *(continued)*

# Umbilical Artery Catheter (UAC)

| Indications for placement UAC[121,122,124] | Catheter size[a] UAC[125] | Infusion solutions UAC[126] | Heparin dose (Units per mL IV fluid) UAC[127] | Medication administration UAC[125, 126, 128, 132, 133] | Contraindications UAC[119, 122] |
|---|---|---|---|---|---|
| 1. To monitor arterial blood pressure.<br><br>2. To allow frequent blood gas analysis.<br><br>Note: If unable to insert a UAC, additional options include cannulation of the radial or posterior tibialis artery.[129] Sodium chloride (0.9%) intravenous infusion or half sodium chloride (0.45%) intravenous infusion with 1 unit heparin per mL may be infused in a peripheral arterial line. | < 1.5 kg: 3.5 French<br><br>>1.5 kg: 5 French | Options:<br>1. Sodium chloride (0.9%) intravenous infusion at 1 to 2 mL/hour to maintain catheter patency.<br><br>2. 5 to 15% dextrose solution ($D_5W$ to $D_{15}W$) with or without amino acids.<br><br>Note: evidence is lacking regarding outcomes or effects related to administration of parenteral nutrition, calcium, medications, (including antibiotics) through the UAC.[130]<br><br>3. Isotonic amino acid solution with a 0.5 normal saline flush regimen.[131] For option 1 and 3, a glucose containing solution should be administered via an alternate intravenous route.<br><br>If unsure which option to select, consult your tertiary center. | 0.5 to 1 unit per mL IV fluid | The UAC is not recommended for medication or blood administration.<br><br>⚠ Do not administer vasopressors (dopamine, dobutamine, or epinephrine), calcium boluses, or blood in the UAC or in any arterial line. | Omphalitis<br><br>Peritonitis<br><br>Omphalocele<br><br>Vascular compromise in the lower limbs or buttocks<br><br>Necrotizing enterocolitis |

[a]Some neonatal texts recommend a 3.5 Fr UAC when the infant weighs less than 1.25 kg.[122,124,134]

**Table 1.6.** Umbilical vein catheter (UVC) tip location and complications related to malposition.

| | | |
|---|---|---|
| **Central location** | On anteroposterior (AP) chest x-ray, the tip should be at the inferior vena cava/right atrial junction (IVC/RA junction).[118,135] If unsure of the location, consider obtaining a cross-table lateral chest x-ray. | 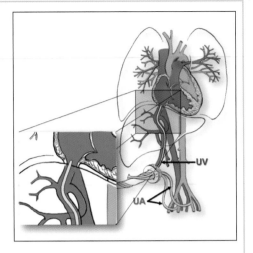 |
| **Emergency placement** | The catheter should be inserted 2 to 4 centimeters, until there is a blood return. This depth usually locates the tip well below the liver.[9]<br><br>◇ The depth of insertion is related to the infant's size.<br><br>⚠ In an emergency, there may not be time to confirm location of the catheter tip by x-ray before infusing hypertonic resuscitation medications. If the catheter tip is located in the liver or portal venous circulation, the liver may be injured by administration of hypertonic solutions. | 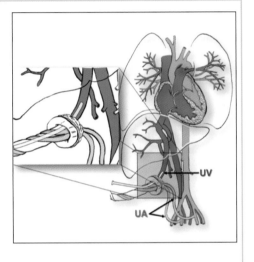 |

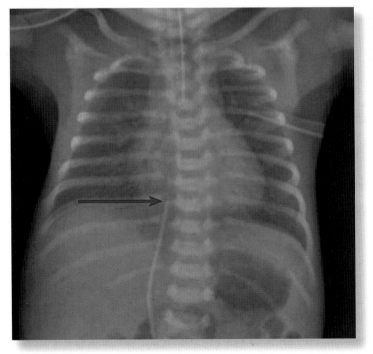

**Figure 1.10. Chest x-ray of an infant showing the Umbilical Vein Catheter (UVC) tip (blue arrow) positioned correctly at the IVC / RA junction.** The ET tube is also in good position in the mid-trachea.

**Table 1.6.** Umbilical vein catheter (UVC) tip location and complications related to malposition.   *(continued)*

| Complications of malposition in the heart[118,134,136,137] | ◇ Arrhythmias<br>◇ Intracardiac thrombus formation<br>◇ Myocardial perforation<br>◇ Pericardial effusion<br>◇ Cardiac tamponade<br>◇ Pulmonary and systemic emboli; infected emboli will result in abscess formation<br>◇ Endocarditis<br>◇ Pulmonary infarction<br>◇ Pulmonary hemorrhage<br><br>⚠ Avoid placement in the right atrium because the tip may easily cross the foramen ovale into the left atrium and increase risk of perforation or release of emboli. Avoid placement in the liver to prevent injury to the liver tissue. | 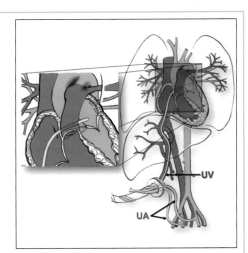 |
|---|---|---|
| Complications of malposition in the liver or portal venous system[118,134-137] | ◇ Hepatic necrosis following thrombus formation or infusion of hypertonic or vasoactive solutions into the liver<br>◇ Portal hypertension<br>◇ Peritoneal perforation<br>◇ Intestinal ischemia<br>◇ Hepatic vessel perforation and hematoma formation; followed by calcification when the hematoma resolves<br>◇ Intravascular thrombus formation<br>◇ Emboli released into the liver | 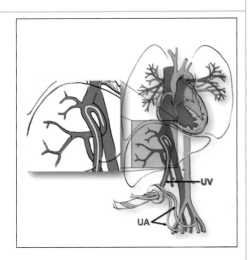 |

## Safe Use of Umbilical Catheters

### Heparin Safety

Heparin, a blood anticoagulant, is frequently added to central line fluids to prevent catheter occlusion by thrombus formation.[125,127] Heparin is supplied in different concentrations; therefore, each time a heparin vial is opened, double check that the correct concentration was selected.

| | |
|---|---|
| **Heparin dose:** | 0.5 to 1 unit per milliliter of IV fluid (0.5 to 1 unit heparin per mL IV fluid). |
| **Indications:** | To heparinize IV fluid that will be infused through a central line. |

| EXAMPLE | |
|---|---|
| **Desired dose** | 1 unit heparin per mL IV fluid administered through a UVC or a UAC |
| **IV solution** | 250 mL bag D$_{10}$W |
| **Heparin concentration** | 1000 units per mL |
| **Dose to draw up** | Use a 1 mL volume syringe<br>Draw up 0.25 mL of heparin (equals 250 units of heparin) and add to a 250 mL bag of D$_{10}$W IV solution |

This will yield a concentration of **1 unit of heparin per mL of IV solution.** If a smaller dose of heparin is desired (0.5 units per mL IV fluid), add the same dose (0.25 mL of heparin) to a 500 mL bag of IV solution.

> ⚠ Ideally, commercially prepared IV fluid containing heparin should be utilized. However, when this is not available the IV fluid should be prepared in the pharmacy under strict aseptic conditions. If this is not possible, the heparin dose (how much was drawn up and the heparin concentration in the vial) must be checked by two registered nurses prior to adding to the IV fluid.

> ⚠ Accidental overdose is a potential hazard when administering heparin. Be aware that it only takes 50 to 100 units of heparin per kg of body weight to "heparinize" an infant, which may lead to excessive bleeding. If a pharmacist is not available to measure and add the heparin to the IV fluid, be certain to double check the following:
> - The heparin concentration
> - The dose and amount that is drawn into the syringe
> - The correct IV fluid volume
>
> Heparin vials may resemble other medication vials used in the nursery, therefore, it is recommended that you discard the heparin vial after use.

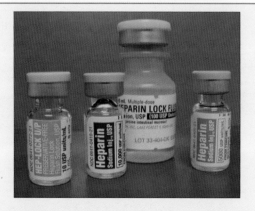

*Photo courtesy of Institute for Safe Medication Practices (ISMP)*

**Table 1.7.** How to calculate the heparin dose to equal 1 unit of heparin per mL of IV solution.

**Figure 1.11 Directions for securing an umbilical catheter using a sterile transparent semipermeable membrane dressing.**

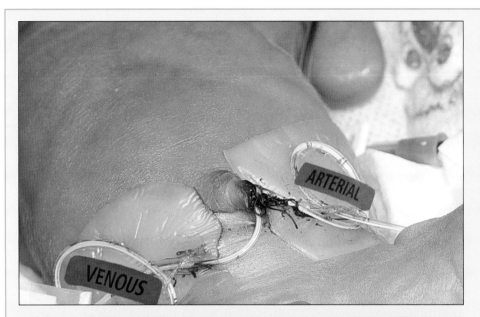

*When possible, first apply a hydrocolloid base layer under the transparent dressing to protect the abdominal skin. This is especially important for premature infants who have immature, fragile skin.*

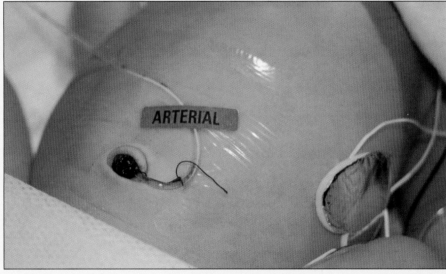

**Step 1.** While the protective backing is still on the transparent dressing, cut a semi-circle in the top of edge of the dressing so that the dressing can be placed as close to the umbilical stump as possible.

**Step 2.** Remove the central backing from the dressing. Position the catheter so it is looped slightly on the abdomen, then hold the catheter in place while the dressing is pressed onto the skin.

**Step 3.** Remove the edges of the backing after the dressing has been pressed onto the skin. The catheter should be held securely under the dressing with as little of the catheter protruding from the umbilical stump as possible. This will help prevent accidental dislodgement. Extra dressing or tape may be used to reinforce the original dressing.

**Step 4.** Always apply a label to the area adjacent to the catheter to identify the type of catheter that is in place.

# SUMMARY

## Umbilical Catheter Safety Guidelines

1. Use sterile technique when placing lines, setting up infusions, drawing labs, and administering fluids.

2. To prevent accidental displacement, suture the catheter in place. Take care to not suture through the skin next to the umbilicus. Further secure the catheter with tape or surgical dressing as shown in Figure 1.11.

3. Do not advance a catheter once the sterile field has been disassembled.

4. Monitor for accidental catheter migration by noting the centimeter marking at the abdominal skin after placement of an umbilical artery or vein catheter, and then at least every 12 hours until the line is removed. Report any changes in the line insertion depth to the medical staff provider. It is important that these catheters do not migrate to an unsafe position.

5. Maintain an air-tight system and do not allow air bubbles to infuse into the baby.

6. Ensure all tubing connections are tight and use a transducer whenever possible on umbilical arterial lines. Significant blood loss, especially with arterial lines, can occur if the tubing is accidentally disconnected.

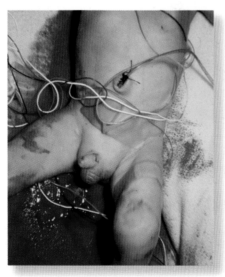

*Massive hemorrhage secondary to accidental disconnection of the arterial line*

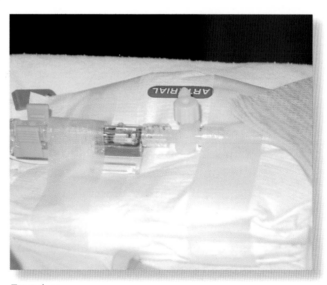

*Transducer*

7. When a UAC is in use, monitor the temperature and color of the infant's toes, legs, groin, abdomen, and buttocks for signs of arterial spasm, clot, or emboli.[138] Any abnormalities in the assessment of the lower body should be reported to the medical staff provider. These complications can occur at any time while the UAC is in place, including just after insertion.

# Additional Information for Neonatal Intensive Care Unit (NICU) Staff

## High versus low positioned umbilical artery catheters: which is best?

A Cochrane review[130] compared high versus low UAC position and frequency of the following adverse events: ischemia, aortic thrombosis, intraventricular hemorrhage (IVH), necrotizing enterocolitis (NEC), and mortality, and supported exclusive use of high positioned UACs because they were associated with a lower incidence of clinically apparent vascular complications. There was no difference in IVH, NEC, or death with low versus high positioned catheters. However, selection of a high versus low UAC position is based on individual and/or institutional preference. Table 1.8 summarizes correct location of high and low catheter tips and Table 1.9 provides guidance for resolving catheter malposition. Figures 1.12 and 1.13 are x-rays of correctly positioned umbilical lines. Figure 1.14 is a cross-table lateral x-ray that shows the pathway of umbilical venous and arterial catheters. Appendices 1.5 and 1.6 contain information about how to estimate catheter insertion depth using a mathematical formula or a graph.

| Umbilical Artery Catheter (UAC) | Tip location | Rationale for this location |
|---|---|---|
| **High line** | On anteroposterior (AP) chest x-ray, the tip should be between thoracic vertebrae 6 and 9 (T6 and T9)[122,124] | To avoid ischemic injury to organs and tissues served by the celiac and superior mesenteric arteries, and to arteries that come off the aorta in the upper chest.<br><br>• The celiac artery originates at the aortic level of T11.<br><br>• The superior mesenteric artery originates at the aortic level of T11–T12.<br><br>• The aortic arch and carotid and subclavian arteries are located above T5. |
| **Low line** | On abdominal x-ray, the tip should be in the lower abdominal aorta, between lumbar vertebrae 3 and 4 (L3 and L4), and above the bifurcation of the iliac arteries.[122,124] | To avoid injury to organs and tissues served by the renal and inferior mesenteric arteries.<br><br>• The renal artery originates at the aortic level of L1.<br><br>• The inferior mesenteric artery originates at the aortic level of L2.<br><br>• The bifurcation of the aorta and iliac arteries is at approximately L4 to L5. |

**Table 1.8.** Umbilical arterial catheter (UAC) tip location.

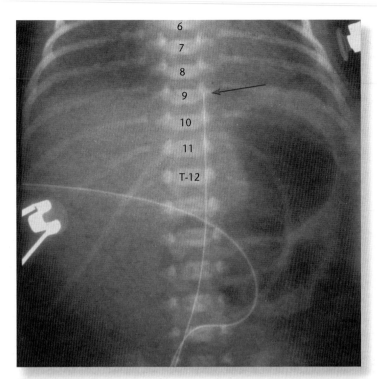

**Figure 1.12. Abdominal x-ray of a term infant showing the Umbilical Artery Catheter (UAC) tip in good position at T9.**

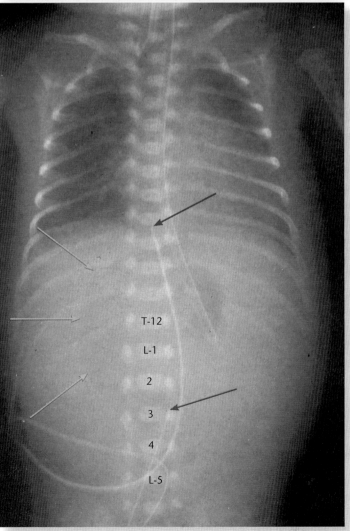

**Figure 1.13. Chest and abdominal x-ray of a preterm infant with a UVC and UAC in correct position.** The UVC tip (blue arrow) is located at the IVC/RA junction and the UAC tip (red arrow) is located at L-3. This infant also had a pneumoperitoneum secondary to an intestinal perforation. The yellow arrows are pointing at the air collection.

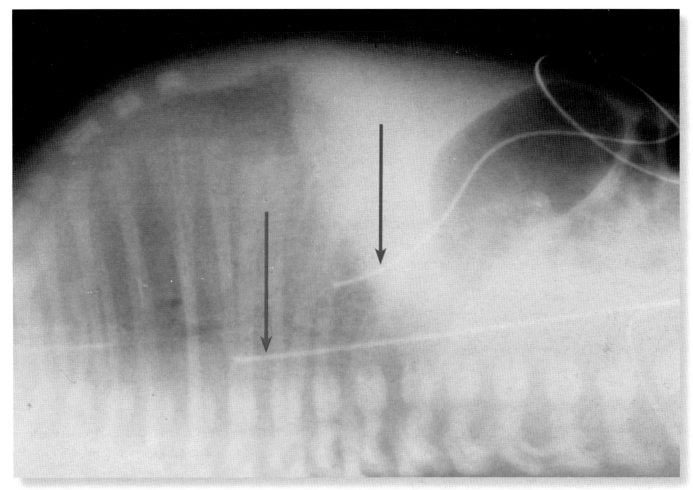

**Figure 1.14. Cross table lateral x-ray showing the pathway of umbilical catheters.** The UAC (red arrow) is in the aorta and the UVC (blue arrow) is in the inferior vena cava. Both catheters are in good position.

**Table 1.9.** Actions to take to when the UAC is malpositioned.

| Catheter position[119,130,139] | Malposition | What to do to correct the malposition |
|---|---|---|
| **High positioned UAC**<br><br>Correct placement is between T6 and T9 | **The UAC tip is higher than T6** | Pull the UAC back until it is between T6 and T9. Repeat the chest x-ray to verify correct position. |
| | **UAC is curved back upon itself** | Try to pull back on the catheter to see if it will straighten out. Repeat the x-ray after the catheter has been repositioned. If the catheter is still curved upon itself further attempts to reposition it will most likely be unsuccessful. Therefore, it should be removed and a new catheter should be inserted using sterile technique. |
| | **UAC tip is below T9** | Pull the catheter back until it is at the level of L3 to L4 (i.e., convert the catheter from a "high" line to a "low" line). |
| **Low positioned UAC**<br><br>Correct placement is between L3 and L4 | **UAC tip is too high for a low line** (the tip is located somewhere between L2 and T10) | The UAC needs to be repositioned to a LOW line at L3 to L4. Once the catheter has been repositioned, repeat an abdominal film to check the new catheter position. |
| | **UAC is curved back upon itself** | Try to pull back on the catheter to see if it will straighten out. Repeat the x-ray after the catheter has been repositioned. If the catheter is still curved upon itself further attempts to reposition it will most likely be unsuccessful. Therefore, it should be removed and a new catheter should be inserted using sterile technique. |
| | **UAC is going down the leg** | Remove the UAC and reinsert a new catheter using sterile technique. |
| | **UAC tip is below L4** | The UAC tip may now be in the iliac artery rather than in the aorta. If the sterile field has been disassembled, do not advance the catheter! Remove the catheter and reinsert a new one using sterile technique. |

# Clinical Tip

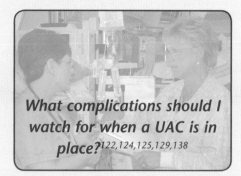

*What complications should I watch for when a UAC is in place?*[122,124,125,129,138]

Arterial spasm or development of emboli from small blood clots that form on the tip or in the circulation adjacent to the tip of the catheter may occur when a UAC or other arterial line is in use. The area distal to the spasm or clot may show signs of impaired skin perfusion. Therefore, monitor the infant frequently for white, blue, or black discoloration of the skin on the back, buttocks, groin, abdomen, legs, feet or toes. If the line is in the radial artery, observe the hand and fingers for the same changes in perfusion and compare the warmth of the fingers to the hand without the arterial line. If there is a difference in skin temperature, this finding is also significant. Document your assessment to include presence of normal findings as well as any abnormal findings.

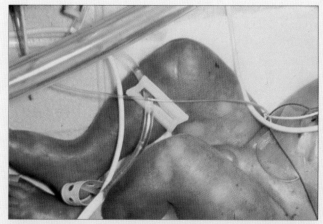

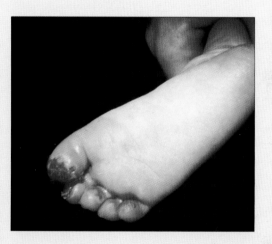

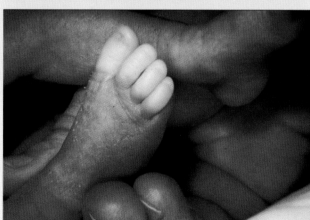

*Examples of impaired perfusion related to arterial lines*

⚠ If any signs of impaired perfusion are observed, immediately notify the medical staff provider to discuss removal of the line. If the catheter stops functioning properly or evidence of vasospasm persists, there may be a thrombus at or near the catheter tip. Once the catheter is removed, monitor closely for improved perfusion. If perfusion does not improve, additional diagnostic studies and treatments should be considered, including: ultrasound, Doppler assessment, angiography, application of systemic or topical vasodilators, and/or treatment with tissue plasminogen activator.[125]

# Clinical Tip

*How fast should I withdraw blood from a high-positioned UAC and how fast should I return blood and flush?*

In most cases, when sampling from a UAC, the removal and return volume is between 1 and 3 milliliters (mL) per lab sampling. Davies et al. (2000) demonstrated a 1.6 mL withdrawal volume was required to clear the UAC sufficiently before obtaining lab samples.[140]

Schulz et al[141] found that withdrawing 2.5 mL of blood from a high-positioned UAC (tip between T6 and T9) over a 40-second interval prevented cerebral hemoglobin desaturation, whereas withdrawing the same volume of blood over a 20-second interval resulted in cerebral hemoglobin desaturation.

Butt et. al[142] found that returning fluid and volume into a low-positioned UAC (catheter tip located between L3 to L4) at a rate of 0.5 mL per five seconds prevented retrograde aortic blood flow and elevation of blood pressure, whereas retrograde aortic blood flow and elevation of blood pressure were observed when faster return times were used.

Gordon et al[143] implemented a practice change in umbilical catheter sampling to withdraw and reinstill at a rate of 1 mL per 30 seconds; viewing this rate as a prudent approach until more research was available that evaluated other withdrawal and re-instillation rates as well as neonatal outcomes.

Roll et al[144] evaluated 40 and 80 second withdrawal sampling times in a population of preterm infants who were smaller and more immature than Schulz's study patients. Both the 40 and 80 second withdrawal rates resulted in similar declines in cerebral desaturation and cerebral blood volume. A re-instillation time of 36 seconds was used to return the 1.6 mL draw-up volume and the 0.6 mL line flushing volume. The clinical significance of these decreases in cerebral desaturation and cerebral blood volume, particularly as regards initiating or worsening intraventricular hemorrhage, has not been established.

# Appendix 1.1 **Bowel Obstruction**

Causes of bowel obstruction include stenosis (narrowing of the lumen) or atresia (complete obstruction) anywhere in the intestinal tract: esophageal, duodenal, jejunal, ileal, anal, or incarcerated hernia. As shown in Figure 1.2 on page 8, volvulus of the bowel will also cause obstruction and if not treated emergently, may result in total bowel necrosis. Functional causes of bowel obstruction include Hirschsprung's disease (absent ganglion cells in a section of the colon which interferes with normal peristaltic movement of stool), meconium plug syndrome, septic ileus, meconium ileus, and hypothyroidism. Acquired causes of bowel obstruction include necrotizing enterocolitis (an intestinal infection that primary affects preterm infants) and peritoneal adhesions that may develop following intestinal infection or surgery. Adhesions can also be congenital; they are usually called "bands".

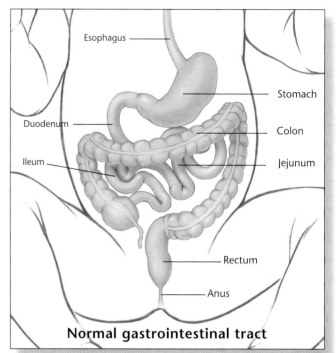

**Normal gastrointestinal tract**

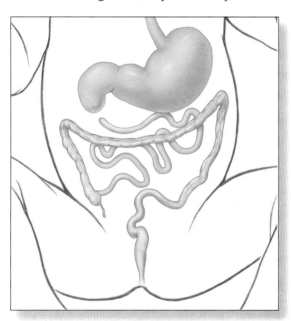

**Duodenal atresia:** complete atresia.

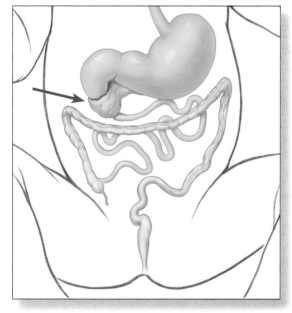

The duodenum may be partially or completely obstructed secondary to an **annular pancreas** (blue arrow).

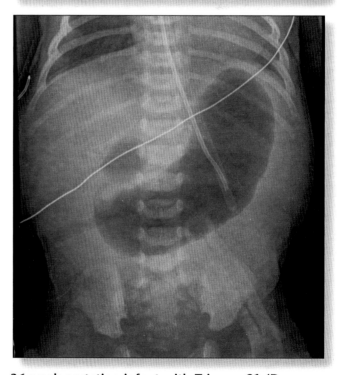

**36 week gestation infant with Trisomy 21 (Down syndrome) with duodenal atresia.** Note the following: distended gas filled stomach, gas in the pyloric channel and mildly distended gas filling the duodenal bulb. No bowel gas is present in the remainder of the bowel. The "double-bubble" sign represents the dilated stomach and obstructed portion of the duodenum.

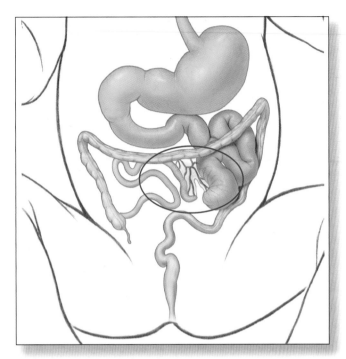

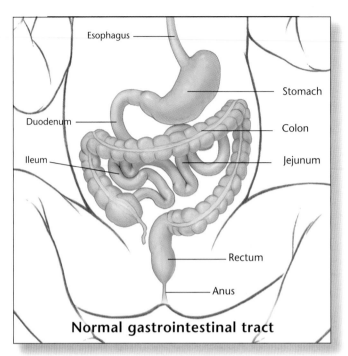

**Normal gastrointestinal tract**

**Jejunoileal atresia.** Atresia may be in the ileum, jejunum or both. There are various forms of jejunoileal atresia. One of the more common, (type IIIa) is illustrated here. Notice the two ends of atretic bowel are separated by a "V" shaped defect in the mesentery. The small bowel is dilated with gas prior to the area of atresia.

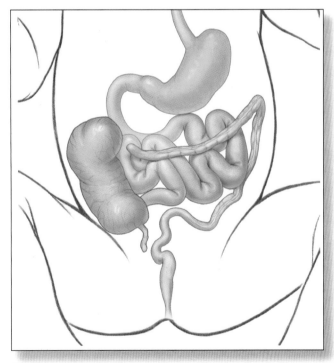

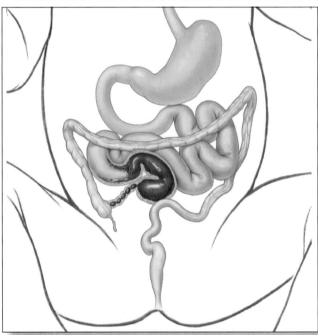

**Colonic atresia.** Notice the dilated small intestine and colon, up to the area of atresia in the colon.

**Meconium ileus.** Inspissated meconium obstructs the terminal ileum just prior to the ileocecal valve. Notice the pellets of hard meconium that prevent any gas or stool to pass. The problem results, in the majority of cases because of a lack of pancreatic enzymes that are necessary to digest intestinal contents, therefore, these infants must be evaluated for cystic fibrosis. If an abdominal x-ray reveals calcifications, this means the infant experienced intestinal perforation in utero.

# Appendix 1.1 **Bowel Obstruction** (continued)

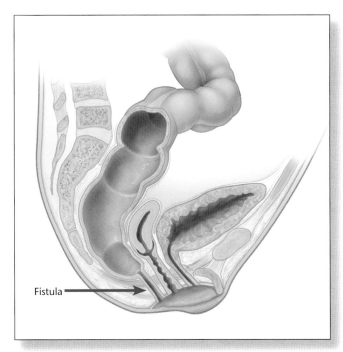

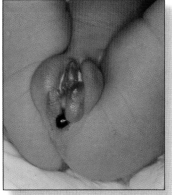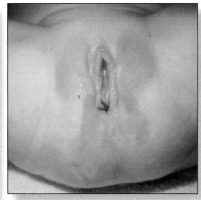

Meconium from a fistula external to the hymen but not on the perineal skin indicates **rectovestibular fistula**. This is the most common type of imperforate anus in females.

**Imperforate anus with rectovestibular fistula in a female infant.** Illustration demonstrates a rectovestibular fistula which is a connection between the rectum and the entroitus external to the hymen and not on the perianal skin.

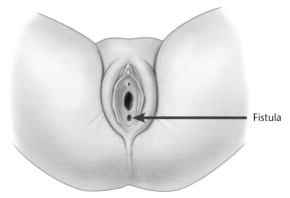

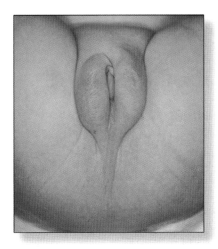

**Female with imperforate anus.** Since there is no evidence of fistula apparent at this time (no meconium is seen exiting the hymen), the differential diagnosis would include rectovestibular fistula and cloaca. Rectovestibular fistula is when there is a connection between the rectum and the entroitus external to the hymen and not on the perineal skin. A cloaca is when the urinary tract, vagina and rectum all meet in a common channel and the rectal fistula is proximal to the hymen. With both of these variants, meconium might be seen draining from the vagina.

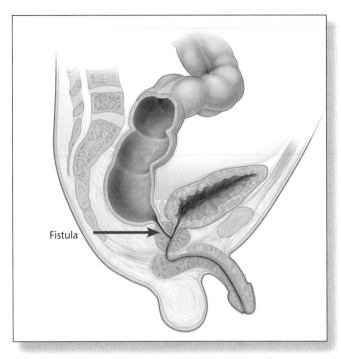

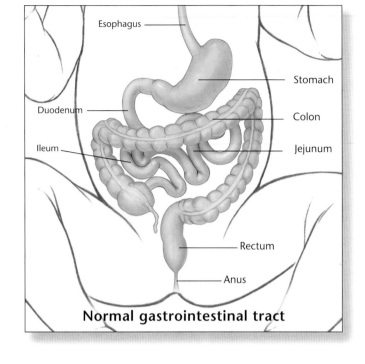

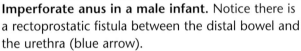

**Normal gastrointestinal tract**

**Imperforate anus in a male infant.** Notice there is a rectoprostatic fistula between the distal bowel and the urethra (blue arrow).

**Photos of two male infants with high imperforate anus.** The most common lesion in a male that would require diversion is the rectoprostatic fistula. Signs of this and more proximal lesions would include the absence of any meconium in the perineum (photo on left), a flat bottom and abnormal sacrum (photo on right), and meconium in the urine or at the tip of the penis (bottom photo). The flat bottom, especially if the sacrum is abnormal is virtually diagnostic of a proximally located rectum which would require diversion.

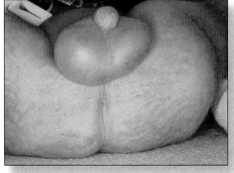

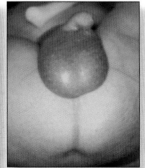

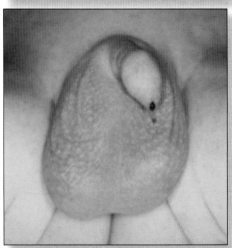

## Appendix 1.1 **Bowel Obstruction** (continued)

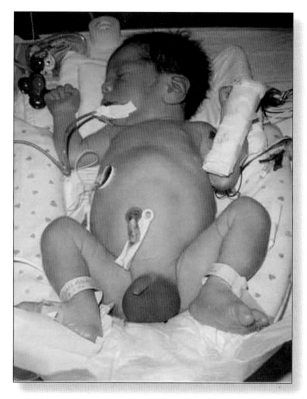

Infant with abdominal distension (gas filled bowel loops) secondary to imperforate anus. Notice the green colored (bilious) drainage in the orogastric tube.

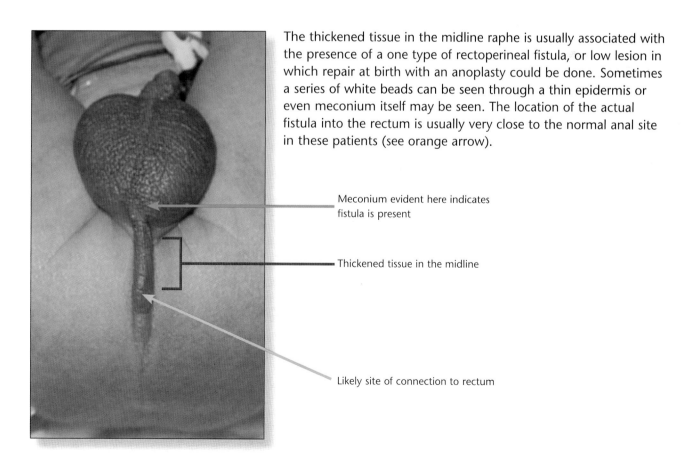

The thickened tissue in the midline raphe is usually associated with the presence of a one type of rectoperineal fistula, or low lesion in which repair at birth with an anoplasty could be done. Sometimes a series of white beads can be seen through a thin epidermis or even meconium itself may be seen. The location of the actual fistula into the rectum is usually very close to the normal anal site in these patients (see orange arrow).

Meconium evident here indicates fistula is present

Thickened tissue in the midline

Likely site of connection to rectum

## Appendix 1.2  **Intrauterine Growth Curves: Female**

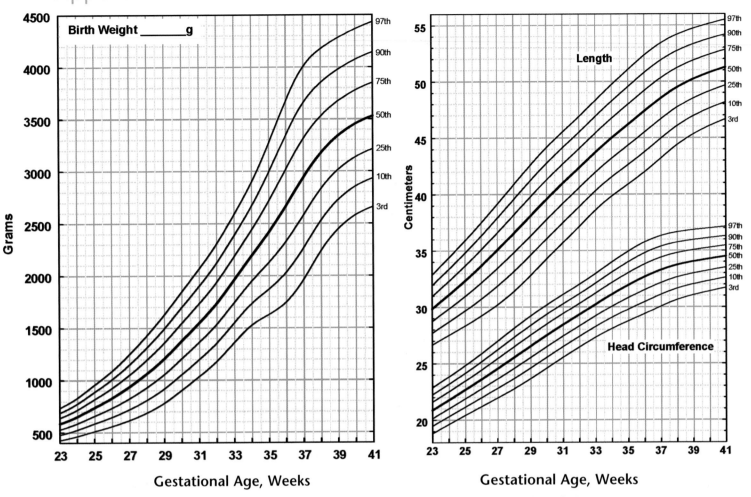

The 3rd and 97th percentiles on all curves for 23 weeks should be interpreted cautiously given the small sample size

### Weekly Growth Assessment

| Date | | | | | | | | | | | | | | | |
|---|---|---|---|---|---|---|---|---|---|---|---|---|---|---|---|
| **GA** (weeks) | | | | | | | | | | | | | | | |
| **WT** (grams) | | | | | | | | | | | | | | | |
| **Length** (cm) | | | | | | | | | | | | | | | |
| **HC** (cm) | | | | | | | | | | | | | | | |

*Reproduced with permission from Pediatrics, Volume 125, Pages e214-e244, Copyright 2010 by the American Academy of Pediatrics.[81]*

| **BIRTH ASSESSMENT:** Classification of Infant | Weight (grams) | Length (cm) | Head (cm) |
|---|---|---|---|
| **LGA:** Large for Gestational age (> 90th percentile) | | | |
| **AGA:** Appropriate for Gestational age (10th to 90th percentile) | | | |
| **SGA:** Small for Gestational Age (< 10th percentile) | | | |

**Directions:** Place an "X" in the appropriate box for the infant's weight, length, and head circumference. At times an infant's measurements may be in the LGA, AGA, or SGA box; not necessarily always in the same weight classification box.

# Appendix 1.3 **Intrauterine Growth Curves: Male**

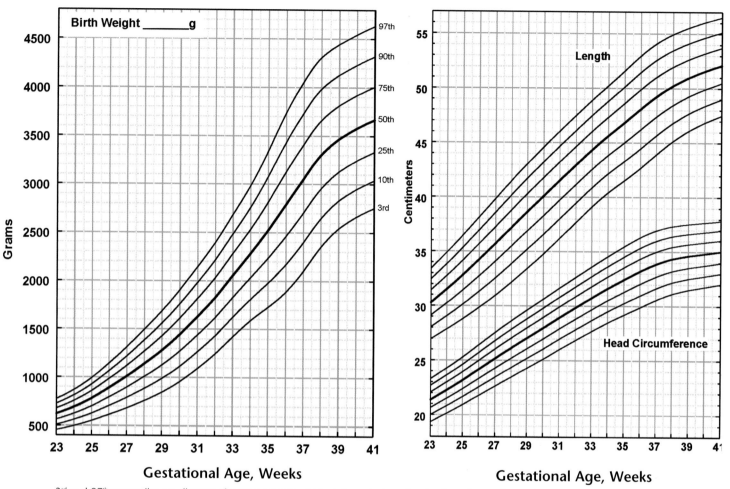

Gestational Age, Weeks

Gestational Age, Weeks

3rd and 97th percentiles on all curves for 23 weeks should be interpreted cautiously given the small sample size. For boys' HC curve at 24 weeks, all percentiles should be interpreted cautiously because the distribution of data is skewed left.

## Weekly Growth Assessment

| Date | | | | | | | | | | | | | | | | | | | | |
|------|--|--|--|--|--|--|--|--|--|--|--|--|--|--|--|--|--|--|--|--|
| GA (weeks) | | | | | | | | | | | | | | | | | | | | |
| WT (grams) | | | | | | | | | | | | | | | | | | | | |
| Length (cm) | | | | | | | | | | | | | | | | | | | | |
| HC (cm) | | | | | | | | | | | | | | | | | | | | |

*Reproduced with permission from Pediatrics, Volume 125, Pages e214-e244, Copyright 2010 by the American Academy of Pediatrics.*[81]

| BIRTH ASSESSMENT: Classification of Infant | Weight (grams) | Length (cm) | Head (cm) |
|---|---|---|---|
| **LGA:** Large for Gestational age (> 90th percentile) | | | |
| **AGA:** Appropriate for Gestational age (10th to 90th percentile) | | | |
| **SGA:** Small for Gestational Age (< 10th percentile) | | | |

**Directions:** Place an "X" in the appropriate box for the infant's weight, length, and head circumference. At times an infant's measurements may be in the LGA, AGA, or SGA box; not necessarily always in the same weight classification box.

# Appendix 1.4  **Dextrose Preparation Chart for IV Infusion**

At times, a higher, or lower dextrose concentration is required for IV infusion. Ideally, commercially prepared concentrations should be used. However if not available, the IV fluid should be prepared in the pharmacy under strict aseptic conditions.

| | **Mixing instructions using a 250 mL bag of $D_{10}W$ or $D_5W$** | | | |
|---|---|---|---|---|
| | Note: there is a 20 mL overfill when using a 250 mL bag, therefore, the starting volume is 270 mL[a] | | | |
| **To Make** | **Dextrose 50% for injection (mL)** | **$D_{10}W$ (mL)** | **$D_5W$ (mL)** | **Final Volume (mL)** |
| $D_5W$ (commercially available) | | | | |
| $D_6W$ | 6 | - | 270 | 276 |
| $D_7W$ | 13 | - | 270 | 283 |
| $D_{7.5}W$ | 16 | - | 270 | 286 |
| $D_8W$ | 19 | - | 270 | 289 |
| $D_9W$ | 26 | - | 270 | 296 |
| $D_{10}W$ (commercially available) | | | | |
| $D_{11}W$ | 7 | 270 | - | 277 |
| $D_{12}W$ | 14 | 270 | - | 284 |
| $D_{12.5}W$ | 18 | 270 | - | 288 |
| Dextrose concentrations exceeding $D_{12.5}W$ should be infused via a central line | | | | |
| $D_{13}W$ | 22 | 270 | - | 292 |
| $D_{14}W$ | 30 | 270 | - | 300 |
| $D_{15}W$ | 39 | 270 | - | 309 |
| $D_{16}W$ | 48 | 270 | - | 318 |
| $D_{17}W$ | 57 | 270 | - | 327 |
| $D_{17.5}W$ | 62 | 270 | - | 332 |
| $D_{18}W$ | 68 | 270 | - | 338 |
| $D_{19}W$ | 78 | 270 | - | 348 |
| $D_{20}W$ | 90 | 270 | - | 360 |

[a]The overfill volume of 20 mLs is based on IV solution bags from Hospira®. If the IV bag is from a different manufacturer, check how much overfill (if any) there is and make appropriate adjustments to the Dextrose 50% volume that is required to make the correct dextrose concentration.

# Appendix 1.4  **Dextrose Preparation Chart for IV Infusion**
(continued)

| To Make | Dextrose 50% for injection (mL) | $D_{10}W$ (mL) | $D_5W$ (mL) | Final Volume (mL) |
|---|---|---|---|---|
| **Mixing instructions using $D_{10}W$ or $D_5W$** | | | | |
| • Because of the smaller final volume, do not round numbers. | | | | |
| • This chart may be utilized if infusing the fluids through a syringe pump using a 50 or 60 mL syringe. | | | | |
| $D_5W$ (commercially available) | | | | |
| $D_6W$ | 1.1 | - | 48.9 | 50 |
| $D_7W$ | 2.2 | - | 47.8 | 50 |
| $D_{7.5}W$ | 2.8 | - | 47.2 | 50 |
| $D_8W$ | 3.3 | - | 46.7 | 50 |
| $D_9W$ | 4.4 | - | 45.6 | 50 |
| $D_{10}W$ (commercially available) | | | | |
| $D_{11}W$ | 1.3 | 48.7 | - | 50 |
| $D_{12}W$ | 2.5 | 47.5 | - | 50 |
| $D_{12.5}W$ | 3.1 | 46.9 | - | 50 |
| Dextrose concentrations exceeding $D_{12.5}W$ should be infused via a central line | | | | |
| $D_{13}W$ | 3.8 | 46.2 | - | 50 |
| $D_{14}W$ | 5 | 45 | - | 50 |
| $D_{15}W$ | 6.3 | 43.7 | - | 50 |
| $D_{16}W$ | 7.5 | 42.5 | - | 50 |
| $D_{17}W$ | 8.8 | 41.2 | - | 50 |
| $D_{17.5}W$ | 9.4 | 40.6 | - | 50 |
| $D_{18}W$ | 10 | 40 | - | 50 |
| $D_{19}W$ | 11.3 | 38.7 | - | 50 |
| $D_{20}W$ | 12.5 | 37.5 | - | 50 |

# Appendix 1.5 **Calculating Umbilical Catheter Depth Using Mathematical Formulas**

## High Umbilical Artery Catheter (UAC)
- Tip is located between thoracic vertebrae 6 and 9 (T6 and T9).[119,122,124]
- **UA catheter length (in centimeters) = [3 X birth weight (in kilograms)] + 9.**[119]
  - ◇ Add the length of the umbilical stump (in centimeters) to the calculation.

## Low Umbilical Artery Catheter (UAC)
- Tip is located between lumbar vertebrae 3 and 4 (L3 and L4).[122,124]
- **UA catheter length (in centimeters) = birth weight (in kilograms) + 7.**[119]
  - ◇ Add the length of the umbilical stump (in centimeters) to the calculation.

## Umbilical Venous Catheter (UVC)
- Tip is located at the junction of the inferior vena cava and right atrium.[118-120,135]
- **UV catheter length (in centimeters) = [0.5 X high line UA length (in centimeters)] + 1.**[119]
  - ◇ Add the length of the umbilical stump (in centimeters) to the calculation.

---

 These formulas are helpful to estimate correct insertion depth, however they may overestimate insertion depth! When the catheter is located too deep or not deep enough, refer to the information in Table 1.9 for guidance on how to correct a malpositioned line.

---

An alternative calculation for:

## High UAC catheter in infants weighing less than 1500 grams
- Tip is located between thoracic vertebrae 6 and 10 (T6 and T10).[148]
- **UA catheter length (in centimeters) = [4 x birth weight (in kilograms)] + 7.**[148]

  Notes:
  1. When using this formula, there was a statistically significant improvement in correctly located UAC catheters, however 11% of the infants had catheters that were sited below T10 (not a statistically significant number of patients, but a clinically important finding).
  2. This study allowed catheter position between T6 and T10, whereas the S.T.A.B.L.E. Program recommends high UAC catheters be located between T6 and T9.
  3. This formula does appear to improve correct catheter location on initial insertion, however, it will be important to use caution when utilizing this formula because a small percentage of catheters may be malpositioned.

**Confirm all catheter placement (or repositioning of catheters) with an x-ray.** It may be necessary to evaluate both a chest and abdominal x-ray to determine whether the catheter was inserted into the umbilical artery or vein. If unsure of the tip location, a cross-table lateral view x-ray may provide additional useful information in addition to the anteroposterior view.

# Appendix 1.6  Determining Umbilical Catheter Tip Location Using a Graph[149]

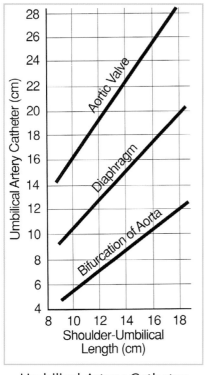

Umbilical Artery Catheter

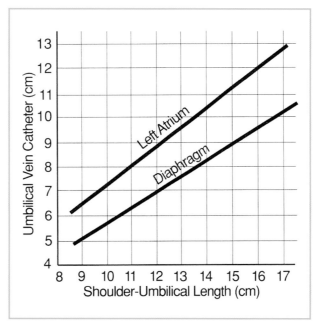

Umbilical Vein Catheter

## Catheter Location:

**High UAC:**  Tip should be above the diaphragm and well below the aortic valve (between T6 and T9). *[preferred]*

**Low UAC:**  Tip should lie just above the aortic bifurcation between L3 to L4.[122,124]

**UVC:**  Tip should be above the diaphragm at the inferior vena cava/right atrial junction. The catheter tip should not be left in the right atrium, liver or ductus venosus.

 These graphs are useful for estimating insertion depth. Confirm all catheter placements (or repositioning of catheters) with an x-ray. It may be necessary to evaluate both a chest and abdominal x-ray to determine whether the catheter was inserted into the umbilical artery or vein. If unsure of the tip location, a cross-table lateral view x-ray may provide additional useful information in addition to the anteroposterior view.

## Procedure:

1. Using a centimeter measuring tape, measure from the top of the shoulder over the lateral end of the clavicle straight down to a point that is level with the center of the umbilicus.[149] [Please note, the measurement is not diagonal from the shoulder to the umbilicus, but straight down from the shoulder to the level of the center of the umbilicus].

2. Find this measurement on the horizontal (bottom) axis of the appropriate umbilical artery or vein graph.

3. Draw a line straight up from this measurement to the desired location on the vertical (side) axis; e.g. for a low UAC, high UAC, or UVC.

4. If the umbilical stump is longer than 0.5 to 1 cm, then add the length of the umbilical stump (in centimeters) to the final measurement.

# Appendix 1.6 Determining Umbilical Catheter Tip Location Using a Graph[149] (continued)

**Example:** How To Use the Shoulder-To-Umbilical-Length Measurement Graph to Calculate Umbilical Artery Catheter Insertion Depth

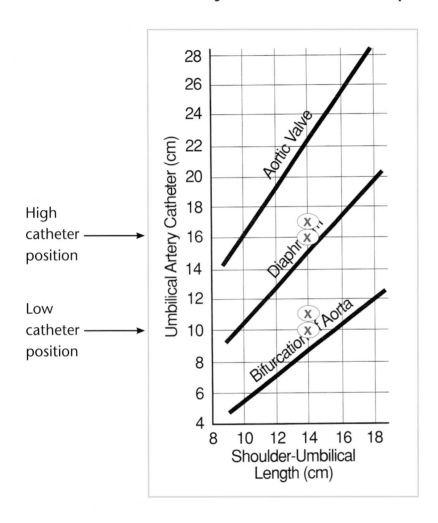

1. Measure the shoulder to umbilical length as previously described (in this example the measurement is 14 centimeters).

2. Next locate 14 cm on the horizontal (bottom) axis of the graph (Shoulder-Umbilical Length cm).

3. To locate the catheter in a low position, move up on the graph from 14 until you reach the Bifurcation of Aorta line.

4. The Bifurcation of Aorta location will be slightly too low so add 1 to 2 cm more which would be about 10 to 11 cms.

5. To place the catheter in a high position, move up on the graph from 14 until you reach the Diaphragm line.

6. The Diaphragm location will be slightly low, so add 1 to 2 cm more which would be about 16 to 17 cms.

7. If there is a long umbilical stump, add the amount of the stump in cm to your calculations.

8. If the catheter is placed low, confirm placement with an abdominal x-ray. If placed high, a chest x-ray should be adequate. If the catheter is repositioned, repeat the x-ray.

*Graphs reproduced with permission from The Harriet Lane Handbook (1993). Procedures. (13th ed., p. 63-65). St. Louis: Mosby-Year Book, Inc. and are based on data from Dunn, P.M. (1966).[149]*

# References

1. Srinivasan C, Sachdeva R, Morrow WR, et al. Standardized management improves outcomes after the Norwood procedure. Congenit Heart Dis 2009;4:329-37.

2. Spector JM, Villanueva HS, Brito ME, Sosa PG. Improving outcomes of transported newborns in Panama: impact of a nationwide neonatal provider education program. J Perinatol 2009;29:512-6.

3. Verónica R, Gallo L, Medina D, et al. Safe neonatal transport in the state of Jalisco: Impact of the S.T.A.B.L.E. program on morbidity and mortality. Bol Med Hosp Infant Mex 2011;68:31-5.

4. Rojas MA, Shirley K, Rush MG. Perinatal Transport and Levels of Care. In: Gardner SL, Carter BS, Enzman-Hines M, Hernandez JA, eds. Merenstein & Gardner's Handbook of Neonatal Intensive Care 7ed. St. Louis: Mosby Elsevier; 2011:39-51.

5. Lockwood CJ, Lemons JA, eds. American Academy of Pediatrics and The American College of Obstetricians and Gynecologists Guidelines for Perinatal Care. 6th ed. Elk Grove Village: American Academy of Pediatrics; 2007.

6. Bellezza F. Mnemonic Devices: Classification, Characteristics, and Criteria. Review of educational research 1981;51:247-75.

7. Kleinman ME, Chameides L, Schexnayder SM, et al. Part 14: Pediatric Advanced Life Support: 2010 American Heart Association Guidelines for Cardiopulmonary Resuscitation and Emergency Cardiovascular Care. Resuscitation 2010;122:S876-S908.

8. Kattwinkel J. Preface. In: Kattwinkel J, McGowan JE, Zaichkin J, eds. Textbook of Neonatal Resuscitation. 6th ed. Elk Grove Village: American Academy of Pediatrics; 2011:vii-x.

9. Kattwinkel J, McGowan JE, Zaichkin J. Textbook of Neonatal Resuscitation. 6th ed. Elk Grove Village: American Academy of Pediatrics; 2011.

10. Clark SL, Miller DD, Belfort MA, Dildy GA, Frye DK, Meyers JA. Neonatal and maternal outcomes associated with elective term delivery. American Journal of Obstetrics and Gynecology 2009;200:156 e1-4.

11. Karlsen KA, Trautman M, Price-Douglas W, Smith S. National survey of neonatal transport teams in the United States. Pediatrics 2011;128:685-91.

12. Schwartz RM, Kellogg R, Muri JH. Specialty newborn care: trends and issues. J Perinatol 2000;20:520-9.

13. Tita AT, Lai Y, Landon MB, et al. Timing of elective repeat cesarean delivery at term and maternal perioperative outcomes. Obstet Gynecol 2011;117:280-6.

14. Wax JR, Pinette MG, Cartin A, Blackstone J. Maternal and newborn morbidity by birth facility among selected United States 2006 low-risk births. American Journal of Obstetrics and Gynecology 2010;202:152 e1-5.

15. Perlman JM, Wyllie J, Kattwinkel J, et al. Neonatal resuscitation: 2010 International Consensus on Cardiopulmonary Resuscitation and Emergency Cardiovascular Care Science with Treatment Recommendations. Pediatrics 2010;126:e1319-44.

16. Taylor RM, Price-Douglas W. The S.T.A.B.L.E. Program: postresuscitation/pretransport stabilization care of sick infants. J Perinat Neonatal Nurs 2008;22:159-65.

17. Gould JB, Medoff-Cooper BS, Donovan EF, Stark AR. Applying Quality Improvement Principles in Caring for the High-risk Infant. In: Berns SD, Kott A, eds. Toward Improving the Outcome of Pregnancy III: Enhancing Perinatal Health Through Quality, Safety and Performance Initiatives. White Plains, NY: March of Dimes Foundation; 2010:76-86.

18. Bradley P. The history of simulation in medical education and possible future directions. Med Educ 2006;40:254-62.

19. Bush MC, Jankouskas TS, Sinz EH, Rudy S, Henry J, Murray WB. A method for designing symmetrical simulation scenarios for evaluation of behavioral skills. Simul Healthc 2007;2:102-9.

20. Ohlinger J, Kantak A, Lavin JP, Jr., et al. Evaluation and development of potentially better practices for perinatal and neonatal communication and collaboration. Pediatrics 2006;118 Suppl 2:S147-52.

21. dos Santos Mezzacappa MA, Collares EF. Gastric emptying in premature newborns with acute respiratory distress. J Pediatr Gastroenterol Nutr 2005;40:339-44.

22. Koenig JS, Davies AM, Thach BT. Coordination of breathing, sucking, and swallowing during bottle feedings in human infants. J Appl Physiol 1990;69:1623-9.

23. Pickler RH. A Model of Feeding Readiness for Preterm Infants. Neonatal Intensive Care 2004;17:31-6.

24. Ferrieri P, Wallen LD. Neonatal Bacterial Sepsis. In: Gleason CA, Devaskar SU, eds. Avery's Diseases of the Newborn. 9th ed. Philadelphia: Elsevier Saunders; 2012:538-50.

25. Puopolo K. Bacterial and Fungal Infections. In: Cloherty JP, Eichenwald EC, Hansen AR, Stark AR, eds. Manual of neonatal care. 7th ed. Philadelphia: Wolters Kluwer / Lippincott Williams & Wilkins; 2012:624-55.

26. Clark DA, Munshi UK. Development of the Gastrointestinal Circulation in the Fetus and Newborn. In: Polin RA, Fox WW, Abman SH, eds. Fetal and Neonatal Physiology. 4th ed. Philadelphia: Elsevier Saunders; 2011:773-7.

27. Phillipps AF. Oxygen Consumption and General Carbohydrate Metabolism of the Fetus. In: Polin RA, Fox WW, Abman SH, eds. Fetal and Neonatal Physiology. 4th ed. Philadelphia: Elsevier Saunders; 2011:535-49.

28. Song C, Upperman JS, Niklas V. Structural Anomalies of the Gastrointestinal Tract. In: Gleason CA, Devaskar SU, eds. Avery's Diseases of the Newborn. 9th ed. Philadelphia: Elsevier Saunders; 2012:979-93.

29. Hackam DJ, Grikscheit TC, Wang KS, Newman KD, Ford HR. Pediatric Surgery. In: Brunicardi FC, Andersen DK, Billiar TR, et al., eds. Schwartz's Principles of Surgery. 9th ed. New York: McGraw Hill Medical; 2010:1409-57.

30. Frost MS, Fashaw L, Hernandez JA, Jones MD. Neonatal Nephrology. In: Gardner SL, Carter BS, Enzman-Hines M, Hernandez JA, eds. Merenstein & Gardner's Handbook of Neonatal Intensive Care. 7th ed. St. Louis: Mosby Elsevier; 2011:717-47.

31. Bates CM, Schwaderer AL. Clinical Evaluation of Renal and Urinary Tract Disease. In: Gleason CA, Devaskar SU, eds. Avery's Diseases of the Newborn. 9th ed. Philadelphia: Elsevier Saunders; 2012:1176-81.

32. Blackburn ST. Carbohydrate, Fat, and Protein Metabolism. In: Blackburn ST, ed. Maternal, fetal, and neonatal physiology: A clinical perspective. St. Louis: Saunders Elsevier; 2007:598-625.

33. Hall JE. Cerebral Blood Flow, Cerebrospinal Fluid, and Brain Metabolism. In: Hall JE, ed. Guyton and Hall textbook of medical physiology 12th ed. Philadelphia: Saunders Elsevier; 2011:743-50.

34. Hall JE. Insulin, Glucagon, and Diabetes Mellitus. In: Hall JE, ed. Guyton and Hall textbook of medical physiology. 12th ed. Philadelphia: Saunders Elsevier; 2011:939-54.

35. Sherwood L. Principals of Endocrinology: The Central Endocrine Glands. In: Sherwood L, ed. Human physiology: From cells to systems 5th ed. Belmont: Brooks/Cole–Thomson Learning; 2004:667-99.

36. Kattwinkel J. Medications. In: Kattwinkel J, McGowan JE, Zaichkin J, eds. Textbook of Neonatal Resuscitation. 6th ed. Elk Grove Village: American Academy of Pediatrics; 2011:211-36.

37. Chameides L. Resources for Management of Circulatory Emergencies. In: Chameides L, Samson RA, Schexnayder SM, Hazinski MF, eds. Pediatric Advanced Life Support Provider Manual. Dallas,: American Heart Association; 2011:109-11.

38. Sax H, Allegranzi B, Uckay I, Larson E, Boyce J, Pittet D. 'My five moments for hand hygiene': a user-centred design approach to understand, train, monitor and report hand hygiene. J Hosp Infect 2007;67:9-21.

39. Deshpande S, Ward Platt M. The investigation and management of neonatal hypoglycaemia. Seminars in fetal & neonatal medicine 2005;10:351-61.

40. Jain V, Chen M, Menon RK. Disorders of Carbohydrate Metabolism. In: Gleason CA, Devaskar SU, eds. Avery's Diseases of the Newborn. 9th ed. Philadelphia: Elsevier Saunders; 2012:1320-9.

41. Angel JL, O'Brien WF, Knuppel RA, Morales WJ, Sims CJ. Carbohydrate intolerance in patients receiving oral tocolytics. American Journal of Obstetrics and Gynecology 1988;159:762-6.

42. Bergman B, Bokstrom H, Borga O, Enk L, Hedner T, Wangberg B. Transfer of terbutaline across the human placenta in late pregnancy. Eur J Respir Dis Suppl 1984;134:81-6.

43. Main EK, Main DM, Gabbe SG. Chronic oral terbutaline tocolytic therapy is associated with maternal glucose intolerance. American Journal of Obstetrics and Gynecology 1987;157:644-7.

44. Buchanan TA, Kitzmiller JL. Metabolic interactions of diabetes and pregnancy. Annu Rev Med 1994;45:245-60.

45. Cheung NW. The management of gestational diabetes. Vasc Health Risk Manag 2009;5:153-64.

46. Elliott BD, Schenker S, Langer O, Johnson R, Prihoda T. Comparative placental transport of oral hypoglycemic agents in humans: a model of human placental drug transfer. American Journal of Obstetrics and Gynecology 1994;171:653-60.

47. Langer O, Conway DL, Berkus MD, Xenakis EM, Gonzales O. A comparison of glyburide and insulin in women with gestational diabetes mellitus. The New England journal of medicine 2000;343:1134-8.

48. Philipps AF, Dubin JW, Raye JR. Response of the fetal and newborn lamb to glucose and tolbutamide infusions. Pediatr Res 1979;13:1375-8.

49. Warburton D, Parton L, Buckley S, Cosico L, Saluna T. Effects of beta-2 agonist on hepatic glycogen metabolism in the fetal lamb. Pediatr Res 1988;24:330-2.

50. Wilker RE. Hypoglycemia and Hyperglycemia. In: Cloherty JP, Eichenwald EC, Hansen AR, Stark AR, eds. Manual of neonatal care. 7th ed. Philadelphia: Wolters Kluwer / Lippincott Williams & Wilkins.; 2012:284-96.

51. Collins R, Yusuf S, Peto R. Overview of randomised trials of diuretics in pregnancy. Br Med J (Clin Res Ed) 1985;290:17-23.

52. Andersohn F, Schade R, Suissa S, Garbe E. Long-term use of antidepressants for depressive disorders and the risk of diabetes mellitus. Am J Psychiatry 2009;166:591-8.

53. Kallen B. Neonate characteristics after maternal use of antidepressants in late pregnancy. Arch Pediatr Adolesc Med 2004;158:312-6.

54. Shrivastava VK, Garite TJ, Jenkins SM, et al. A randomized, double-blinded, controlled trial comparing parenteral normal saline with and without dextrose on the course of labor in nulliparas. American Journal of Obstetrics and Gynecology 2009;200:379 e1-6.

55. Luna B, Feinglos MN. Drug-induced hyperglycemia. Jama 2001;286:1945-8.

56. McGowan JE, Rozance PJ, Price-Douglas W, Hay WW. Glucose Homeostasis. In: Gardner SL, Carter BS, Enzman-Hines M, Hernandez JA, eds. Merenstein & Gardner's Handbook of Neonatal Intensive Care. 7th ed. St. Louis: Mosby Elsevier; 2011:353-77.

57. Ward Platt M, Deshpande S. Metabolic adaptation at birth. Seminars in fetal & neonatal medicine 2005;10:341-50.

58. Stanley C, Hardy O. Pathophysiology of Hypoglycemia. In: Polin RA, Fox WW, Abman SH, eds. Fetal and Neonatal Physiology. 4th ed. Philadelphia: Elsevier Saunders; 2011:568-75.

59. Kliegman RM. Problems in Metabolic Adaptation: Glucose, Calcium, and Magnesium. In: Klaus MH, Fanaroff AA, eds. Care of the high-risk neonate. 5th ed. Philadelphia: Saunders; 2001:301-23.

60. Engle WA. Infants born late preterm: definition, physiologic and metabolic immaturity, and outcomes. NeoReviews 2009;10:e280-e6.

61. Shapiro-Mendoza CK. Infants born late preterm: Epidemiology, trends, and morbidity risk. NeoReviews 2009;10:e287-e94.

62. Hibbard JU, Wilkins I, Sun L, et al. Respiratory morbidity in late preterm births. Jama 2010;304:419-25.

63. Loftin RW, Habli M, Snyder CC, Cormier CM, Lewis DF, Defranco EA. Late preterm birth. Rev Obstet Gynecol 2010;3:10-9.

64. Radtke JV. The paradox of breastfeeding-associated morbidity among late preterm infants. J Obstet Gynecol Neonatal Nurs 2011;40:9-24.

65. Yoder BA, Gordon MC, Barth WH, Jr. Late-preterm birth: does the changing obstetric paradigm alter the epidemiology of respiratory complications? Obstet Gynecol 2008;111:814-22.

66. Lubow JM, How HY, Habli M, Maxwell R, Sibai BM. Indications for delivery and short-term neonatal outcomes in late preterm as compared with term births. American Journal of Obstetrics and Gynecology 2009;200:e30-3.

67. McGowan JE, Alderdice FA, Holmes VA, Johnston L. Early childhood development of late-preterm infants: a systematic review. Pediatrics 2011;127:1111-24.

68. Morse SB, Zheng H, Tang Y, Roth J. Early school-age outcomes of late preterm infants. Pediatrics 2009;123:e622-9.

69. Simmons R. Abnormalities of Fetal Growth. In: Gleason CA, Devaskar SU, eds. Avery's Diseases of the Newborn. 9th ed. Philadelphia: Elsevier Saunders; 2012:51-9.

70. Styne DM. Endocrine Factors Affecting Neonatal Growth. In: Polin RA, Fox WW, Abman SH, eds. Fetal and Neonatal Physiology. 4th ed. Philadelphia: Elsevier Saunders; 2011:310-23.

71. Kliegman RM. Intrauterine Growth Restriction. In: Martin RJ, Fanaroff AA, Walsh MC, eds. Fanaroff and Martin's Neonatal-Perinatal Medicine: Diseases of the Fetus and Infant. 9th ed. St. Louis: Elsevier Mosby; 2011:245-75.

72. Bhat MA, Kumar P, Bhansali A, Majumdar S, Narang A. Hypoglycemia in small for gestational age babies. Indian J Pediatr 2000;67:423-7.

73. Mejri A, Dorval VG, Nuyt AM, Carceller A. Hypoglycemia in term newborns with a birth weight below the 10th percentile. Paediatr Child Health 2010;15:271-5.

74. Smith VC. The High-Risk Newborn: Anticipation, Evaluation, Management, and Outcome. In: Cloherty JP, Eichenwald EC, Hansen AR, Stark AR, eds. Manual of neonatal care. 7th ed. Philadelphia: Wolters Kluwer / Lippincott Williams & Wilkins; 2012:74-90.

75. Subhani M. Intrauterine Growth Restriction. In: Spitzer AR, ed. Intensive care of the fetus & neonate. 2nd ed. Philadelphia: Elsevier Mosby; 2005:135-48.

76. Das UG, Sysyn GD. Abnormal fetal growth: intrauterine growth retardation, small for gestational age, large for gestational age. Pediatric Clinics of North America 2004;51:639-54, viii.

77. De Santis M, Carducci B, Cavaliere AF, De Santis L, Straface G, Caruso A. Drug-induced congenital defects: strategies to reduce the incidence. Drug Saf 2001;24:889-901.

78. Lubchenco LO, Bard H. Incidence of hypoglycemia in newborn infants classified by birth weight and gestational age. Pediatrics 1971;47:831-8.

79. Townsend SF. The Large-for-Gestational-Age and the Small-for-Gestational-Age Infant. In: Thureen PJ, Deacon J, Hernandez JA, Hall DM, eds. Assessment and care of the well newborn. 2nd ed. St. Louis: Elsevier; 2005:267-78.

80. Trotter CW. Gestational Age Assessment. In: Tappero EP, Honeyfield ME, eds. Physical assessment of the newborn: A comprehensive approach to the art of physical examination. 4th ed. Santa Rosa: NICU Ink; 2009:21-39.

81. Olsen IE, Groveman SA, Lawson ML, Clark RH, Zemel BS. New intrauterine growth curves based on United States data. Pediatrics 2010;125:e214-24.

82. Persson B. Neonatal glucose metabolism in offspring of mothers with varying degrees of hyperglycemia during pregnancy. Seminars in fetal & neonatal medicine 2009;14:106-10.

83. Katz LL, Stanley CA. Disorders of glucose and other sugars. In: Spitzer AR, ed. Intensive care of the fetus & neonate. Philadelphia: Elsevier Mosby; 2005:1167-78.

84. Lee-Parritz A, Cloherty JP. Diabetes Mellitus. In: Cloherty JP, Eichenwald EC, Hansen AR, Stark AR, eds. Manual of neonatal care. 7th ed. Philadelphia: Wolters Kluwer / Lippincott Williams & Wilkins; 2012:11-23.

85. Nodine PM, Arruda J, Hastings-Tolsma M. Prenatal Environment: Effect on Neonatal Outcome. In: Gardner SL, Carter BS, Enzman-Hines M, Hernandez JA, eds. Merenstein & Gardner's Handbook of Neonatal Intensive Care. 7th ed. St. Louis: Mosby Elsevier; 2011:13-38.

86. Vora N, Bianchi DW. Genetic considerations in the prenatal diagnosis of overgrowth syndromes. Prenat Diagn 2009;29:923-9.

87. Metzger BE, Lowe LP, Dyer AR, et al. Hyperglycemia and Adverse Pregnancy Outcome (HAPO) Study: associations with neonatal anthropometrics. Diabetes 2009;58:453-9.

88. ADA. Diagnosis and classification of diabetes mellitus. Diabetes Care 2010;33 Suppl 1:S62-9.

89. Gabbe SG, Landon MB, Warren-Boulton E, Fradkin J. Promoting health after gestational diabetes: a national diabetes education program call to action. Obstet Gynecol 2012;119:171-6.

90. ADA. Standards of medical care in diabetes--2011. Diabetes Care 2011;34 Suppl 1:S11-61.

91. Heideman WH, Middelkoop BJ, Nierkens V, et al. Changing the odds. What do we learn from prevention studies targeted at people with a positive family history of type 2 diabetes? Prim Care Diabetes 2011;5:215-21.

92. Bellamy L, Casas JP, Hingorani AD, Williams D. Type 2 diabetes mellitus after gestational diabetes: a systematic review and meta-analysis. Lancet 2009;373:1773-9.

93. ACOG. Committee opinion no. 504: screening and diagnosis of gestational diabetes mellitus. Obstet Gynecol 2011;118:751-3.

94. Catalano PM. Management of obesity in pregnancy. Obstet Gynecol 2007;109:419-33.

95. Yogev Y, Metzger BE, Hod M. Establishing diagnosis of gestational diabetes mellitus: Impact of the hyperglycemia and adverse pregnancy outcome study. Seminars in Fetal & Neonatal Medicine 2009;14:94-100.

96. Catalano PM, Ehrenberg HM. The short- and long-term implications of maternal obesity on the mother and her offspring. Bjog 2006;113:1126-33.

97. Cowett RM, Farrag HM. Selected principles of perinatal-neonatal glucose metabolism. Semin Neonatol 2004;9:37-47.

98. Hall JE. Red Blood Cells, Anemia, and Polycythemia. In: Hall JE, ed. Guyton and Hall textbook of medical physiology 12th ed. Philadelphia: Saunders Elsevier; 2011:413-22.

99. Kahn R, Fonseca V. Translating the A1C Assay. Diabetes Care 2008;31:1704-7.

100. Metzger BE, Gabbe SG, Persson B, et al. International association of diabetes and pregnancy study groups recommendations on the diagnosis and classification of hyperglycemia in pregnancy. Diabetes Care 2010;33:676-82.

101. Weindling AM. Offspring of diabetic pregnancy: Short-term outcomes. Seminars in Fetal & Neonatal Medicine 2009;14:111-8.

102. Eriksson UJ. Congenital anomalies in diabetic pregnancy. Seminars in fetal & neonatal medicine 2009;14:85-93.

103. Yang J, Cummings EA, O'Connell C, Jangaard K. Fetal and neonatal outcomes of diabetic pregnancies. Obstet Gynecol 2006;108:644-50.

104. Landon MB, Spong CY, Thom E, et al. A multicenter, randomized trial of treatment for mild gestational diabetes. The New England journal of medicine 2009;361:1339-48.

105. Hall JE. Metabolism of Carbohydrates, and Formation of Adenosine Triphosphate. In: Hall JE, ed. Guyton and Hall textbook of medical physiology. 12th ed. Philadelphia: Saunders Elsevier; 2011:809-18.

106. Sherwood L. Cellular Physiology. In: Sherwood L, ed. Human physiology: From cells to systems. 5th ed. Belmont: Brooks/Cole-Thomson Learning.; 2004:23-55.

107. Rozance PJ, Hay WW. Hypoglycemia in newborn infants: Features associated with adverse outcomes. Biol Neonate 2006;90:74-86.

108. Hay Jr WW, Raju TNK, Higgins RD, Kalhan SC, Devaskar SU. Knowledge Gaps and Research Needs for Understanding and Treating Neonatal Hypoglycemia: Workshop Report from Eunice Kennedy Shriver National Institute of Child Health and Human Development. J Pediatr 2009;155:612-7.

109. Rozance PJ, Hay WW, Jr. Describing hypoglycemia—definition or operational threshold? Early Human Development 2010;86:275-80.

110. Williams AF. Neonatal hypoglycaemia: clinical and legal aspects. Seminars in fetal & neonatal medicine 2005;10:363-8.

111. Koh TH, Eyre JA, Aynsley-Green A. Neonatal hypoglycaemia--the controversy regarding definition. Arch Dis Child 1988;63:1386-8.

112. Hawdon JM, Ward Platt MP, Aynsley-Green A. Patterns of metabolic adaptation for preterm and term infants in the first neonatal week. Arch Dis Child 1992;67:357-65.

113. Hall JE. Lipid Metabolism. In: Hall JE, ed. Guyton and Hall Textbook of medical physiology. 12th ed. Philadelphia: Saunders Elsevier; 2011:819-30.

114. Doherty EG. Fluid and Electrolyte Management. In: Cloherty JP, Eichenwald EC, Hansen AR, Stark AR, eds. Manual of neonatal care. 7th ed. Philadelphia: Wolters Kluwer / Lippincott Williams & Wilkins; 2012:269-83.

115. Lilien LD, Pildes RS, Srinivasan G, Voora S, Yeh TF. Treatment of neonatal hypoglycemia with minibolus and intravenous glucose infusion. J Pediatr 1980;97:295-8.

116. Ellard DM, D.M. A. Nutrition. In: Cloherty JP, Eichenwald EC, Hansen AR, Stark AR, eds. Manual of Neonatal Care. 7th ed. Philadelphia: Wolters Kluwer / Lippincott Williams & Wilkins; 2012:230-68.

117. ElHassan NO, Kaiser JR. Parenteral nutrition in the neonatal intensive care unit. NeoReviews 2011;12:e130-e40.

118. Wortham BM, Rais-Bahrami K. Umbilical Vein Catheterization. In: MacDonald M, G., Ramasethu J, eds. Atlas of Procedures in Neonatology. 4th ed. Philadelphia: Wolters Kluwer / Lippincott Williams & Wilkins; 2007:177-85.

119. Sigman LJ. Procedures. In: Tschudy MM, Arcara KM, eds. The Harriet Lane Handbook. 19th ed. Philadelphia: Elsevier Mosby; 2012:57-88.

120. Gomella TL. Venous Access: Umbilical Vein Catheterization. In: Gomella TL, Cunningham MD, Eyal FG, Tuttle D, eds. Neonatology: Management, Procedures,On-call Problems, Diseases, and Drugs. New York: McGraw Hill Medical; 2009:243-6.

121. Ringer SA, Gray JE. Common Neonatal Procedures. In: Cloherty JP, Eichenwald EC, Hansen AR, Stark AR, eds. Manual of neonatal care. 7th ed. Philadelphia: Wolters Kluwer / Lippincott Williams & Wilkins; 2012:851-69.

122. Wortham BM, Gaitatzes CG, Rais-Bahrami K. Umbilical Artery Catheterization. In: MacDonald M, G., Ramasethu J, eds. Atlas of Procedures in Neonatology. 4th ed. Philadelphia: Lippincott Williams & Wilkins; 2007:157-76.

123. Revenis ME. Intraosseous Infusions. In: Macdonald M, G., Ramasethu J, eds. Atlas of Procedures in Neonatology. Philadelphia: Wolters Kluwer / Lippincott Williams & Wilkins; 2007:362-5.

124. Gomella TL. Arterial Access: Umbilical Artery Catheterization. In: Gomella TL, Cunningham MD, Eyal FG, Tuttle D, eds. Neonatology: Management, Procedures,On-call Problems, Diseases, and Drugs. 6th ed. New York: McGraw Hill Medical; 2009:203-7.

125. Durand DJ, Mickas NA. Blood Gases: Technical Aspects and Interpretation. In: Goldsmith JP, Karotkin EH, eds. Assisted Ventilation of the Newborn. 5th ed. St. Louis: Elsevier Saunders; 2011:292-305.

126. Smith L, Dills R. Survey of medication administration through umbilical arterial and venous catheters. Am J Health Syst Pharm 2003;60:1569-72.

127. Barrington KJ. Umbilical artery catheters in the newborn: effects of heparin. Cochrane Database Syst Rev 2000:CD000507.

128. Young TE, Mangum B. In: Neofax 2010. 23rd ed. Montvale: Thomson Reuters; 2010.

129. Massaro AN, Rais-Bahrami K, Eichelberger MR. Peripheral Arterial Cannulation. In: MacDonald M, G., Ramasethu J, eds. Atlas of Procedures in Neonatology. Philadelphia: Wolters Kluwer / Lippincott Williams & Wilkins; 2007:186-98.

130. Barrington KJ. Umbilical artery catheters in the newborn: effects of position of the catheter tip. Cochrane Database Syst Rev 2000:CD000505.

131. Jackson JK, Biondo DJ, Jones JM, et al. Can an alternative umbilical arterial catheter solution and flush regimen decrease iatrogenic hemolysis while enhancing nutrition? A double-blind, randomized, clinical trial comparing an isotonic amino acid with a hypotonic salt infusion. Pediatrics 2004;114:377-83.

132. Brown MS, Phibbs RH. Spinal cord injury in newborns from use of umbilical artery catheters: report of two cases and a review of the literature. J Perinatol 1988;8:105-10.

133. Zenk KE, Noerr B, Ward R. Severe sequelae from umbilical arterial catheter administration of dopamine. Neonatal network : NN 1994;13:89-91.

134. Bradshaw WT, Tanaka DT. Physiologic Monitoring. In: Gardner SL, Carter BS, Enzman-Hines M, Hernandez JA, eds. Merenstein & Gardner's Handbook of Neonatal Intensive Care. 7th ed. St. Louis: Mosby Elsevier; 2011:134-52.

135. Schlesinger AE, Braverman RM, DiPietro MA. Pictorial essay. Neonates and umbilical venous catheters: normal appearance, anomalous positions, complications, and potential aid to diagnosis. AJR Am J Roentgenol 2003;180:1147-53.

136. Nash P. Umbilical catheters, placement, and complication management. J Infus Nurs 2006;29:346-52.

137. Bradshaw WT, Furdon SA. A nurse's guide to early detection of umbilical venous catheter complications in infants. Advances in neonatal care : official journal of the National Association of Neonatal Nurses 2006;6:127-38; quiz 39-41.

138. Furdon SA, Horgan MJ, Bradshaw WT, Clark DA. Nurses' guide to early detection of umbilical arterial catheter complications in infants. Advances in neonatal care : official journal of the National Association of Neonatal Nurses 2006;6:242-56; quiz 57-60.

139. Gomella TL. Neonatal Radiology. In: Gomella TL, Cunningham MD, Eyal FG, Tuttle D, eds. Neonatology: Management, Procedures,On-call Problems, Diseases, and Drugs. 6th ed. New York: McGraw Hill Medical; 2009:108-30.

140. Davies MW, Mehr S, Morley CJ. The effect of draw-up volume on the accuracy of electrolyte measurements from neonatal arterial lines. Journal of paediatrics and child health 2000;36:122-4.

141. Schulz G, Keller E, Haensse D, Arlettaz R, Bucher HU, Fauchere JC. Slow blood sampling from an umbilical artery catheter prevents a decrease in cerebral oxygenation in the preterm newborn. Pediatrics 2003;111:e73-6.

142. Butt WW, Gow R, Whyte H, Smallhorn J, Koren G. Complications resulting from use of arterial catheters: retrograde flow and rapid elevation in blood pressure. Pediatrics 1985;76:250-4.

143. Gordon M, Bartruff L, Gordon S, Lofgren M, Widness JA. How fast is too fast? a practice change in umbilical arterial catheter blood sampling using the Iowa Model for Evidence-Based Practice. Advances in neonatal care : official journal of the National Association of Neonatal Nurses 2008;8:198-207.

144. Roll C, Huning B, Kaunicke M, Krug J, Horsch S. Umbilical artery catheter blood sampling volume and velocity: impact on cerebral blood volume and oxygenation in very-low-birthweight infants. Acta Paediatr 2006;95:68-73.

145. Ringer SA, Hansen AR. Surgical Emergencies in the Newborn. In: Cloherty JP, Eichenwald EC, Hansen AR, Stark AR, eds. Manual of Neonatal Care. 7th ed. Philadelphia: Lippincott, Williams & Wilkins; 2012:808-30.

146. Lovvorn HN, Glenn JB, Pacetti AS, Carter BS. Neonatal Surgery. In: Gardner SL, Carter BS, Enzman-Hines M, Hernandez JA, eds. Merenstein & Gardner's Handbook of Neonatal Intensive Care. 7th ed. St. Louis: Mosby Elsevier; 2011:812-47.

147. Barksdale EM, Chwals WJ, Magnuson DK, Parry RL. Selected Gastrointestinal Anomalies. In: Martin RJ, Fanaroff AA, Walsh MC, eds. Fanaroff & Martin's Neonatal-Perinatal Medicine: Diseases of the Fetus and Infant. 9th ed. St. Louis: Elsevier Mosby; 2011:1400-31

148. Wright IM, Owers M, Wagner M. The umbilical arterial catheter: a formula for improved positioning in the very low birth weight infant. Pediatr Crit Care Med 2008;9:498-501.

149. Dunn PM. Localization of the umbilical catheter by post-mortem measurement. Arch Dis Child 1966;41:69-75.

# **S**ugar and **S**afe Care
# **T**emperature
# **A**irway
# **B**lood Pressure
# **L**ab Work
# **E**motional Support

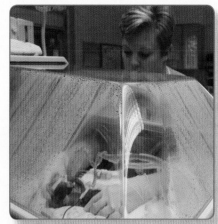

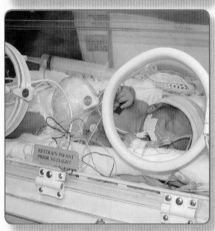

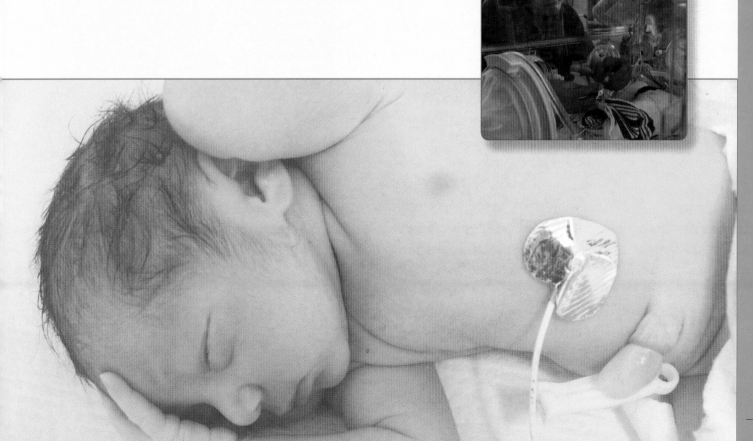

## Temperature – Module Objectives

Upon completion of this module, participants will gain an increased understanding of:

1.  Infants at increased risk for hypothermia.

2.  The normal physiologic response to cold stress for term infants.

3.  Mechanisms of heat gain and loss.

4.  The physiologic response to hypothermia for term and preterm infants.

5.  Candidates for therapeutic neuroprotective hypothermia.

6.  Methods to rewarm hypothermic infants and how to monitor hypothermic infants during rewarming.

## Introduction

Hypothermia is a **preventable** condition that has well documented impact on morbidity and mortality, especially in preterm infants.[1-6] Therefore, assisting the infant to maintain a normal body temperature and preventing hypothermia *and* hyperthermia during resuscitation and stabilization is critically important.

## Key Concepts

### I. Maintenance of a normal body temperature must be a priority whether infants are well or sick.

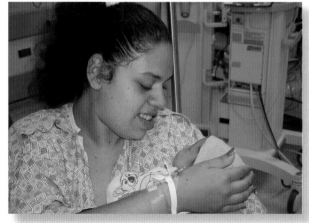

Routine care following birth and throughout the neonatal period includes many activities aimed at conserving the infant's body heat. For healthy term infants, these activities include removing wet linens, bundling in warm blankets, laying the infant skin-to-skin on the mother's chest, covering the infant's head with a hat, and keeping the infant clothed.[7,8] When infants are acutely sick or preterm however, normal care procedures are replaced with activities aimed at resuscitation and stabilization. Infants are usually left undressed and placed on open radiant warming beds to permit observation and performance of intensive care procedures. During resuscitation and stabilization, the risk of cold stress and hypothermia dramatically increases; therefore, extra care should be directed at preventing hypothermia.[3,8-10]

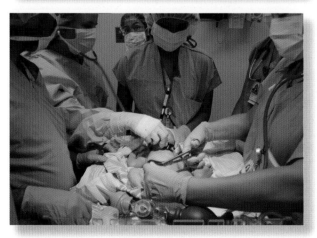

## What is a normal core temperature for infants and what is considered hypothermic?

A normal core temperature is between 36.5 and 37.5°C (97.7 and 99.5°F).[5,11] The World Health Organization[5] defines levels of mild, moderate, and severe hypothermia in infants as follows:

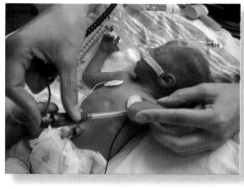

- **Mild:** core temperature is between 36 and 36.4°C (96.8 and 97.6°F).

- **Moderate:** core temperature is between 32 and 35.9°C (89.6 and 96.6°F).

- **Severe:** core temperature is less than 32°C (less than 89.6°F).

It is very possible that preterm infants experience the effects of hypothermia sooner than term infants; however, preterm specific ranges for mild, moderate, and severe hypothermia have not yet been defined. In small preterm infants (weight less than 1000 grams), the lower end of the thermal range that defines severe hypothermia may start at ≤ 35°C.[12]

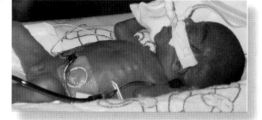

In addition, infants with concurrent illness including sepsis, respiratory distress, hypoxia or shock may experience the negative effects of hypothermia more quickly and severely.[6] Of major importance is the recognition that significant deterioration can and does occur in all infants well before they reach the severely hypothermic range.[10] Furthermore, in tiny preterm infants, this temperature may be higher than for their larger counterparts.

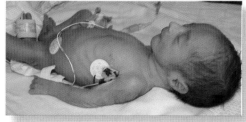

## II. Infants at highest risk for hypothermia include:

- Preterm, low-birth-weight infants.

- Small for gestational age (SGA) infants.

- Infants who require prolonged resuscitation.

- Infants who become acutely ill with infectious, cardiac, neurologic, and endocrine problems.

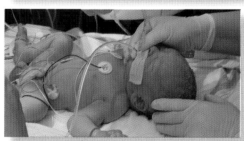

- Infants with surgical problems – especially infants with open body wall defects (such as gastroschisis [shown], omphalocele, or exposed spinal defects), where heat loss is more rapid.

- Infants who have decreased activity or are hypotonic from sedatives, analgesics, paralytics, or anesthetics.

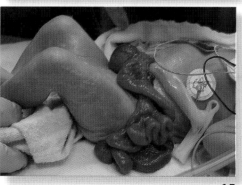

### III. Term infants who are "cold-stressed" will physiologically respond in an effort to conserve and generate body heat.

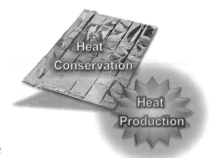

Cold and warm temperature receptors in the skin and deep tissues play an integral role in the maintenance of a normal body temperature. In response to cold stress, a series of reactions are activated for the purpose of decreasing heat loss and increasing heat production.[12] These include constriction of blood vessels in the arms and legs (peripheral vasoconstriction), increased muscle flexion and activity (to decrease surface area for heat loss and generate heat by moving the muscles), and metabolism of brown fat (also called chemical or non-shivering thermogenesis). To mount these responses, the metabolic rate must increase which, in turn, increases utilization of both oxygen and glucose.[10,12-14]

## Physiologic Response to Cold Stress

### Vasoconstriction – Decreases heat loss

When an infant experiences cold stress, blood vessels in the arms and legs constrict. This vasoconstriction prevents blood from reaching the skin surface where heat loss occurs; blood stays in the core of the body.[13,15,16] In the presence of prolonged vasoconstriction, blood flow and oxygen delivery to the tissues is reduced. This increases the risk for developing anaerobic metabolism and lactic acidosis, resulting in organ and tissue damage.[13]

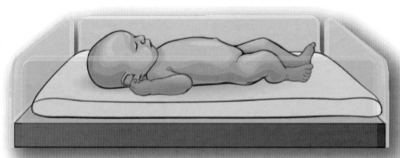

### Brown fat metabolism – Increases heat production

Brown fat is a substance that is accumulated in increasing amounts as the infant advances through gestation, especially in the last part of the third trimester. At term gestation, brown fat accounts for approximately 2 to 7 percent of the infant's total body weight.[10] Brown fat is located around the kidneys, adrenal glands, mediastinum, subscapular and axillary regions and the nape of the neck. In response to cold stress, norepinephrine is released into the nerve endings in brown fat, directing it to be metabolized or "burned."[17] When signaled to burn, brown fat cells generate more energy than any other tissue in the body! This highly metabolic activity produces heat in the core regions of the body and warms the blood as it circulates past. This process of generating heat is called "non-shivering thermogenesis."

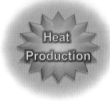

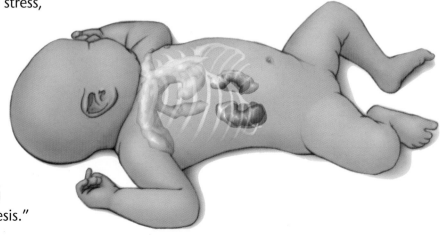

## Physiologic Response to Cold Stress (continued)

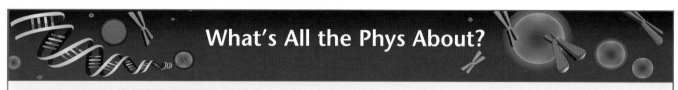

# What's All the Phys About?

### What factors affect ability to metabolize brown fat?

Brown fat metabolism requires oxygen and glucose as substrates, therefore, an infant who is hypoglycemic, has poor or depleted glycogen stores, and/or is hypoxic (insufficient tissue oxygenation to meet cellular demands), will not be able to metabolize brown fat.[12,18] In addition, if an infant is neurologically impaired, the hypothalamus, which is the part of the brain that regulates temperature, may not respond appropriately and fail to signal brown fat to burn, blood vessels to constrict, or muscle activity to increase.

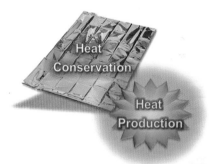

### Increased muscle activity and flexion – Increases heat production and decreases heat loss

In response to cold stress, infants have poor to no capacity to shiver. Instead, they increase their activity level by crying and flexing their arms and legs, which generates some heat in the muscles. Flexion of the arms and legs also reduces the surface area for heat loss.

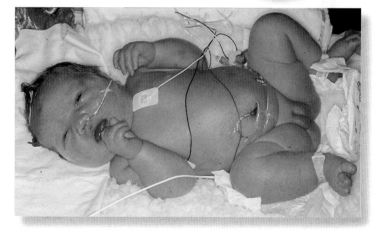

Depressed, severely ill, and preterm infants often are hypotonic and flaccid – lying with their limbs extended. This posture increases the surface area for heat loss.[13]

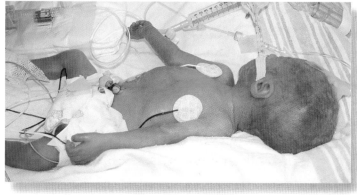

# REVIEW

## Infants at increased risk for hypothermia:

Infants who undergo prolonged resuscitation or become acutely ill

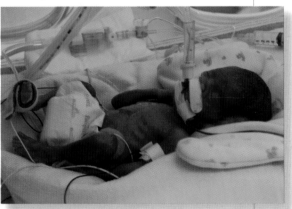

⬥ Infants who require prolonged resuscitation have a period of hypoxia; therefore, they are unable to metabolize brown fat.[12,14,18] Following fetal asphyxia, newborn infants who are exposed to a cold stimulus have a delayed metabolic response. This inability to mount a normal response to cold stress increases the risk for becoming hypothermic.[12]

⬥ Acutely ill infants, such as those with infections or cardiac problems, are often hypothermic when they present to the healthcare provider.

⬥ Infants with open abdominal defects, such as gastroschisis and omphalocele are at increased risk for convective, conductive, and evaporative heat loss because of their increased body surface area for losing heat and the close proximity of their blood vessels to the environment.[19,20]

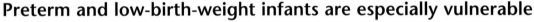

## Preterm and low-birth-weight infants are especially vulnerable

⬥ Infants often have difficulty balancing heat loss with heat production; this problem is further amplified in preterm and small for gestational age infants. When infants are born weighing less than 1500 grams, the problem is further accentuated.

⬥ Main factors contributing to this problem include:[8,10,13,14,16,21,22]

- A larger surface area to body mass ratio

- Weak muscle tone / poor flexion

- Thinner immature skin – diminished barrier to water evaporation

- Increased evaporative water loss

- Poor ability to vasoconstrict in the first few days of life

- Decreased amounts of insulating fat

- Reduced amounts or no brown fat

## Extra vigilance and protection from heat loss should be provided at all times!

# Temperature and Effect on Metabolic Rate and Oxygen Consumption

Figure 2.1 illustrates the effects of temperature on metabolic rate and oxygen consumption. With the onset of even mild hypothermia, defined as a core temperature below 36.5°C or 97.7°F, the infant's metabolic rate increases in an effort to produce *and* conserve heat, which in turn increases oxygen consumption and glucose utilization.[12,15] If the infant is already experiencing respiratory distress, increased oxygen demand from hypothermia may lead to hypoxemia (low blood oxygen levels). There is significant risk that the infant will convert to anaerobic metabolism which will increase lactic acid production.

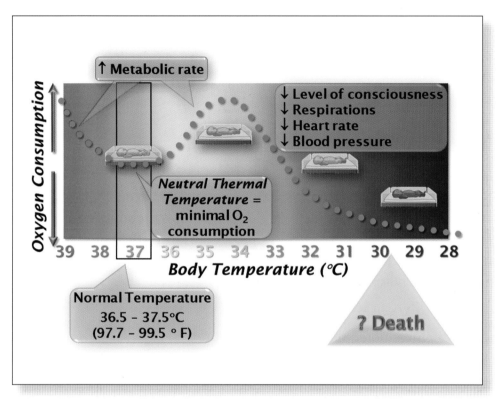

**Figure 2.1. Effect of body temperature on metabolic rate and oxygen consumption.** As body temperature rises or falls outside of the normal range of 36.5 to 37.5°C (97.7 to 99.5°F), metabolic rate and oxygen consumption increase.[12,15,21] With progressive hypothermia, the infant will exhibit a decreased level of consciousness, hypoventilation, bradycardia, and hypotension.[23] Hypoxia and hypothermia eventually lead to a decrease in oxygen consumption. This is thought to be an adaptive response to save oxygen that would otherwise be used to generate heat.[12,18] If left untreated, the risk of dying from hypothermia is very high. Increasing temperature above 37.5°C (99.5°F) drives the metabolism faster (van't Hoff's law),[12] hypermetabolism exceeds substrate supply, eventually resulting in death at around 42 to 43°C (107.6 to 109.4°F).[24]

## Clinical Tip

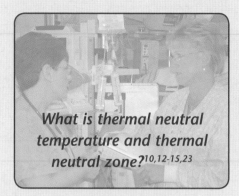

*What is thermal neutral temperature and thermal neutral zone?*[10,12-15,23]

minimal energy is expended, oxygen consumption is also lowest.

**A thermal neutral zone** is the environmental temperature that permits the infant to expend the least amount of energy to maintain a normal body temperature (in other words, the metabolic rate is minimal). Preterm infants nursed in incubators require higher environmental temperatures than term infants. As the preterm infant grows and matures, the environmental temperature required for a thermal neutral zone can be reduced. Eventually the infant is large enough and mature enough to grow and thrive outside of the incubator. See reference Brown and Landers[13] (page 123) for a neutral thermal environmental temperature chart.

**Thermal neutral temperature** is the body temperature at which minimal energy is expended by the infant in order to maintain a normal body temperature. When

# Detrimental Effects of Hypothermia: Term and Preterm Infants

In response to cold stress and progression to hypothermia, a cascade of events occurs that explain the increased morbidity and mortality in these infants. Temperature regulation is controlled by the hypothalamus. When peripheral and core temperature sensors detect cold stress, they send signals to the hypothalamus. The hypothalamus in turn activates norepinephrine release. The effects of norepinephrine throughout the body are numerous.

## Norepinephrine and Peripheral Vasoconstriction

In response to cold stress and hypothermia, norepinephrine causes peripheral blood vessels to constrict. This is a protective mechanism to keep blood in the core of the body and away from the skin where heat is dissipated.[15] With prolonged vasoconstriction however, tissue perfusion and oxygenation can become impaired and result in conversion to anaerobic metabolism in these tissues. In this setting, lactic acid will increase and the pH will drop. Acidosis also contributes to pulmonary vasoconstriction and right-to-left shunting.[13]

Preterm infants become hypothermic even faster than term infants. Main factors contributing to this include their larger surface area to body mass ratio, decreased amounts of insulating fat, thinner immature skin (diminished barrier to water evaporation), increased insensible water loss, poor muscle tone and little, if any, brown fat.

## Norepinephrine and Pulmonary Vasoconstriction

Norepinephrine also causes the pulmonary blood vessels to constrict, which increases vascular resistance in the lungs (i.e., increased pulmonary vascular resistance or PVR).[25] In the presence of increased PVR, blood that would normally enter the lungs may shunt through pathways less resistant to blood flow. That is, blood shunts from right-to-left through the ductus arteriosus and/or foramen ovale. Right-to-left shunting means that deoxygenated blood ejected from the right ventricle will pass through the ductus arteriosus into the aorta (instead of into the lungs) and out to the body as shown in Figure 2.2. When deoxygenated blood enters the aorta, the infant will become hypoxemic (i.e., have a low blood oxygen level). Hypoxemia also causes pulmonary vasoconstriction and may further worsen right-to-left shunting at the ductus arteriosus and/or foramen ovale.

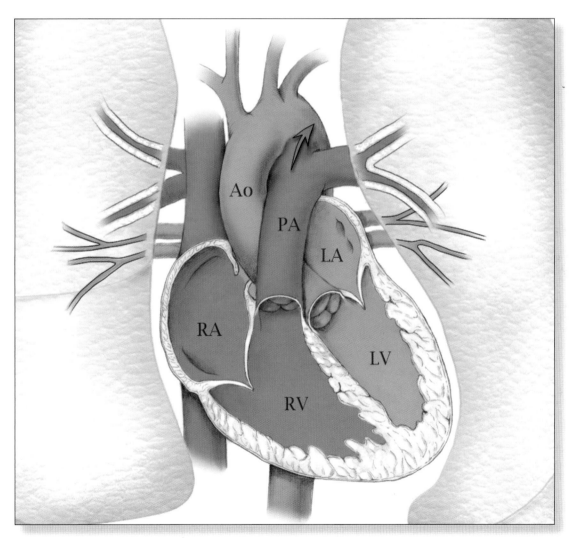

**Figure 2.2. Right-to-left shunting of blood at the ductus arteriosus.** When the blood vessels in the lungs constrict, blood will flow via pathway of least resistance, which is often right-to-left across the ductus arteriosus. Deoxygenated blood will enter the arterial circulation and the infant will become hypoxemic.

The response to hypothermia for term infants is different than the response for preterm infants, as illustrated in Figures 2.3 and 2.4.

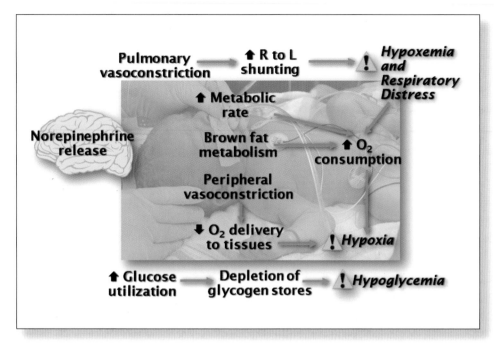

**Figure 2.3. Response to hypothermia for term infants.** Norepinephrine release from the hypothalamus causes pulmonary and peripheral vasoconstriction, increased metabolic rate, and increased oxygen and glucose consumption. Right-to-left shunting secondary to pulmonary vasoconstriction leads to hypoxemia.[25] Increased oxygen consumption and poor tissue oxygenation secondary to prolonged peripheral vasoconstriction can lead to hypoxia.[13]

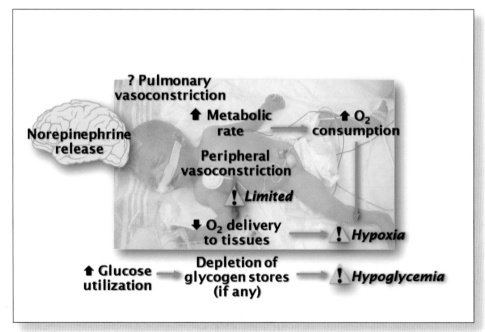

**Figure 2.4. Response to hypothermia for preterm infants.** Norepinephrine release from the hypothalamus causes the metabolic rate to increase, which increases oxygen consumption and glucose utilization.[12] Increased oxygen consumption can lead to hypoxemia and, if severe, progression to hypoxia. Peripheral vasoconstriction is limited in very low-birth-weight infants in the first 48 hours of life, thus increasing heat loss at the skin level.[16,26] The effect of norepinephrine release on pulmonary vasoconstriction in the preterm infant is not well described. In preterm infants, heat loss occurs at a faster rate than their ability to produce or conserve heat. If left unprotected from heat loss, the preterm infant will decrease his body temperature to the same temperature as the surrounding environment.[15]

# Detrimental Effects of Hypothermia

As illustrated in Figure, 2.5, the end result of hypothermia is similar for both term and preterm infants. When infants become hypothermic, metabolic rate, oxygen consumption, and glucose utilization increase. If the infant is already experiencing respiratory distress, he may not be able to meet the increased tissue demand for oxygen. This may lead to, or worsen hypoxemia, which in turn can trigger or worsen pulmonary vasoconstriction.[10] In addition, hypothermia can impair surfactant production, which may worsen respiratory distress syndrome in preterm infants.[10,13] Whether because of norepinephrine release, hypoxemia, acidosis, or a combination of these, pulmonary vasoconstriction has the same overall effect as follows:

> Severe *hypoxemia* may progress to hypoxia, which means there is reduced oxygen supply to the tissues below physiological levels required for normal cell functioning. There is significant risk that the infant will need to rely on anaerobic metabolism, which will increase lactic acid accumulation and glucose consumption.

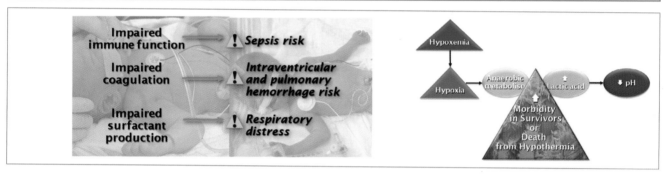

**Figure 2.5. The detrimental effects of hypothermia for both term and preterm infants.** Survivors of hypothermia experience additional harmful side effects including impaired immune function, impaired coagulation and impaired surfactant production. Severe hypoxemia may progress to hypoxia which may lead to anaerobic metabolism. During anaerobic metabolism, lactic acid accumulates rapidly and the pH of the blood drops quickly. If not reversed, there is significant risk of cell damage and even death.

During hypothermia, hypoglycemia may result from increased glucose utilization and depletion of glycogen stores.[22] Since glucose is the primary energy source for the brain, the infant's level of consciousness will decline, respirations will slow, and oxygenation may suffer. Survivors of hypothermia experience additional harmful side effects including impaired coagulation (which may result in intraventricular or pulmonary hemorrhage), impaired surfactant production, worsened respiratory distress, patent ductus arteriosus, increased incidence of infection and acute renal failure.[3,11,13,27-29]

**Protect the infant from heat loss and maintain the body temperature at 37°C (98.6°F).** Check the temperature every 15 to 30 minutes until it is within a normal range and then at least every hour until the infant is transported or transferred to the neonatal intensive care unit (NICU). When the body temperature remains consistently in the normal range, temperature measurement intervals can be extended.

> ## Remember!
> *Preventing hypothermia is much easier than overcoming the detrimental effects of hypothermia once they have occurred.*

# Mechanisms of Heat Loss

Body temperature is lost (and gained) via four mechanisms: **conduction, convection, evaporation, and radiation.**[13,14]

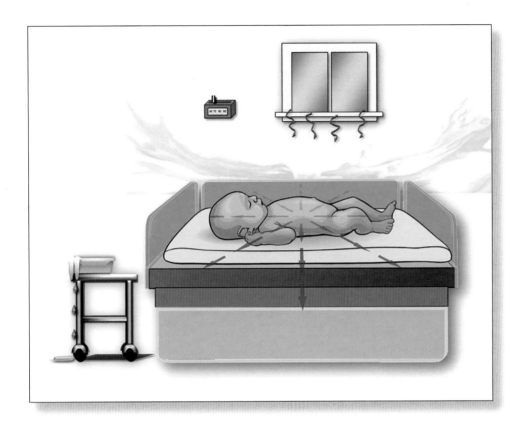

**Concept #1. Heat is lost on a gradient from warmer to cooler.** The larger the gradient, the faster heat is lost. For example, if a person dressed only in a short-sleeved shirt and pants stands in a windy field with an outside temperature of 10°C (50°F), that person will lose heat much faster than if standing in the same windy field with an outside temperature of 25°C (77°F).

**Concept #2. Heat loss is faster when there is more than one mechanism of heat loss present.** Take the person in the previous example. If it suddenly starts to rain and that person becomes wet, then the combination of water plus wind, plus a cool environmental temperature, will dramatically increase the rate of heat loss.[30]

 If not protected from heat loss, the infant's body temperature may drop as quickly as 0.2 to 1°C per minute.[10,15]

## Heat Loss by Conduction[11,14,31]

Conductive heat loss involves the transfer of heat between two solid objects that are in contact with each other. For example, the infant's body and another solid object like a mattress, scale, or x-ray plate. The larger the temperature gradient between the two surfaces, the faster the heat loss.

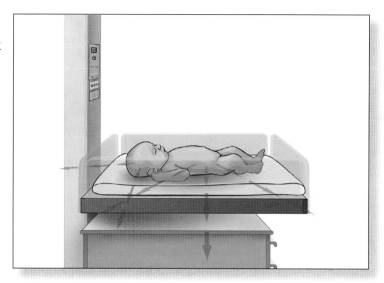

### What you can do to help reduce conductive heat loss:

- Pre-warm objects before they come in contact with the infant. This includes (but is not limited to), the mattress, your hands, stethoscope, x-ray plates, and blankets.

- Provide some form of insulation between the infant's body and the cooler surface. For example, if weighing an infant, place a warm blanket on the scale, re-zero the scale, and then weigh the baby.

- Clothing and hats serve as good insulators, however, it is usually not practical to clothe the critically ill infant. Cover the infant's head with a hat whenever possible.

- If the infant is very preterm, place a chemical thermal mattress underneath the infant.[32] Be sure to place a thin cover over the mattress before lying the infant on it.

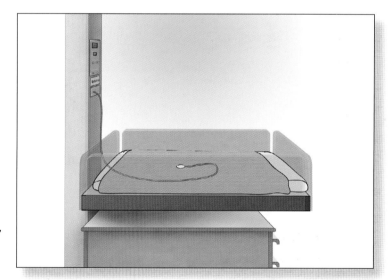

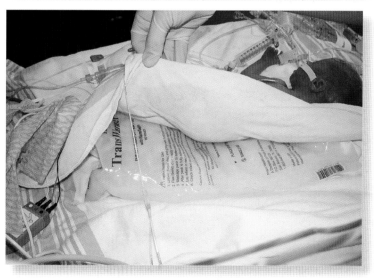

**To reduce the risk of HYPERthermia and burns:**

- Radiant warmers should be used in servo-control mode. Manual control mode should be avoided.

- Do not overheat surfaces or place an infant on a surface hotter than the infant's skin temperature. The exception is when using warming mattresses (Porta-Warm™, TransWarmer®, etc.) which warm to 40°C (104°F); follow manufacturers guidelines for safe use.

- Never place hot water bottles or gloves filled with hot water next to the infant's skin.

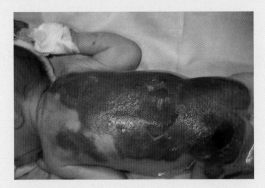

**Preterm baby burned by gloves
filled with hot water**

- Heat blankets in a temperature-controlled blanket warmer.

- Heat distribution is uneven and the risk of fire is increased when:

  ◇ Blankets are heated in a microwave.

  ◇ Blankets are placed on the top of a radiant warmer heating unit for the purpose of warming the blankets.

- Microwave heating may superheat liquids and with boiling; there is increased risk of scalding injury to staff or infants. In addition, fluids heated in a microwave have uneven heat distribution; some areas are extremely hot, and therefore, fluids should not be heated in this manner.

- Do not apply heat directly to extremities that are poorly perfused.

## Heat Loss by Convection[11,14,31]

Convective heat loss occurs when the infant's body heat is swept away by air currents, such as when the infant is exposed to drafts from air vents, air conditioners, windows, doors, heaters, fans, open incubator portholes, and traffic around the bed. Heat loss will be accelerated when the environmental air temperature is colder and/or when the air flow velocity is higher.

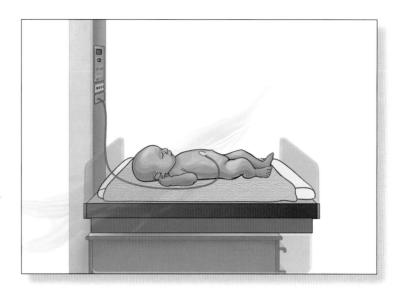

## What you can do to help reduce convective heat loss:

- Keep warmer sides up and incubator portholes closed.

- If it is anticipated that a preterm infant will be born, especially if the infant is less than or equal to 28 weeks gestation, increase the delivery room temperature to 26 to 28°C (78.8 to 82.4°F).[5,8,33,34] This will decrease the gradient for heat loss. In other words, a warm draft is much less chilling to the infant than a cold draft.

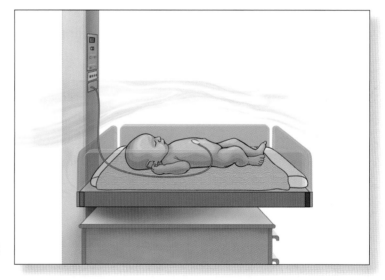

- Cover the preterm infant with a piece of food grade plastic. The use of plastic coverings may not be as helpful for infants who weigh more than 1.5 kg.

⚠ Do not cover the face or obstruct the airway with the plastic covering. If the infant is active, monitor closely to be sure the plastic does not get displaced onto the face.

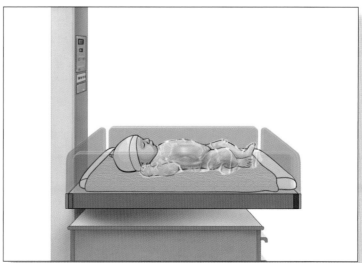

## What you can do to help reduce convective heat loss: (continued)

- Transport the sick and/or preterm infant between the delivery room and the nursery in a closed, pre-warmed incubator.[8] If this is not possible, cover the infant with pre-warmed blankets before moving the infant into drafty hallways.

- An incubator reduces convective heat loss by providing a warmer environment within an enclosed space. Pre-warm the incubator to an appropriate environmental temperature before moving the infant into it.

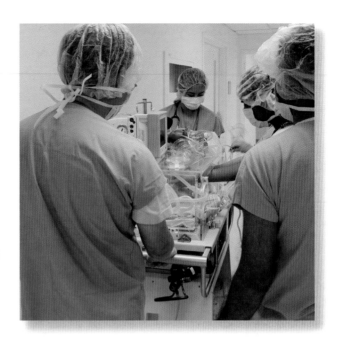

- Cold oxygen gas blown at the infant's face will stimulate cold receptors and norepinephrine release, which will increase metabolic rate and oxygen consumption. Cold gases inhaled directly into the lungs will cool the blood flowing through the lungs and into the body. Minimize such exposures to cold gases by utilizing a heated humidified system.

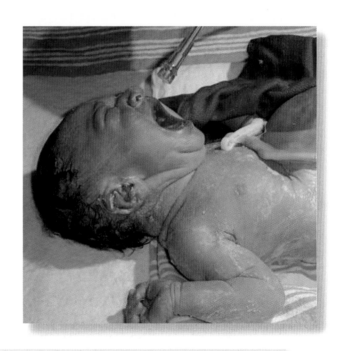

## Clinical Tip

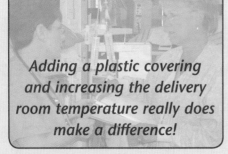

*Adding a plastic covering and increasing the delivery room temperature really does make a difference!*

One study[33] evaluated NICU admission temperature in preterm infants (< 29 weeks gestation) and found statistically significant higher temperatures in infants who were cared for in delivery rooms with a temperature > 26°C (78.8°F). When a plastic bag was also used (leaving the face uncovered), the mean admission temperature was no longer in the hypothermic (< 36.4°C) range.

## Heat Loss by Evaporation[11,14,31]

Evaporative heat loss occurs when moisture on the skin surface or respiratory tract mucosa is converted into vapor. The process of evaporation is always accompanied by a cooling effect. Once again, the colder the environment, the more rapid the heat loss. Most commonly, infants experience evaporative heat loss in the form of insensible losses, that is, passive evaporation from the skin and respiration. Sensible losses are the type that occur with sweating, however newborns don't sweat.

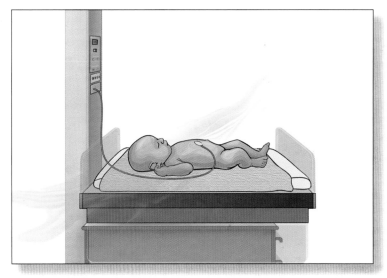

### What you can do to help reduce evaporative heat loss:

- Quickly dry the infant after delivery or bathing with pre-warmed blankets or towels and immediately remove any wet or damp linens. After thoroughly drying the infant's head, apply a hat.

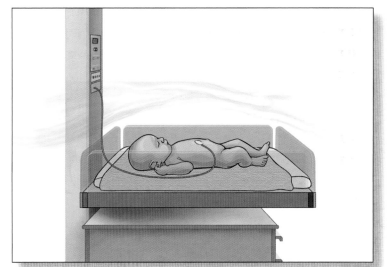

⚠ Do not bathe infants who are hypothermic or show other signs of instability. These infants may be at increased risk for developing a clinical problem called "persistent pulmonary hypertension" which is illustrated in Figure 2.2 and explained in more detail in the Airway module.

### What you can do to help reduce evaporative heat loss: (continued)

- Preterm infants have thin, translucent skin which is an ineffective barrier to heat loss. Cover or wrap the very low-birth-weight infant (less than 1500 grams) immediately after birth with polyethylene (plastic), from neck to feet, to reduce both evaporative and convective heat loss. Monitor the temperature closely to prevent hyperthermia and do not cover the face with the plastic.[32]

- Increase the room temperature to reduce the environmental air temperature gradient.[33,34]

- Air turbulence past the infant will increase evaporative losses; therefore sources of air turbulence should be minimized or eliminated.

- Heat and humidify oxygen as soon as possible.

- If possible, carefully warm solutions that come in contact with the infant's skin. For example, if an umbilical line is placed, warm the antiseptic solution before applying it to the skin (maintain sterility of the solution). Be careful not to over-warm fluids or the infant may be burned.

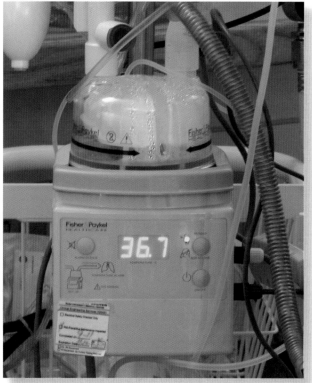

## Heat Loss by
## Radiation[11,14,31]

Radiant heat loss is the transfer of heat between solid surfaces that are not in contact with each other. The infant's skin temperature is usually warmer than surrounding surfaces, so the direction of heat transfer will be from the exposed parts of the infant's body to the adjacent solid surfaces. The cooler those surfaces, the greater the heat loss. The size of the two solid surfaces also affects the amount of heat loss; therefore, it is easy to see that a small infant will potentially lose heat very quickly to a large cool window or wall.

### What you can do to help reduce radiant heat loss:

- Move the infant away from cold windows or walls.

- Use thermal shades over windows.

- Cover the incubator to insulate it from a cold wall or window.

- Use a double-walled incubator to provide a warmer internal surface closest to the infant.

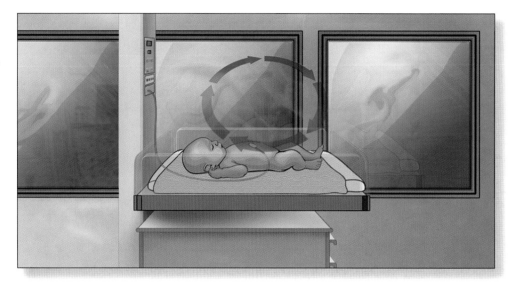

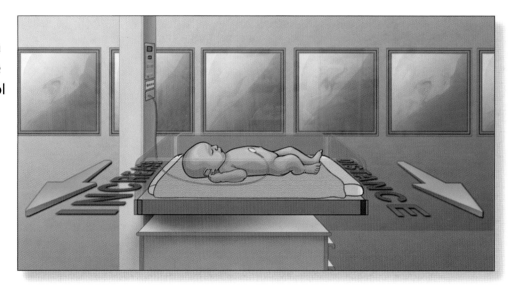

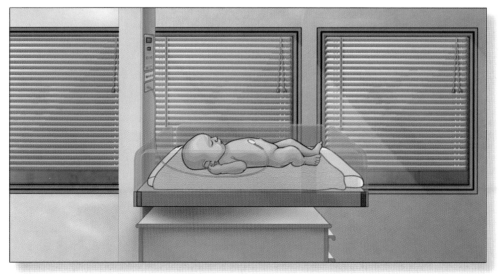

## Radiant Heat Gain[11,31]

- Radiant heat gain occurs when the surrounding surfaces are warmer than the infant's skin temperature. For example, when an infant is placed under a radiant warmer, the temperature under the heating element and projected over the infant's body is higher than the temperature a few feet away from the warmer.

- It should be remembered that during resuscitation, radiant warmer heat is obstructed when caregivers are working over an infant. Remember to keep the area below the heating unit clear.

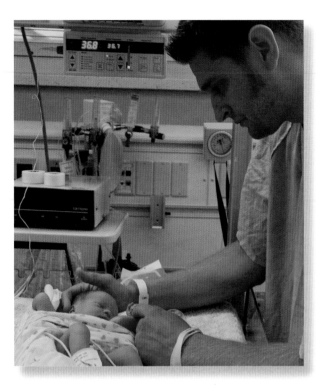

### What you can do to help reduce unwanted radiant heat gain:

- Whenever an infant is placed on a radiant warming bed, ensure the skin temperature control is set on servo-control, not manual.

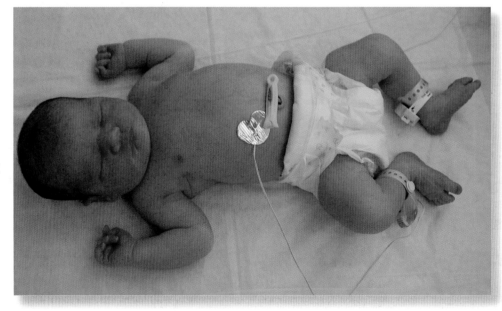

- Place the temperature sensor probe over the right upper quadrant of the abdomen (liver location).[13] If the temperature sensor has loose contact with the skin, the radiant heating device will increase heat output and the infant will overheat. Ensure the temperature sensor is well secured and that the infant is not lying on it.

**What you can do to help reduce unwanted radiant heat gain:** (continued)

- Sunlight directly on the infant, or into an incubator may cause significant overheating; therefore, this should be prevented.

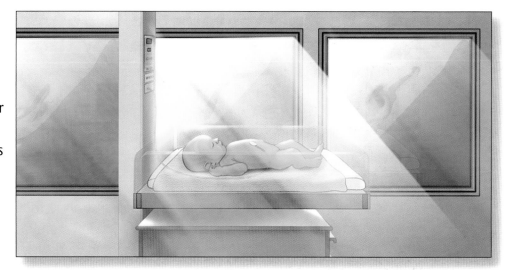

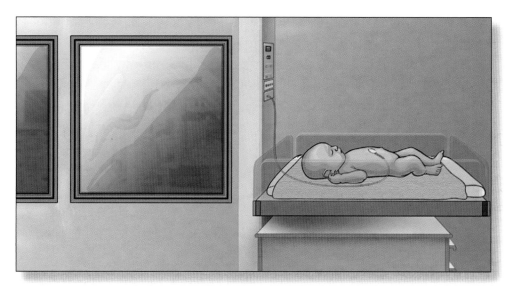

- If a radiant warmer is not available during resuscitation and/or stabilization, an infrared heat lamp may be used. But, extreme caution should be used to prevent burning the baby!

⚠ **Infrared heat lamp precautions.** Provide extra care to keep the lamp bulb a safe distance from the baby. The closer the infant is to the radiant heat source, the higher the temperature. Remember that most heat lamps are not servo-controlled to the skin temperature; therefore, the risk that the infant can overheat or be burned is increased. Closely monitor the infant's temperature and move the infant to an incubator or radiant warmer with servo-control as soon as possible. Also, be aware that heat lamp bulbs have different lamp wattage, with some capable of causing burns in a very short period of time. Each time a bulb is changed, be sure that the lamp wattage is appropriate for infant use.

# Therapeutic / Neuroprotective Hypothermia to Treat Hypoxic-Ischemic Encephalopathy (HIE)

At times, infants experience very stressful births secondary to acute perinatal events, such as placental abruption, uterine rupture, prolapsed or ruptured cord, or maternal collapse that requires cardiopulmonary resuscitation. With impaired placental – fetal perfusion, the fetal cardiac output is markedly diminished. This results in poor perfusion and oxygenation of all organs, including the vulnerable immature brain. The term "ischemia" is used to describe this process of impaired perfusion and oxygenation.[35]

The term *asphyxia* is used to describe impaired gas exchange that results in hypoxemia (low blood oxygen levels) and hypercarbia (elevated $CO_2$ levels).[35] Severe hypoxemia may lead to anaerobic glycolysis. Lactic acid that is produced during anaerobic glycolysis diffuses into the blood stream and causes metabolic acidosis ➡ blood pH drops and the base deficit increases.[35,36] The term *birth asphyxia* may be applied when there is a known perinatal sentinel event that is capable of impairing perfusion and oxygen delivery to the fetus or newborn, and that results in hypoxia, acidemia, and metabolic acidosis.[37,38] Severe metabolic acidosis may lead to end organ and brain damage.[36] This form of neonatal brain damage or injury is most commonly referred to as *hypoxic-ischemic encephalopathy* (HIE). However some neonatal experts promote the use of the term *neonatal encephalopathy* so as to encompass other etiologies that may be the reason for the neurologic findings.[39,40]

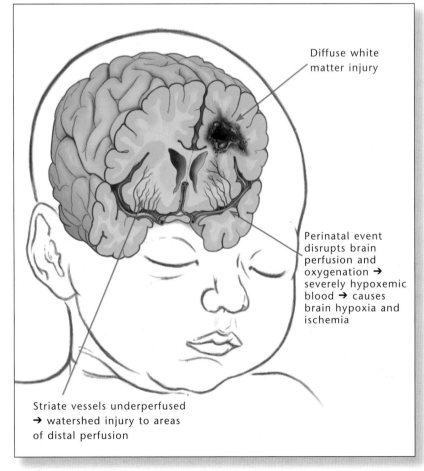

Diffuse white matter injury

Perinatal event disrupts brain perfusion and oxygenation ➔ severely hypoxemic blood ➔ causes brain hypoxia and ischemia

Striate vessels underperfused ➔ watershed injury to areas of distal perfusion

## Incidence of HIE

In developed parts of the world, the incidence of HIE is approximately 3 to 5 per 1000 live births.[41] In the United States, the incidence of neonatal encephalopathy (caused by brain hemorrhage, cerebral infarction and HIE) is estimated at 2 to 3 per 1000 live births. Based on the current annual U.S. birth rate, this represents as many as 8600 to 12,900 infants per year who will be afflicted with this condition.[42] In less developed nations where obstetric and perinatal care is less advanced, the rate is appreciably higher.[36,43] For survivors of this insult, the neurologic impact of HIE includes cerebral palsy, cognitive and motor deficits, epilepsy, deafness and learning problems when the child is school age.[35,36,40]

# Therapeutic / Neuroprotective Hypothermia

Following the initial ischemic insult to the brain, a series of events lead to death of neurons. The most promising therapy available to treat infants with HIE is intentional body cooling – also called *therapeutic* or *neuroprotective hypothermia*. Therapeutic hypothermia reduces mortality rate and in survivors, decreases the chance that the infant will have major disability.[44,45]

 **Two factors that are associated with worsened outcomes in neonates with HIE include hypoglycemia and hyperthermia.**

During resuscitation and stabilization of the infant who has experienced an asphyxial insult, take extra care to prevent hyperthermia (temperature > 37.5°C or 99.5°F), or to reduce fever if it occurs, since an elevated body temperature may worsen damage to neurons.[42,46-48] In addition, an infant afflicted with HIE who becomes hypoglycemic may have worse neurologic outcomes. Monitor the blood sugar closely and treat the infant promptly with $D_{10}W$ glucose boluses to maintain the blood sugar between 50 and 110 mg/dL (2.8 to 6.1 mmol/L). In one study, infants with HIE who had blood sugars below 46 mg/dL (2.6 mmol/L) had worse neurodevelopmental outcomes compared with infants who were normoglycemic.[40]

# Candidates for Therapeutic Hypothermia

At present, therapeutic hypothermia must be started within **six hours of birth** and is limited to infants who are **greater than or equal to 36 weeks gestation** and **greater than or equal to 1800 grams**.These infants must also have an abnormal neurologic exam.[40,41] There are ongoing studies evaluating therapeutic hypothermia for smaller infants as well as initiating hypothermia therapy beyond the current 6-hour therapeutic window (i.e., 6 to 24 hours after birth) [see https://neonatal.rti.org/studies.cfm] Each tertiary center has specific inclusion and exclusion criteria and some centers may be involved in these new studies. Therefore, it is important to consult your tertiary center quickly to determine patient eligibility.

## Passive cooling prior to arrival of the transport team

In addition, it is important to inquire whether the tertiary center wants "passive" cooling started prior to transport. This involves turning the radiant warmer off and monitoring the temperature very closely (at least every 15 minutes) to ensure the temperature does not drop too low (below 33.5°C or 92.3°F).[49-51] Only initiate passive cooling if instructed by the tertiary center. See Figure 2.6 for guidance in evaluating candidacy for therapeutic therapy. After completing the checklist in Figure 2.6, proceed to Figure 2.7 for help with the neurologic exam. Completing both components prior to calling the tertiary center will assist in accurately and rapidly identify candidates for therapeutic hypothermia.

# CANDIDACY FOR THERAPEUTIC / NEUROPROTECTIVE HYPOTHERMIA CHECKLIST
## Directions: Start at the top and work through each numbered component

*Note: if patient is less than six hours old and meets the gestation, weight and blood gas criteria and has a witnessed seizure, patient is eligible for hypothermia regardless of additional exam findings. Consult the tertiary center where cooling is offered to discuss any questions or concerns.

TIME of birth: _____ a.m./p.m.     CURRENT AGE in hours/minutes: _____ h. _____ min.

If current age > 6 hours, call tertiary center before proceeding. There are ongoing studies evaluating therapeutic hypothermia for infants 6 to 24 hours old and your tertiary facility may be participating.

| Clinical information | Criteria (place a check in the box that corresponds to the patient information) | Instructions |
|---|---|---|
| **Gestation** | **1** ≥ 36 weeks gestation ☐ | Go to ➡ 2 *Weight* |
| | < 36 weeks gestation ☐ | Not eligible |
| **Weight** | **2** ≥1800 grams ☐ | Go to ➡ 3 *Blood gas* |
| | < 1800 grams ☐ | Not eligible |
| **Blood gas**<br><br>pH = ___ Base deficit (BD) = ___<br><br>Source: Cord ☐<br>_ _ _ _ _ _ _ _ _ _ _<br>*Or 1st baby blood gas at < 1 hour of life.*<br>Time obtained: ___ : ___<br>Arterial ☐  Capillary ☐  Venous ☐ | **3** pH ≤ 7.0 ☐<br>*or*<br>Base deficit > 16 ☐ | Criteria met thus far.<br>Go to **EXAM**\* |
| | No gas obtained ☐<br>Or pH 7.01 to 7.15 ☐<br>Or Base deficit 10 to 15.9 ☐ | Go to ➡ 4 *History of acute perinatal event* |
| | pH > 7.15  or Base deficit < 10 ☐ | May not be eligible;<br>Go to ➡ 4 *History of acute perinatal event* |
| **Acute perinatal event**<br><br>(check all that apply) | **4**<br>Variable / late fetal HR decelerations ☐<br>Prolapsed / ruptured or tight nuchal cord ☐<br>Uterine rupture ☐<br>Maternal hemorrhage / placental abruption ☐<br>Maternal trauma (e.g. vehicle accident) ☐<br>Mother received CPR ☐ | Any checked,<br>Go to ➡ 5 *Apgar score* |
| | No perinatal event<br>*Or*<br>Indeterminate what the event was because of home birth or missing information | May not be eligible;<br>Go to ➡ 5 *Apgar score* |
| **Apgar score at**<br>    1 minute _____<br>    5 minutes _____<br>    10 minutes _____ | **5** Apgar ≤ 5 at 10 minutes (yes) ☐ | Criteria met thus far.<br>Go to **EXAM**\* |
| | Apgar ≤ 5 at 10 minutes (no) ☐<br>(no, was 6 or greater at 10 minutes) | Go to ➡ 6<br>*Resuscitation after delivery* |
| **Resuscitation after delivery**<br>(check all that apply)<br>___ PPV / intubated at 10 minutes<br>___ CPR<br>___ Epinephrine administered | **6** Continued need for PPV or intubated at 10 minutes? **(yes)** ☐ | Criteria met thus far.<br>Go to **EXAM**\* |
| | PPV / intubated at 10 minutes? **(no)** ☐ | May not be eligible;<br>Go to **EXAM**\* |

**Figure 2.6. Evaluating candidacy for therapeutic/neuroprotective hypothermia.** Start at the top and work through each numbered component. When directed to proceed to the exam, refer to the exam found in Figure 2.7. If there is missing data, such as a known perinatal event and/or Apgar scores, and you are in doubt whether the patient qualifies for cooling, consult the tertiary center promptly to discuss the patient.

Decision tree template courtesy of Neonatology-Neurology Program at Children's National Medical Center, Washington, D.C. Adapted with permission.

| Circle findings for each domain. | | |
|---|---|---|
| Patient is eligible for hypothermia if 3 or more domains with findings in columns 2 or 3. | | |
| **Domain** | **1** | **2** | **3** |

| Domain | 1 | 2 | 3 |
|---|---|---|---|
| **Seizures** | None | Common: focal or multifocal seizures<br><br>Note: If the infant is < 6 hours old and meets gestation, weight, and blood gas criteria and has a witnessed seizure, patient is eligible for hypothermia regardless of the rest of these exam findings. | Uncommon (excluding decerebration)<br><br>*Or*<br><br>Frequent seizures |
| **Level of consciousness** | Normal<br><br>Hyperalert | *Lethargic*<br>Decreased activity in an infant who is aroused and responsive<br><br>• Can be irritable to external stimuli (i.e., touch) | *Stuporous / Comatose*<br>Not able to arouse and unresponsive to external stimuli |
| **Spontaneous activity when awake or aroused** | Active<br><br>Vigorous, doesn't stay in one position | Less than active, not vigorous | No activity whatsoever |
| **Posture** | Moving around and does not maintain only one position | Distal flexion, complete extension, or "frog-legged" position | Decerebrate with or without stimulation (all extremities extended) |
| **Tone** | Normal – resists passive motion<br><br>Hypertonic, jittery | Hypotonic or floppy, either focal or general | Completely flaccid like a rag doll |
| **Primitive reflexes** | *Suck:*<br>Vigorously sucks finger or ET tube<br><br>Moro – normal:<br><br>Extension of limbs followed by flexion with stimulus | *Suck:*<br>Weak<br><br>Moro:<br><br>Incomplete | *Suck:*<br>Completely absent<br><br>Moro:<br><br>Completely absent |
| **Autonomic system** | *Pupils:*<br>• Normal size (~1/3 iris diameter)<br>• Reactive to light<br><br>*Heart rate:*<br>Normal, > 100 bpm<br><br>*Respirations:*<br>• Regular spontaneous breathing | *Pupils:*<br>• Constricted (<3 mm estimated), but react to light<br><br>*Heart rate:*<br>• Bradycardia (< 100 bpm, variable up to 120 bpm)<br><br>*Respirations:*<br>• Periodic, irregular breathing effort | *Pupils:*<br>• Skew gaze, fixed, dilated, not reactive to light<br><br>*Heart rate:*<br>• Variable, inconsistent rate, irregular heart rate, may be bradycardic<br><br>*Respirations:*<br>• Completely apneic, requiring positive pressure ventilation (PPV) and/or ET intubation and ventilation |

**Figure 2.7. Neurological exam to evaluate candidacy for therapeutic/ neuroprotective hypothermia.** If in doubt whether the patient qualifies for cooling, consult the tertiary center promptly to discuss the patient.

Neurologic Exam template courtesy of Neonatology-Neurology Program at Children's National Medical Center, Washington, D.C. Adapted with permission.

# Rewarming the Hypothermic Infant after Unintentional (accidental) Hypothermia

There is little research that has investigated the safest way and the speed with which to rewarm severely hypothermic infants following unintentional hypothermia.[7,11,28,52-54] Methods for rewarming hypothermic infants are largely based on practical approaches and best opinion. Published studies on rewarming after therapeutic, or intentional hypothermia for hypoxic ischemic encephalopathy (a treatment reserved for term and near-term infants), recommend rewarming speeds not exceed 0.5°C per hour to avoid sudden vasodilatation and hypotension, and that volume expanders and blood pressure medications be readily available during rewarming.[44] However, this rate of rewarming (0.5°C per hour) after *unintentional or accidental hypothermia* has not been scientifically evaluated and may be too slow or impractical.[14]

The best recommendation is to rewarm the infant while closely monitoring vital signs, level of consciousness, and acid-base status. Adjust the rewarming speed to the infant's stability and tolerance of the procedure.[13,14,55]

## Several concepts should guide rewarming care:

**Concept #1**  When rewarming hypothermic infants, the skin temperature will be higher than rectal temperature, therefore, it may be helpful to monitor the rectal temperature until the temperature is in a normal range. If the infant is preterm, then avoid rectal temperatures since the risk for injury is higher.[32] The axillary temperature may be 0.2 to 0.5°C higher than the rectal temperature.

**Concept #2.**  Rewarming too rapidly can result in clinical deterioration.[56]

**Concept #3.**  Either an incubator or a radiant warmer can be used for rewarming the infant. An incubator will allow for more control over the rewarming rate.

**Concept #4.**  Adding humidity while rewarming will help reduce ongoing heat loss from evaporation.[11] This may be achieved by adding warm humidified mist into the incubator, placing the infant into a warm humidified mist tent, increasing the humidification setting on the incubator if it has this capacity, and covering the infant with a sheet of plastic (but do not cover the face).[32]

## Incubator Method of Rewarming

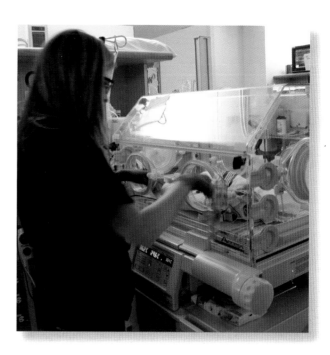

- Set the incubator on air temperature mode and set the air temperature so that it is 1 to 1.5°C above the infant's core temperature in Celsius.[14]

- Some infants may need a higher gradient than this in order to see any appreciable increase in the core temperature.

- Table 2.1 identifies what to monitor while rewarming the infant.

- As the infant's core temperature reaches the air temperature set point, and if the infant is not showing any signs of deterioration from overly rapid rewarming as outlined in Table 2.2, increase the air temperature again by 1 to 1.5°C above the infant's core temperature (in Celsius).

- This process should continue until the infant's temperature is in the normal range.

---

### Closely monitor the following during rewarming:

- ✧ Core temperature (rectal or esophageal).
  - If the infant is preterm monitor the axillary temperature instead of a rectal temperature
  - Once the infant is normothermic, the axillary temperature may be monitored
- ✧ Heart rate and rhythm
- ✧ Blood pressure, pulses, and perfusion
- ✧ Respiratory rate and effort
- ✧ Oxygen saturation
- ✧ Acid/base status
- ✧ Blood glucose

**Table 2.1.** Monitoring during rewarming of severely hypothermic infants. The rewarming speed after unintentional hypothermia should be based on the infant's tolerance and response to rewarming efforts.

✧ Tachycardia
  • May indicate a compensatory mechanism because of a decrease in cardiac output
✧ Hypotension
✧ Development of a cardiac arrhythmia
✧ Onset of hypoxemia or increased oxygen requirement as evidenced by desaturation and cyanosis
✧ Worsening respiratory distress
  • May include apnea, tachypnea, retractions
✧ Worsening acidosis
  • Metabolic or mixed

**Table 2.2.** Signs of deterioration when rewarming a severely hypothermic infant.

## Radiant Warmer Method of Rewarming

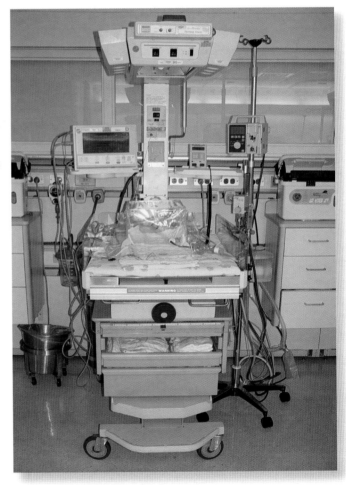

- Place the hypothermic infant supine on a radiant warmer with the servo-temperature probe located over the liver and the servo-control temperature set at 36.5°C.[11] Alternatively, to slow the rate of rewarming, set the skin temperature 1°C higher than the body temperature.[11] However, the lowest servo-control skin temperature setting on a radiant warmer may not be low enough to reach 1°C higher than the body temperature.

- Monitor the infant closely as outlined in Tables 2.1 and 2.2.

- The skin blood vessels are very sensitive to heat, so one risk with this method of rewarming is that the radiant warmer, in response to a low skin temperature, will operate on full heater output. This may cause the blood vessels to dilate suddenly and cause a rapid drop in blood pressure.

- If the infant deteriorates during rewarming the rate of rewarming may need to be slowed.

⚠ Be prepared to institute full cardiopulmonary resuscitative measures described in the Airway and Blood pressure modules in this manual.

# TEMPERATURE MODULE — Key Points

**Be vigilant – prevent hypothermia in the first place!**

✧ Infants who are most vulnerable for becoming hypothermic include:

- Preterm infants - especially infants who are less than 32 weeks gestation.

- Small for gestational age infants.

- Those who undergo prolonged resuscitation.

- Acutely ill infants.

- Infants with open skin defects (abdomen, chest, bladder, spine).

✧ Remember the basics!

- Use warm, humidified oxygen as soon as possible.

- Warm instruments and objects before they come in contact with the infant.

- Use a radiant warmer on servo-control, not manual.

✧ Quickly recognize the infant who qualifies for neuroprotective / therapeutic hypothermia and initiate cooling therapy prior to six hours of life.

✧ Rewarm hypothermic infants cautiously and be prepared to resuscitate during or after rewarming.

# References

1. Day RL, Caliguiri L, Kamenski C, Ehrlich F. Body Temperature and Survival of Premature Infants. Pediatrics 1964;34:171-81.

2. Silverman WA, Fertig JW, Berger AP. The influence of the thermal environment upon the survival of newly born premature infants. Pediatrics 1958;22:876-86.

3. Laptook AR, Salhab W, Bhaskar B. Admission temperature of low birth weight infants: predictors and associated morbidities. Pediatrics 2007;119:e643-9.

4. Mullany LC, Katz J, Khatry SK, LeClerq SC, Darmstadt GL, Tielsch JM. Risk of mortality associated with neonatal hypothermia in southern Nepal. Arch Pediatr Adolesc Med 2010;164:650-6.

5. WHO. Thermal protection of the newborn: A practical guide. In: Maternal and Newborn Health/Safe Motherhood Unit DoRH, ed. Geneva: World Health Organization; 1997:1-68.

6. Mathur NB, Krishnamurthy S, Mishra TK. Evaluation of WHO classification of hypothermia in sick extramural neonates as predictor of fatality. J Trop Pediatr 2005;51:341-5.

7. Chandra S, Baumgart S. Fetal and neonatal thermal regulation. In: Spitzer AR, ed. Intensive Care of the Fetus & Neonate. 2nd ed. Philadelphia: Elsevier Mosby; 2005:495-513.

8. Laptook AR, Watkinson M. Temperature management in the delivery room. Seminars in Fetal & Neonatal Medicine 2008;13:383-91.

9. Knobel R, Holditch-Davis D. Thermoregulation and heat loss prevention after birth and during neonatal intensive-care unit stabilization of extremely low-birthweight infants. J Obstet Gynecol Neonatal Nurs 2007;36:280-7.

10. Blackburn ST. Thermoregulation. In: Blackburn ST, ed. Maternal, fetal, and neonatal physiology: A clinical perspective. 3rd ed. St. Louis: Saunders Elsevier; 2007:700-23.

11. Sedin G. Physical environment. In: Martin RJ, Fanaroff AA, Walsh MC, eds. Fanaroff & Martin's Neonatal-Perinatal Medicine: Diseases of the Fetus and Infant. 9th ed. St. Louis: Elsevier Mosby; 2011:555-76.

12. Sahni R, Schulze K. Temperature control in newborn infants. In: Polin RA, Fox WW, Abman SH, eds. Fetal and Neonatal Physiology. 4th ed. Philadelphia: Elsevier Saunders; 2011:624-48.

13. Brown VD, Landers S. Heat balance. In: Gardner SL, Carter BS, Enzman-Hines M, Hernandez JA, eds. Merenstein & Gardner's Handbook of Neonatal Intensive Care. 7th ed. St. Louis: Mosby Elsevier; 2011:113-33.

14. Baumgart S, Chandra S. Temperature regulation of the premature neonate. In: Gleason CA, Devaskar SU, eds. Avery's Diseases of the Newborn. 9th ed. Philadelphia: Elsevier Saunders; 2012:357-66.

15. Baumgart S. Iatrogenic hyperthermia and hypothermia in the neonate. Clin Perinatol 2008;35:183-97, ix-x.

16. Lyon AJ, Pikaar ME, Badger P, McIntosh N. Temperature control in very low birthweight infants during first five days of life. Arch Dis Child Fetal Neonatal Ed 1997;76:F47-50.

17. Nedergaard J, Cannon B. Brown adipose tissue: development and function. In: Polin RA, Fox WW, Abman SH, eds. Fetal and Neonatal Physiology. Philadelphia: Elsevier Saunders; 2011:470-82.

18. Power GG, Blood AB. Perinatal thermal physiology. In: Polin RA, Fox WW, Abman SH, eds. Fetal and Neonatal Physiology. 4th ed. Philadelphia: Elsevier Saunders; 2011:615-24.

19. Poenaru D. Abdominal wall problems. In: Gleason CA, Devaskar SU, eds. Avery's Diseases of the Newborn. 9th ed. Philadelphia: Elsevier Saunders; 2012:1007-21.

20. Barksdale EM, Chwals WJ, Magnuson DK, Parry RL. Selected Gastrointestinal Anomalies. In: Martin RJ, Fanaroff AA, Walsh MC, eds. Fanaroff & Martin's Neonatal-Perinatal Medicine: Diseases of the Fetus and Infant. 9th ed. St. Louis: Elsevier Mosby; 2011:1400-31.

21. Klaus MH, Fanaroff AA. The physical environment. In: Klaus MH, Fanaroff AA, eds. Care of the High-Risk Neonate. 5th ed. Philadelphia: W.B. Saunders Company; 2001:130-46.

22. Mohan SS, Jain L. Care of the late preterm infant. In: Gleason CA, Devaskar SU, eds. Avery's Diseases of the Newborn 9th ed. Philadelphia: Elsevier Saunders; 2012.

23. Chatson K. Temperature control. In: Cloherty JP, Eichenwald EC, Hansen AR, Stark AR, eds. Manual of Neonatal Care. 7th ed. Philadelphia: Wolters Kluwer / Lippincott Williams & Wilkins; 2012:178-84.

24. Bettaieb A, Averill-Bates DA. Thermotolerance induced at a fever temperature of 40 degrees C protects cells against hyperthermia-induced apoptosis mediated by death receptor signalling. Biochem Cell Biol 2008;86:521-38.

25. Steinhorn RH, Abman SH. Persistent pulmonary hypertension. In: Gleason CA, Devaskar SU, eds. Avery's Diseases of the Newborn. 9th ed. Philadelphia: Elsevier Saunders; 2012.

26. Knobel RB, Holditch-Davis D, Schwartz TA, Wimmer JE, Jr. Extremely low birth weight preterm infants lack vasomotor response in relationship to cold body temperatures at birth. J Perinatol 2009;29:814-21.

27. Bartels DB, Kreienbrock L, Dammann O, Wenzlaff P, Poets CF. Population based study on the outcome of small for gestational age newborns. Arch Dis Child Fetal Neonatal Ed 2005;90:F53-9.

28. Sofer S, Yagupsky P, Hershkowits J, Bearman JE. Improved outcome of hypothermic infants. Pediatr Emerg Care 1986;2:211-4.

29. Sofer S, Benkovich E. Severe infantile hypothermia: short- and long-term outcome. Intensive Care Med 2000;26:88-92.

30. Hall JE. Body temperature regulation, and fever. In: Hall JE, ed. Guyton and Hall textbook of medical physiology. 12th ed. Philadelphia: Saunders Elsevier; 2011:867-77.

31. Sedin G. Physics and physiology of human neonatal incubation. In: Polin RA, Fox WW, Abman SH, eds. Fetal and Neonatal Physiology. 4th ed. Philadelphia: Elsevier Saunders; 2011.

32. McCall EM, Alderdice F, Halliday HL, Jenkins JG, Vohra S. Interventions to prevent hypothermia at birth in preterm and/or low birthweight infants. Cochrane Database Syst Rev 2010:CD004210.

33. Knobel RB, Wimmer JE, Jr., Holbert D. Heat loss prevention for preterm infants in the delivery room. J Perinatol 2005;25:304-8.

34. Bhatt DR, White R, Martin G, et al. Transitional hypothermia in preterm newborns. J Perinatol 2007;27 Suppl 2:S45-7.

35. Levene MI, deVries LS. Hypoxic-Ischemic Encephalopathy. In: Martin RJ, Fanaroff AA, Walsh MC, eds. Fanaroff & Martin's Neonatal-Perinatal Medicine: Diseases of the Fetus and Infant. 9th ed. St. Louis: Elsevier Mosby; 2011:952-76.

36. Dilenge ME, Majnemer A, Shevell MI. Long-term developmental outcome of asphyxiated term neonates. J Child Neurol 2001;16:781-92.

37. ACOG Committee Opinion No. 348, November 2006: Umbilical cord blood gas and acid-base analysis. Obstet Gynecol 2006;108:1319-22.

38. ACOG. Neonatal Encephalopathy and Cerebral Palsy: Defining the Pathogenesis and Pathophysiology. Washington DC: The American College of Obstetricians and Gynecologists and the American Academy of Pediatrics; 2003.

39. Dammann O, Ferriero D, Gressens P. Neonatal encephalopathy or hypoxic-ischemic encephalopathy? Appropriate terminology matters. Pediatr Res 2011;70:1-2.

40. Wachtel EV, Hendricks-Munoz KD. Current management of the infant who presents with neonatal encephalopathy. Curr Probl Pediatr Adolesc Health Care 2011;41:132-53.

41. Gonzalez FF, Ferriero DM. Neuroprotection in the newborn infant. Clin Perinatol 2009;36:859-80, vii.

42. Wyatt JS, Gluckman PD, Liu PY, et al. Determinants of outcomes after head cooling for neonatal encephalopathy. Pediatrics 2007;119:912-21.

43. Sahni R, Sanocka UM. Hypothermia for hypoxic-ischemic encephalopathy. Clin Perinatol 2008;35:717-34, vi.

44. Jacobs SE, Hunt R, Tarnow-Mordi WO, Inder TE, Davis PG. Cooling for newborns with hypoxic ischaemic encephalopathy. In: Cochrane Database of Systematic Reviews 2007: John Wiley & Sons, Ltd.; 2008:1-56.

45. Hoehn T, Hansmann G, Buhrer C, et al. Therapeutic hypothermia in neonates. Review of current clinical data, ILCOR recommendations and suggestions for implementation in neonatal intensive care units. Resuscitation 2008;78:7-12.

46. Yager JY, Armstrong EA, Jaharus C, Saucier DM, Wirrell EC. Preventing hyperthermia decreases brain damage following neonatal hypoxic-ischemic seizures. Brain Res 2004;1011:48-57.

47. Gressens P, Huppi PS. The central nervous system. In: Martin RJ, Fanaroff AA, Walsh MC, eds. Fanaroff & Martin's Neonatal-Perinatal Medicine: Diseases of the Fetus and Infant. 9th ed. St. Louis: Elsevier Mosby; 2011:887-1036.

48. Laptook A, Tyson J, Shankaran S, et al. Elevated temperature after hypoxic-ischemic encephalopathy: risk factor for adverse outcomes. Pediatrics 2008;122:491-9.

49. Akula VP, Davis AS, Gould JB, Van Meurs K. Therapeutic hypothermia during neonatal transport: current practices in California. Am J Perinatol 2012;29:319-26.

50. Fairchild K, Sokora D, Scott J, Zanelli S. Therapeutic hypothermia on neonatal transport: 4-year experience in a single NICU. J Perinatol 2010;30:324-9.

51. Laptook AR. Brain Cooling for Neonatal Encephalopathy: Potential Indications for Use. In: Perlman JM, Polin RA, eds. Neurology: Nenatology Questions and Controversies. Philadelphia: Saunders Elsevier; 2008:66-78.

52. Naulaers G, Cossey V, Morren G, Van Huffel S, Casaer P, Devlieger H. Continuous measurement of cerebral blood volume and oxygenation during rewarming of neonates. Acta Paediatr 2004;93:1540-2.

53. Motil KJ, Blackburn MG, Pleasure JR. The effects of four different radiant warmer temperature set-points used for rewarming neonates. J Pediatr 1974;85:546-50.

54. Kaplan M, Eidelman AI. Improved prognosis in severely hypothermic newborn infants treated by rapid rewarming. J Pediatr 1984;105:470-4.

55. Blackburn ST. Thermoregulation. In: Blackburn ST, ed. Maternal, fetal, & neonatal physiology: A clinical perspective. 2nd ed. St. Louis: Saunders; 2003:707-30.

56. Thoresen M, Whitelaw A. Cardiovascular changes during mild therapeutic hypothermia and rewarming in infants with hypoxic-ischemic encephalopathy. Pediatrics 2000;106:92-9.

**S**ugar and **S**afe Care

**T**emperature

**A**irway

**B**lood Pressure

**L**ab Work

**E**motional Support

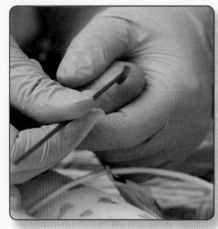

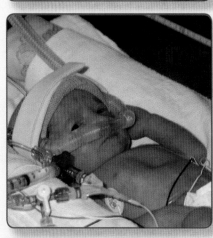

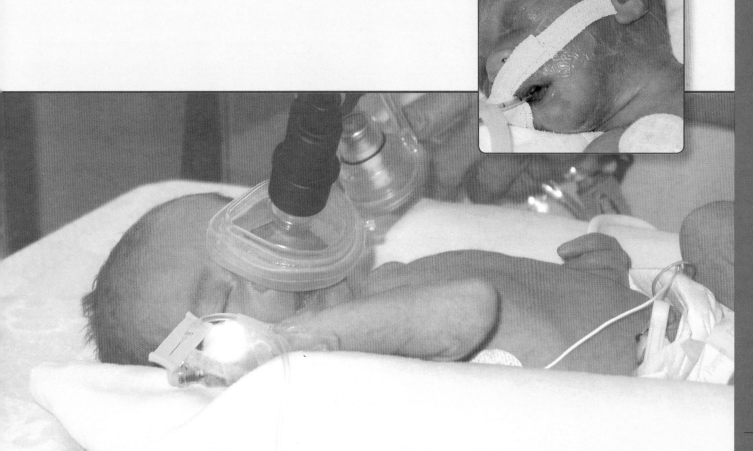

# Airway – Module Objectives

Upon completion of this module, participants will gain an increased understanding of:

1.  Labs and tests to obtain during the post-resuscitation / pre-transport period.

2.  Signs of neonatal respiratory distress and how to distinguish between mild, moderate, and severe distress.

3.  Blood gas interpretation and treatment of respiratory and metabolic acidosis.

4.  Signs of respiratory failure.

5.  Principles of assisted ventilation, including candidates for continuous positive airway pressure (CPAP), bag and mask or T-piece resuscitator positive pressure ventilation (PPV), assisting with endotracheal (ET) intubation, securing the ET tube, chest x-ray evaluation for ET tube position, and initial ventilatory support.

6.  Respiratory illnesses and airway challenges that present in the neonatal period.

7.  Identification and treatment of pneumothorax.

8.  How to safely use analgesics to treat pain.

## Airway — General Guidelines

### I. Determining the reason for respiratory distress begins with information gathering.

Infants with respiratory distress from a variety of causes represent the largest population of infants who are referred to the neonatal intensive care unit.[1-3]

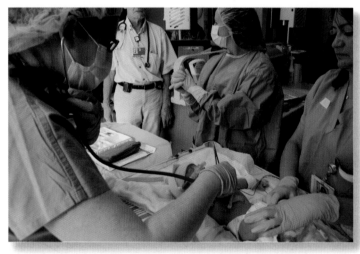

Determining the reason for respiratory distress begins with information gathering—maternal history: pre-pregnancy, pregnancy, labor and delivery; infant history: presenting signs, timing of presentation, physical exam, and laboratory and x-ray evaluation. In the post-resuscitation period and/or while preparing an infant for transport, caregivers must continuously evaluate the degree of respiratory distress the infant is experiencing so that appropriate support can be provided.

## II. Respiratory failure can occur rapidly.

In most cases, respiratory failure can be prevented by providing an appropriate level of respiratory support to meet the infant's needs. Respiratory support ranges from providing supplemental oxygen via a hood or nasal cannula, to increased levels of support via high flow nasal cannula, continuous positive airway pressure, noninvasive ventilation,[4,5] or endotracheal intubation with positive pressure ventilation.[6,7]

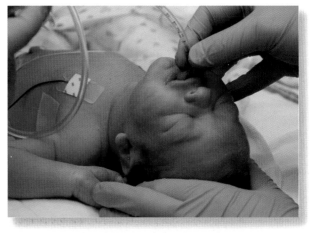

# Patient Evaluation and Monitoring

Evaluate the infant's condition frequently and record your observations. Some infants require re-assessment every few minutes while others may be less ill and can be assessed every one to three hours.

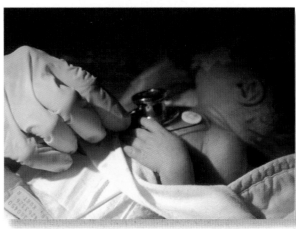

Evaluate and record:

- Vital signs

  - Temperature

  - Heart rate and rhythm

  - Respiratory rate and effort

  - Blood pressure

- Color

- Oxygen ($O_2$) saturation and location of the probe

- How much oxygen is being provided and how the oxygen is being delivered (i.e., cannula, hood, etc.)

- Other signs of well-being

  - Neurologic status

  - Skin perfusion

  - Strength of the pulses

  - Urine output

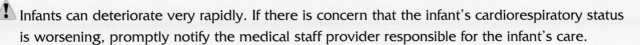

⚠ Infants can deteriorate very rapidly. If there is concern that the infant's cardiorespiratory status is worsening, promptly notify the medical staff provider responsible for the infant's care.

Labs and tests to obtain in the pre-transport / post-resuscitation period, are listed in Table 3.1. If the infant is being transported to another facility, write a detailed transfer note and copy all of the maternal and infant records and the infant's x-rays. These records are invaluable to the clinicians at the receiving hospital.

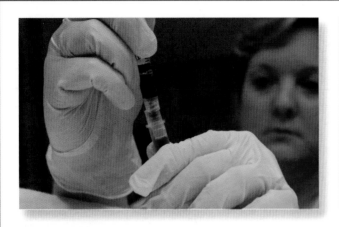
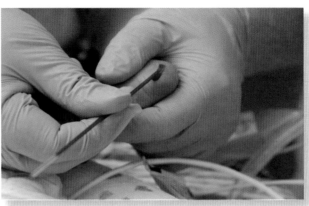

✧ Blood glucose

✧ Blood gas

✧ Complete blood count (includes white blood cell differential and platelet count)

✧ Blood culture

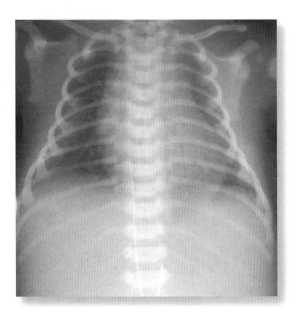
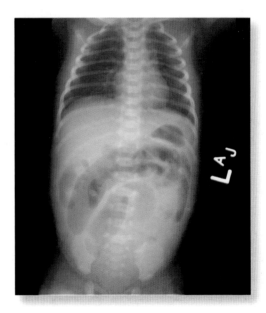

✧ Chest x-ray (if the infant is experiencing respiratory distress)

✧ Abdominal x-ray (if the infant has gastrointestinal signs such as abdominal distension, vomiting, or a history of not stooling)

**Table 3.1.** Labs and tests to obtain in the post-resuscitation / pre-transport period.

# Respiratory Distress Evaluation

When determining the severity of respiratory distress, evaluate the following:[1,8,9]

- Respiratory rate
- Work of breathing (nasal flaring, grunting, retractions)
- Presence of cyanosis
- Oxygen ($O_2$) saturation
- $O_2$ requirement
- Blood gas
- Chest x-ray
- Neurologic status

## Severity of Respiratory Distress: Mild, Moderate, Severe

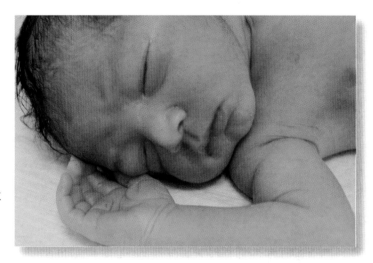

Respiratory distress may be *mild*, consisting of a rapid respiratory rate with or without the need for supplemental oxygen and with or without signs of distress such as nasal flaring; to *moderate*, where the infant is cyanotic on room air, and has additional signs of respiratory distress, such as grunting and retractions; to *severe*, where the infant is struggling to breathe and has increasing difficulty maintaining an acceptable $O_2$ saturation despite supplemental oxygen, has an abnormal blood gas indicative of respiratory failure, shows exhaustion and worsening hypoxia, and has altered mental status that usually presents as hypotonia and poor or no response to stimulation.[2,9]

 It is important to recognize that infants may progress from mild to moderate to severe respiratory distress very rapidly and that constant vigilance is required so that increased levels of support can be provided in a timely manner.

# Respiratory Rate

The **normal respiratory** rate in the young infant is between 30 and 60 breaths per minute. The infant should be breathing without difficulty – no nasal flaring, grunting, retractions, or cyanosis and there should be clear breath sounds and equal air entry.[10]

A **fast respiratory rate,** greater than 60 breaths per minute, is called **tachypnea.** Similar to why the heart rate increases when an infant is trying to compensate for decreased cardiac output (explained further in the Blood pressure module), an infant will also breath faster in response to $CO_2$ that builds up in the arterial blood. This occurs when the infant has lung pathology that interferes with effective inhalation and exhalation (tidal volume).

## A few definitions help to understand this concept:[8,9,11,12]

- **Tidal volume** ($V_T$) is the amount of air that is breathed in and out with each breath.

- **Minute ventilation** is the volume of air that is *inhaled and exhaled* over a period of one minute.

- The calculation for minute ventilation is: Tidal volume ($V_T$) multiplied by respiratory rate (R) or $V_T$ x R.

For example, an infant with pneumonia will have congestion in the alveoli which causes decreased tidal volume and blocks effective gas exchange. Impaired gas exchange leads to increasing $PaCO_2$ levels and the development of respiratory acidosis (further explained later in this module). In response to this evolving respiratory acidosis, the respiratory center will be stimulated to increase respiratory rate as well as the size (or volume) of each breath to try to bring the $PaCO_2$ back to normal – that is, to *increase minute ventilation.* The attempt to increase the volume of each breath is often evidenced by use of accessory muscles of respiration – nasal flaring and retractions.

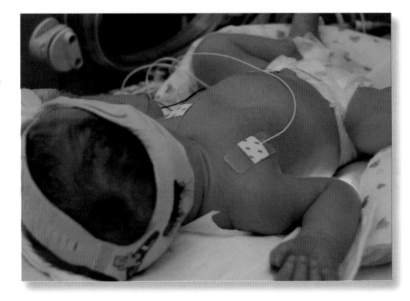

An infant may also become tachypneic for non-pulmonary reasons.[1] For example, if an infant is in shock and the pH in the blood is worsening, the respiratory center will be stimulated to increase minute ventilation (to breathe off $CO_2$) to help correct or *compensate* for the metabolic acidosis.

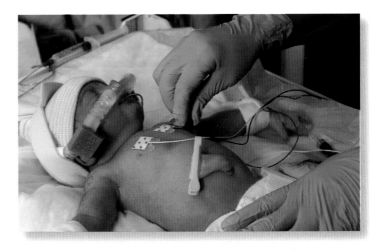

A **slow respiratory rate**, less than 30 breaths per minute is called **bradypnea**. In association with labored breathing, a slow respiratory rate may be a sign that the infant is becoming exhausted. A slow respiratory rate may be secondary to a decrease in central respiratory drive because of brain injury (for example, hypoxic ischemic encephalopathy, cerebral edema, or intracranial hemorrhage), a metabolic disorder, medications (for example, opioids), neuromuscular disease, or severe shock. A very depressed or sick infant may develop *gasping* respirations, which almost always progresses to apnea (breathing stops completely).[13]

> ⚠ **Gasping respirations are a sign of impending cardio-respiratory arrest!** When an infant is gasping, ventilation and air exchange is ineffective. This extremely critical state should be treated the same as if the infant were apneic. Immediately provide positive pressure ventilation (PPV) via a bag and mask.[13,14] If the infant's heart rate is low, and not rising, endotracheal intubation or insertion of a laryngeal mask airway (LMA) should be considered. If proceeding with intubation or LMA, continue to provide PPV while preparing to insert a more advanced airway and then continue PPV once it has been inserted.[13]

Respiratory Rate

## Work of Breathing

Oxygen Saturation

Oxygen Requirement

Blood Gas

# Increased Work of Breathing

In addition to an abnormal respiratory rate, other signs of respiratory distress include nasal flaring, grunting, wheezing, chest retractions, and cyanosis. Stridor may be heard if there is upper airway obstruction.[1,2,9]

**Nasal flaring** is a sign of air hunger as the infant attempts to decrease airway resistance and increase airway diameter by flaring the nostrils.[1,9]

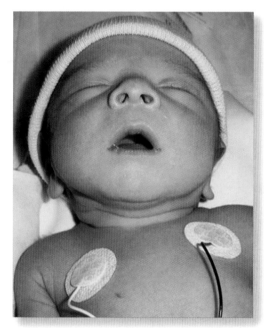

**Grunting** is the infant's attempt to increase functional residual capacity (lung volume) when there is collapse of alveoli. The infant will partially close his vocal cords to try and trap air in the lungs when exhaling. The grunting sound is made when the infant exhales through the partially closed vocal cords. Grunting 'splints open' the small airways and helps to maintain functional residual capacity in the alveoli. Until the infant tires too much, grunting serves as a mechanism to improve oxygenation and ventilation.[1,9,10,15]

Older infants and children who grunt are usually severely ill, however, this rule may not apply to all newborns with grunting respirations. Most late preterm and term infants who have grunting respirations will begin grunting within 30 minutes after birth and will stop grunting by two hours after birth.[16] When grunting is observed, evaluate the infant for other signs of respiratory distress (tachypnea, nasal flaring, cyanosis, and retractions). If grunting does not stop after a few hours following birth, or if grunting appears for the first time several hours after birth, this is a warning sign that merits further evaluation. As a rule, the louder and more continuous the grunting, the more severe the respiratory distress.

⚠ Beware of the grunting late-preterm or term infant – they are trying to tell you something!

**Retractions** occur with inspiration and reflect abnormal inward movement of the chest wall as the infant tries to increase tidal volume (the amount of air that is breathed in and out with each breath). Retractions become evident because of a combination of diaphragm contraction and accessory use of respiratory muscles.[1] Retractions are graded as *mild, moderate* or *severe* to communicate the degree to which accessory muscles are being used. Varying degrees of lung disease cause the lungs to become stiffer, and the stiffer the lungs (less compliant), the worse the retractions.

Intercostal retractions alone usually signal mild respiratory distress. When retractions become severe, (deeper and/or more areas are involved), the infant should be thoroughly assessed for causes including airway obstruction, pneumothorax, displaced or plugged endotracheal tube or worsening atelectasis because of progression of lung disease.[1,17] Retractions may be observed in one or more of the following locations:

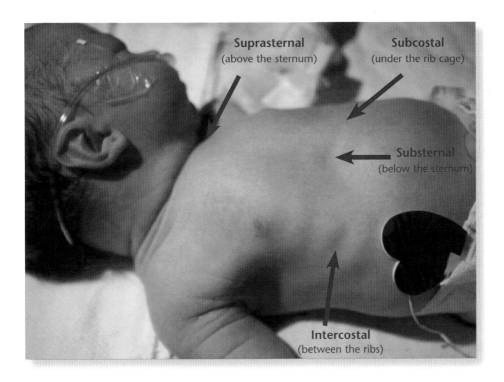

Respiratory Rate

Work of Breathing

### Oxygen Saturation
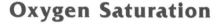

Oxygen Requirement

Blood Gas

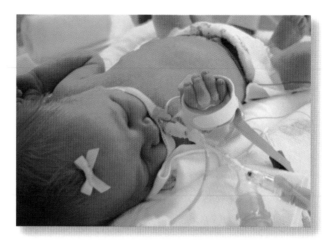

## Oxygen Saturation

Oxygen is transported to the tissues bound to the hemoglobin in red blood cells.

- **Oxygen saturation (SaO$_2$)** is the percentage of hemoglobin carrying oxygen.

- **Pulse oximetry** is the method of monitoring used to estimate the O$_2$ saturation in the arterial blood.[18] The oximeter probe can be attached to the palm, wrist, or foot. To start, attach the oximeter probe to the **right palm**. This will provide information about the **pre-ductal** O$_2$ saturation. Figure 3.1 contains information about pre- and post-ductal O$_2$ saturation monitoring.

Once the probe is attached to the infant, the blood pulsating beneath the oximeter probe should register as a heart rate on the monitor. If a cardio-respiratory monitor is also being used, compare the two heart rates to ensure they match. The saturation reading will range from 0 (no hemoglobin is carrying oxygen) to 100 (all of the hemoglobin is saturated with oxygen). For healthy late preterm and term infants, **by 24 hours of life**, O$_2$ saturation on room air at sea level ranges between 95.6 and 98.8% (median 97%).[19]

> **By 24 hours of life, O$_2$ saturation on room air at sea level** for healthy late preterm and term infants is 95 to 99% (median 97%)

## Clinical Tip

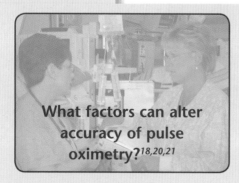

**What factors can alter accuracy of pulse oximetry?**[18,20,21]

- A low perfusion state (pulsations are not strong enough to be picked up).

- Securing the probe too tightly (pulsations are cut off).

- Securing the probe too loosely such that light can strike the sensor (optical interference).

- Movement of the extremity that the probe is secured to (motion artifact).

- Severe edema (pulsations are not picked up adequately).

- Presence of abnormal forms of hemoglobin (methemoglobin, carboxyhemoglobin; oximeter reading will be falsely high as these forms of hemoglobin are also included in the saturation calculation)

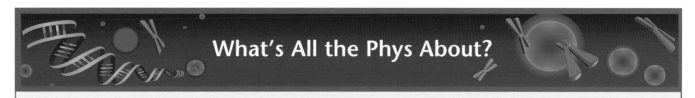

## What's All the Phys About?

### How does altitude affect $O_2$ saturation?

As altitude increases, both barometric pressure and partial pressure of oxygen in the air decreases.[22] Therefore, normal values of $O_2$ saturation are less as altitude increases. This fact will become important to recognize as universal pulse oximetry screening is performed more frequently in hospitals. See page 108 for more information on this form of screening. Two studies are summarized in the table below. Full results may be found in the publications cited.

| | Altitude in feet (meters) | Mean $O_2$ saturation % Right upper extremity (range) | Mean $O_2$ saturation % Left lower extremity (range) |
|---|---|---|---|
| **Healthy infants, at 12 to 24 hours old**[23] | 4498 (1371) | 96.67 (88–100) | 96.29 (90–100) |
| | 8150 (2484) | 93.69 (79–99) | 94.43 (77–100) |
| **Healthy infants 24 hours old**[24] | 5380 (1640) | 95.4 (91–98) | Not measured at 24 hours |

It should be noted that pulse oximetry equipment and the algorithms used to derive saturation values are continually being improved. Therefore, saturation values reported in various studies may be somewhat different or variable because of the technology available when the study was conducted.[19,23-28]

At times, it is of diagnostic value to evaluate the $O_2$ saturation in two locations at the same time. Figure 3.1 illustrates the concept of this form of monitoring, which helps determine whether there is a *right-to-left shunt* at the ductus arteriosus. A right-to-left shunt refers to the direction that blood is diverting away from its normal path; in this case deoxygenated blood is not going to the lungs (to become oxygenated), but instead is being 'shunted' through the ductus arteriosus and directly into the system circulation.

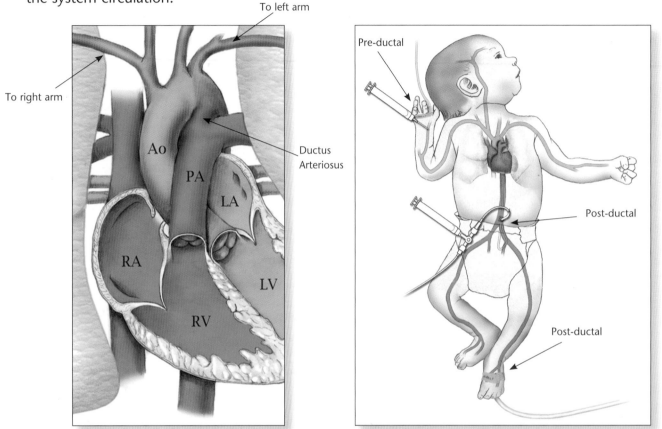

**Figure 3.1. Pre- and post-ductal blood gas and $O_2$ saturation monitoring sites.** Pre-ductal saturation is monitored on the right hand, and a pre-ductal blood gas is obtained from the right radial artery. Post-ductal saturation is monitored on either foot, and a post-ductal blood gas is obtained from the umbilical artery or either posterior tibialis artery.[1]

## Procedure for monitoring pre- and post-ductal $O_2$ saturation.

Two pulse oximeters are needed to evaluate pre and post-ductal saturation. If two monitors are not available, place the oximeter probe on the right hand (pre-ductal) for several minutes, record the saturation values, and then move the probe to either foot (post-ductal) for several minutes, and record the saturations. If there is greater than a 10% saturation difference between the two sites in either direction, meaning if the pre-ductal is 10% higher or 10% lower than the foot, then report this observation to the infant's medical staff provider. If there is a right-to-left shunt at the foramen ovale, there will not be much, if any, difference between the pre- and post-ductal sites. See the information under universal pulse oximetry screening on page 108 for different pre- and post-ductal saturation values that should be reported to the infant's medical staff provider.[29]

# Clinical Tip

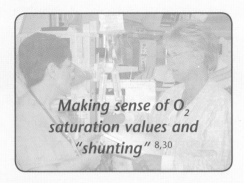

*Making sense of O₂ saturation values and "shunting"* [8,30]

- **No evidence of right-to-left shunt at the ductus arteriosus** – right hand and foot saturation values are nearly equal. For example, structurally normal heart and blood flow.

- **Evidence of right-to-left shunt at the ductus arteriosus** – right hand saturation is approximately 10% higher (or more) than the saturation in the foot. For example, persistent pulmonary hypertension (see illustration in Appendix 3.2), or left-sided structural heart obstructive lesions like coarctation of the aorta or interrupted aortic arch.

- **Right-to-left shunt at the foramen ovale, with or without shunting at the ductus arteriosus** – right hand and foot saturation values are nearly equal, but both are lower than normal. For example, persistent pulmonary hypertension with shunting at both locations (see illustration in Appendix 3.2), or right-sided structural heart obstructive lesions like tricuspid or pulmonary atresia.

- Transposition of the great arteries – when the ductus arteriosus is widely open, the right hand saturation may be lower than the saturation in the foot (usually by 10% or more). This is called reverse differential cyanosis and is further explained in Figure 3.2.

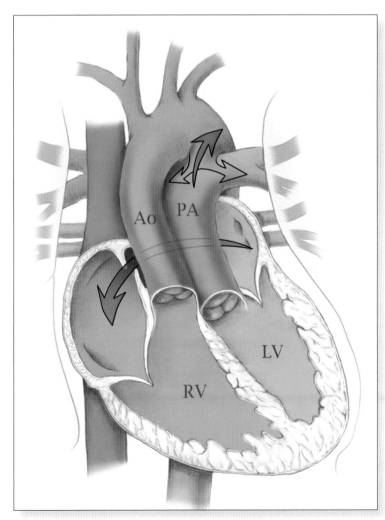

**Figure 3.2. Illustration of the blood flow pattern seen with Transposition of the Great Arteries (with intact ventricular septum).** With this severe form of congenital heart disease, the aorta originates from the right ventricle and the pulmonary artery originates from the left ventricle.[31,32] Once prostaglandin E₁ is started and the ductus arteriosus is widely open, the O₂ saturation in the right hand may be *lower* than the O₂ saturation in the foot. This is called *reverse differential cyanosis*[31] and is opposite of what is observed when there is a right-to-left shunt at the ductus arteriosus secondary to persistent pulmonary hypertension of the newborn (PPHN).

## Universal Pulse Oximetry Screening

Pulse oximetry screening for **critical congenital heart disease** (CCHD) is being performed in many hospitals worldwide.[29,33-37] The purpose of screening is to detect *lower than normal $O_2$ saturation values* secondary to previously undiagnosed CCHD. The goal is to screen healthy-appearing infants prior to discharge to home since there is significant risk of morbidity or even mortality if the infant is home when the symptoms of heart disease appear.[38,39] Some clinicians also recommend screening of infants in intermediate care nurseries especially when discharge to home is within the first week of life.[29] This is because some of the severe forms of CCHD do not present initially. One study[39] found infants were as old as six weeks when the CCHD presented.

Specific heart lesions that may be detected by pulse oximetry screening include, but are not limited to, hypoplastic left heart syndrome, critical coarctation of the aorta, pulmonary atresia, tetralogy of Fallot, total anomalous pulmonary venous return, transposition of the great arteries, tricuspid atresia, and truncus arteriosus.[29] Pulse oximetry screening has also revealed infants who have a lower $O_2$ saturation secondary to non-cardiac problems with pulmonary or infectious etiologies.[33,40]

### How is the test done?

After birth, fetal shunts (foramen ovale and ductus arteriosus) begin to close. Therefore, to prevent false positive results (meaning it is determined the infant has a problem when in fact, he does not), it is best to wait until the infant is at least 24 hours old to perform screening. One method of screening involves measuring and comparing $O_2$ saturations in both the right hand (pre-ductal) and either foot (post-ductal). See reference Kemper[29] Figure 1 for a pulse-oximetry monitoring protocol that uses pre- and post-ductal measurements. If pre- and post-ductal screening is performed, then the following abnormalities should be reported to the infant's medical staff provider:[29]

- A difference of greater than 3% between the pulse oximeter readings of the pre- and post-ductal sites.

- Any saturation value less than 90%.

- Pre- and post-ductal $O_2$ saturations between 90 and 95% on three separate measures taken 1 hour apart.

---

Notes:[29,41]

1. Not all CCHD is detected by this method of screening.

2. The saturation value determined as "normal" may vary from state to state and hospital to hospital.

3. Staff should be properly trained in how to perform pulse oximetry screening so that both false negative and false positive results are avoided. A false positive result means a problem was detected, when in fact, there was no problem.

4. At times, the results of oximetry screening will lead to a delay in discharge or possibly a neonatal transport to another facility if additional diagnostic testing is required. This creates a financial and emotional burden since neonatal transport is expensive and it results in separation of the infant from his or her family.

5. The effect of altitude on lowering the normal range for saturation must be considered when interpreting results (see What's all the Phys About: How does altitude affect $O_2$ saturation for references and more information).

6. When the test result is positive (abnormal), additional follow-up, including a thorough physical exam and possibly an echocardiogram is indicated.

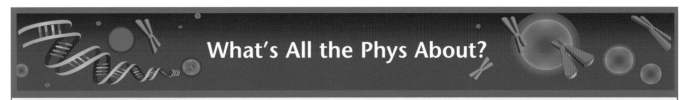

## What's All the Phys About?

### The Oxygen-Hemoglobin Dissociation Curve: what is shift to the left and shift to the right?[30]

Oxygen is transported to the tissues bound to hemoglobin and $O_2$ saturation ($SaO_2$) is the **percentage of hemoglobin carrying oxygen**. The oxygen-hemoglobin dissociation curve (shown below) rises rapidly from a starting point of zero for both $PO_2$ and percent $O_2$ saturation. When the saturation of fetal hemoglobin, which is the predominant hemoglobin in the neonate, reaches 50%, the $PO_2$ is 20 mmHg; at 75% saturation, the $PO_2$ is 30; at 95% saturation the $PO_2$ is 70; and at 98%, the $PO_2$ is 100. If alveolar oxygenation is high, which may occur when the infant is breathing supplemental oxygen, the saturation will change by only one or two percent, to a maximum of 100%, but the amount of dissolved oxygen will increase substantially such that the $PO_2$ may reach 300 or 400 mmHg.

### Shift to the left or shift to the right

A shift in the oxygen-hemoglobin dissociation curve to the left or right affects the saturation at an given $PO_2$ level and affects the ability of hemoglobin to release oxygen to the tissues. **When the curve is shifted to the left**, as in the presence of fetal hemoglobin, alkalemia, hypocarbia, and hypothermia, the saturation will be higher for any given $PO_2$, but the hemoglobin will less readily release oxygen to the tissues. **When the curve is shifted to the right**, as seen with acidemia, hypercarbia, and hyperthermia, the saturation will be lower for any given $PO_2$, but the hemoglobin will more readily release oxygen to the tissues.

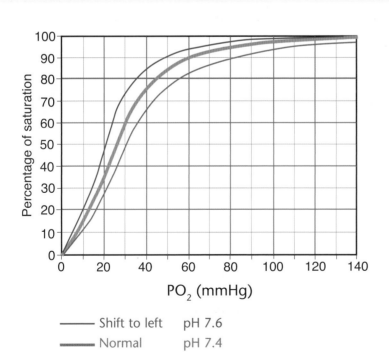

**Shift-to-left curve:**

1. Fetal hemoglobin
2. Decreased hydrogen ions (higher pH)
3. Decreased $CO_2$
4. Decreased temperature

**Shift-to-right curve:**

1. Increased hydrogen ions (lower pH)
2. Increased $CO_2$
3. Increased temperature
4. Increased 2,3-diphosphoglycerate (DPG)

——— Shift to left    pH 7.6

——— Normal    pH 7.4

——— Shift to right   pH 7.2

Respiratory Rate

Work of Breathing

Oxygen Saturation

**Oxygen Requirement**

Blood Gas

**Central cyanosis** represents desaturation of arterial blood secondary to respiratory and/or cardiac dysfunction

# Oxygen Requirement

**Cyanosis** is the term used to describe bluish discoloration of the skin.[9,42] If the tongue and mucous membranes are cyanotic, then the infant has *central* cyanosis. In the first few days of life, *acrocyanosis* (blue color of the hands and/or feet) is often a normal finding,[9,43] however, cold stress should be ruled out.

**Central cyanosis** represents desaturation of arterial blood secondary to respiratory and/or cardiac dysfunction.[30] The color of *reduced* hemoglobin, or hemoglobin that is not carrying oxygen, is **purple**. It takes approximately 3 to 5 grams/dL of reduced hemoglobin for cyanosis to be apparent.[42] This has implications for infants with both low and high hemoglobin levels. Especially important is to realize that by the time cyanosis is apparent, an anemic infant will be more severely hypoxemic and desaturated than an infant with a normal or elevated hemoglobin level.[44]

## What to do if the Infant is Cyanotic

In the post-resuscitation period, if the infant is cyanotic when breathing room air, then the $O_2$ saturation should be evaluated and the infant should be given supplemental oxygen. Whenever possible, administer oxygen using an $O_2$ / air blender. Starting with 21% oxygen, slowly increase the amount of inspired oxygen until the saturation remains around 90%. Remember, oxygen is a drug and administration should follow the same rules and precautions as any drug. That is, the dose should be regulated and monitored while in use (by pulse oximetry), and side effects can occur from overdose.[9]

 If it is necessary to increase the oxygen concentration to 100% and the infant's saturation is still not rising above 90%, it is helpful to consider the infant may have **cyanotic congenital heart disease** (CHD) or persistent pulmonary hypertension of the newborn (PPHN; explained later in this module). Seek guidance from a neonatologist or pediatric cardiologist if the infant is not improving satisfactorily and especially if concerned that the infant might have CHD.

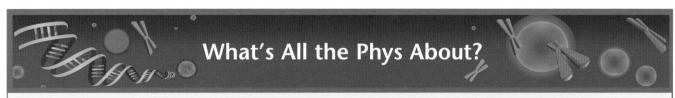

## What's All the Phys About?

How does the amount of hemoglobin affect when cyanosis will be apparent? [30]

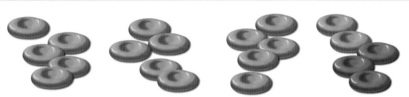

**Hgb 20 gm/dL** — O₂ saturation 85% and cyanosis is apparent

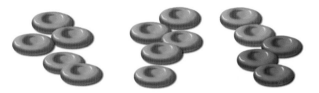

**Hgb 15 gm/dL** — O₂ saturation 80% and cyanosis is apparent

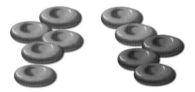

**Hgb 10 gm/dL** — O₂ saturation 70% and cyanosis is apparent

Red RBCs represent 1 gram of saturated hemoglobin

~~Red~~ Purple RBCs represent 1 gram of ~~saturated~~ desaturated hemoglobin

When an infant is *polycythemic* (hemoglobin > 20 gm/dL or a venous hematocrit of >60%)[45] cyanosis will be apparent when there is desaturation of 3 grams/dL of hemoglobin (15% of the infant's total hemoglobin). Using an example of fetal hemoglobin 20 gm/dL, the infant will appear cyanotic when the O₂ saturation is 85%. Yet, the infant will have an adequate O₂ content since each gram of hemoglobin binds 1.34 mL of O₂. The total O₂ content at 85% saturation will be 22.8 mL/dL.

When an infant is *anemic* (hemoglobin ≤ 10 gm/dL or ≤ a hematocrit of 30%)[46] the infant will not appear cyanotic until there is desaturation of 3 grams/dL of hemoglobin (30 percent of the infant's total hemoglobin). This means the infant's O₂ saturation will be 70% before cyanosis is apparent. The oxygen content in this infant, when the saturation is 70% will only be 9.4 mL/dL. **Therefore, it is important to interpret saturation values and cyanosis in the context of how much hemoglobin the infant has.** This is further explained in Table 3.2.

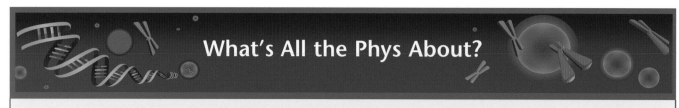

# What's All the Phys About?

## What is Retinopathy of Prematurity (ROP) and are Term Infants also at Risk for ROP?

Retinopathy of prematurity (ROP) refers to abnormal growth of developing vessels in the retina. The more preterm the infant, the higher the risk the infant will develop severe forms of ROP.[47,48] Worldwide, ROP is one of the most common causes of blindness, therefore, preventing severe forms of ROP is of utmost importance.[49] Development of ROP has been attributed to various environmental factors which include prolonged or excessive administration of oxygen and a complicated hospital course.[48] Several studies to date have evaluated the incidence and severity of ROP (and other outcomes including mortality rates) when $O_2$ saturation is maintained in the following ranges: 83 to 93%[50], 85 to 89% versus 91 to 95%[51] and 89 to 94% versus 96 to 99%.[52] The science is emerging, and the problem is complicated. At present, it is clear that effort should be directed at limiting exposure to higher saturations that lead to an elevated $PO_2$ (beyond 100 mmHg).[9,48,49] .

### Key Points:

- For the vast majority of infants, the retina is fully vascularized by the time the infant reaches term gestation. Therefore, **term infants are at very low risk for developing ROP.**[47] Infants born late preterm are also at much reduced risk for developing ROP.[9] The infants who are at most risk for ROP are the very low birth weight preterm infants.[48]

- **For all gestation infants, excessive oxygen administration** may lead to a high $PO_2$ *(hyperoxia)*. Excessive $O_2$ administration should be avoided whenever possible because hyperoxia causes *oxidant injury* which has a detrimental

- Target saturation has been studied in very preterm infants (24 to 27 completed weeks).[51] Although the incidence of severe ROP was reduced when $O_2$ saturation was maintained between 85 and 89% versus between 91 and 95%, the mortality rate was significantly higher in the infants with the lower saturation target. Therefore, until more definitive data is available, including the safety of lower saturation targets for infants 28 weeks gestation and greater, it is prudent to recommend regulating oxygen concentration to keep the saturation between 91 and 95%.

**Until more definitive data is available, when giving oxygen to infants, the S.T.A.B.L.E. Program recommends maintaining the $O_2$ saturation between 91 and 95%. This is particularly important for any gestation preterm infant.**

Note: other conditions such as congenital heart disease and pulmonary hypertension may require adjustment of this saturation target.

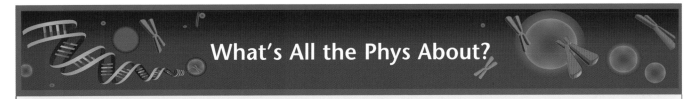

# What's All the Phys About?

## The Process of Gas Exchange

### Key Concept 1

**Adequate respiration and cardiac function is necessary for oxygenation and ventilation.** With respiration (inspiration and expiration), oxygen in the air that is inhaled diffuses from the alveoli through the interstitium of the lung into the pulmonary capillary blood, where it is bound by hemoglobin. The heart pumps oxygen-rich blood through the arterial system to the tissue capillaries. Oxygen diffuses from the tissues capillaries, through cell membranes and into the cells. Deoxygenated blood is returned to the heart along with $CO_2$ produced in the cells. The lungs inhale and exhale, thus repeating the cycle of oxygenation and removal of $CO_2$.

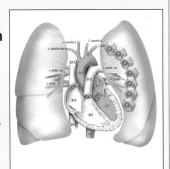

Respiration → → Breath taken → → $PO_2$ in the alveoli rises → → $O_2$ diffuses through the interstitium of the lung to the plasma in pulmonary capillary blood → → $O_2$ moves from the plasma into the red blood cells → → $O_2$ binds with hemoglobin molecules contained in the red blood cells → → hemoglobin becomes saturated with $O_2$ → → blood is returned to the 🫀 where it is pumped via the arterial system to the body → → hemoglobin releases $O_2$ to the tissues → → $O_2$ diffuses into the tissues, through cell membranes, and into the cells → → $O_2$ is supplied to the cells for normal cellular function → → $CO_2$ diffuses from the cells into the capillaries to veins → → to lungs → → $CO_2$ removed from the lung by ventilation → → process is repeated. . .

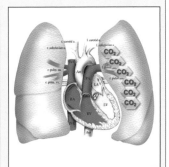

### Key Concept 2

**Movement of oxygen from one point to the next occurs across a partial pressure gradient, from higher to lower.** The gradient needs to be high enough to allow oxygen to move from the alveoli to the pulmonary capillary blood to the peripheral arterial blood and systemic capillaries to the tissue cells.[56-58] For diffusion to occur, the $PO_2$ in arterial blood must be higher than the $PO_2$ in tissue capillaries. Figure 3.3 illustrates the changes in $PO_2$ from 100 mmHg in the pulmonary alveolus to 40 mmHg in the tissue capillaries, to less than 30 mmHg in the cells. Note that the cells only require a $PO_2$ between 1 and 3 mmHg to carry out their normal chemical processes.[58] Therefore, under conditions of near complete lack of oxygen delivery to the cells, as seen with severe shock, ATP to maintain cell life may be generated by anaerobic glycolysis. For very short periods of time (minutes), this type of metabolism will be sufficient to support cellular function. After that, failure to provide oxygen to the cells will result in death.

Alveolar $PO_2$ 100 mmHg → → systemic capillary $PO_2$ 40 mmHg → → intracellular $PO_2$ averages 23 mmHg

**Figure 3.3. Changes in average $PO_2$ from the alveolar space to the cell.**

## Hypoxemia, Hypoxia and Anaerobic Metabolism

**Hypoxemia** is the term used to describe a low arterial blood oxygen content.[20]

**Hypoxia** is the term used to describe an inadequate oxygen level in the tissues, below physiologic levels required for normal cell functioning.[42,59]

Hypoxemia, combined with poor cardiac output or the presence of factors cited in Table 3.2, can lead to hypoxia. For a very short period of time, cells can survive with reduced or no oxygen supply by relying on **anaerobic metabolism**. During periods of anaerobic metabolism, tremendous amounts of glucose are consumed (thus increasing risk for hypoglycemia) and significant amounts of lactic acid accumulate in the blood. In the extreme, this may lead to cellular death.[60] See Figures 1.4 and 1.5 in the Sugar module for illustrations of aerobic and anaerobic metabolism. In the face of significant hypoxia and acidosis there is a significantly increased risk that organs, including the brain, may be damaged and if severe enough, the infant could die.

> ⚠ If the oxygen requirement is rapidly increasing, whether or not the respiratory distress is worsening, then this may be a sign of impending respiratory or cardiac failure and should be reported immediately to the infant's medical staff provider.

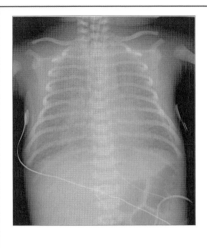

**Lung disease:**
Blood goes to the lungs to become oxygenated. Lung diseases, such as pneumonia, meconium aspiration syndrome, and respiratory distress syndrome interfere with normal oxygenation of the pulmonary capillary blood. Poorly oxygenated blood returns to the heart and is then ejected by the left ventricle into the aorta. The necessary gradient for diffusion of oxygen (from the lung to the tissue level) is therefore impaired and oxygen delivery to the tissues may be insufficient.

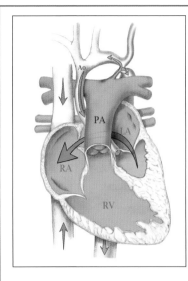

**Cardiac failure:**
Interferes with pumping of oxygenated blood to the tissues which decreases $O_2$ delivery to the tissues. Cardiac failure often also leads to development of pulmonary edema which increases the diffusion barrier for oxygenation (alveoli to red blood cells). Examples include cardiomyopathy, myocarditis, post-asphyxia cardiac dysfunction, and left-sided obstructive lesions. The illustration shows hypoplastic left heart syndrome.

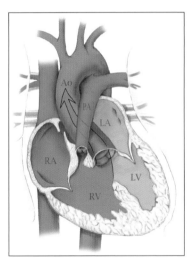

**Intracardiac mixing of blood:**
Deoxygenated blood is returned from the body to the heart for oxygenation. However, instead of the blood going to the lungs to become oxygenated, it is shunted to the left side of the heart. This lowers the $PO_2$ of the arterial blood that is ejected through the aorta to the body. This occurs with cyanotic congenital heart disease, specifically right-sided obstructive lesions. The illustration shows tetralogy of Fallot with significant pulmonary stenosis.

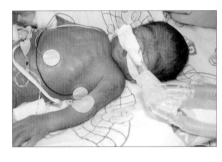

**Increased metabolic rate or demand:**
Increases oxygen consumption at the cellular level. For example, sepsis. Photo is of a preterm infant with sepsis and hypotension.

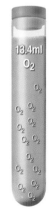

10 gm hgb

**Anemia or abnormal hemoglobin type:** Inadequate hemoglobin level or altered hemoglobin-oxygen affinity (as occurs with hypothermia, hypocarbia, alkalosis and fetal hemoglobin, or an abnormal type of hemoglobin, such as methemoglobin) lowers oxygen content in the blood. To support metabolism, the tissues require approximately 5 mL of $O_2$ per 100 mL of blood perfusing them.

**Table 3.2.** Factors that interfere with oxygenation of the blood and $O_2$ delivery to the tissues.[20,42,61]

Respiratory Rate

Work of Breathing

Oxygen Saturation

Oxygen Requirement

**Blood Gas**

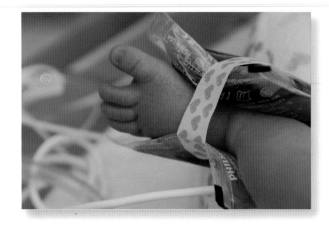

# Blood Gas Evaluation

Evaluation and interpretation of blood gases is important for evaluating the degree of distress an infant is experiencing, and to aid in the diagnosis and treatment of sick infants. When an arterial sample is obtained, acid-base balance and oxygenation can be assessed simultaneously.[9] If a capillary sample is obtained, pH, $PCO_2$ and acid-base balance can be assessed[20] and oxygenation is evaluated by pulse oximetry ($O_2$ saturation).

Blood gas values commonly observed in very young infants are summarized in Table 3.3. The newly born infant (less than 48 hours old) is slightly acidemic, but with retention of bicarbonate and removal of $CO_2$, the pH rises to the normal range of 7.35 to 7.45 by approximately 48 hours of life. Figure 3.4 contains an acid-base alignment nomogram that is useful for interpreting blood gas results. Appendix 3.1 is a blood gas interpretation practice session that may be useful for applying these principles to patient care.

|  | **Arterial** | **Capillary*** |
|---|---|---|
| pH | 7.30 – 7.45 | 7.30 – 7.45 |
| $PCO_2$ | 35 – 45 mmHg | 35 – 50 mmHg |
| $PO_2$ (on room air) | 60 – 80 mmHg | — — — (not useful for assessing oxygenation) |
| Bicarbonate ($HCO_3$) | 19 – 26 mEq/L | 19 – 26 mEq/L |
| Base Excess | -4 to +4 | -4 to +4 |

**Table 3.3.** Blood gas values in young infants.[20,61,62]

*Prior to obtaining a capillary blood gas, warm the foot/heel area for 3 to 5 minutes to improve blood flow to the area.*

Notes:

- Lower limits of normal for pH and bicarbonate values are 7.35 and 22 respectively after the first few days of life.

- Arterial samples are the gold standard for assessing oxygenation, ventilation and pH.

- Capillary samples are useful for evaluating all parameters on the blood gas except $PO_2$.

- Capillary blood gas values may be inaccurate if the infant is hypotensive or hypothermic (i.e., if there is poor blood flow to the heel), or if the heel was not warmed properly.

- $PO_2$ and $O_2$ saturation will vary with altitude and body temperature.

- The $O_2$ saturation reported on the blood gas report is calculated from a nomogram based on adult hemoglobin. This is inaccurate for the infant because of the presence of fetal hemoglobin. The pulse oximeter saturation is accurate and should be used to assess oxygenation.

- It is also important to note that blood gas values for $HCO_3$ and base deficit/excess are calculated based on the measured pH and measured $pCO_2$. Too much heparin in the sample can markedly decrease sample pH resulting in spurious calculations for base excess and $HCO_3$.

- If the blood gas cannot be analyzed immediately, place the sample on ice. This will slow down ongoing $O_2$ consumption and $CO_2$ production that occurs once the sample is drawn.

# Blood Gas Interpretation Using a Modified Acid-Base Alignment Nomogram[63] and S.T.A.B.L.E. Blood Gas Rules©

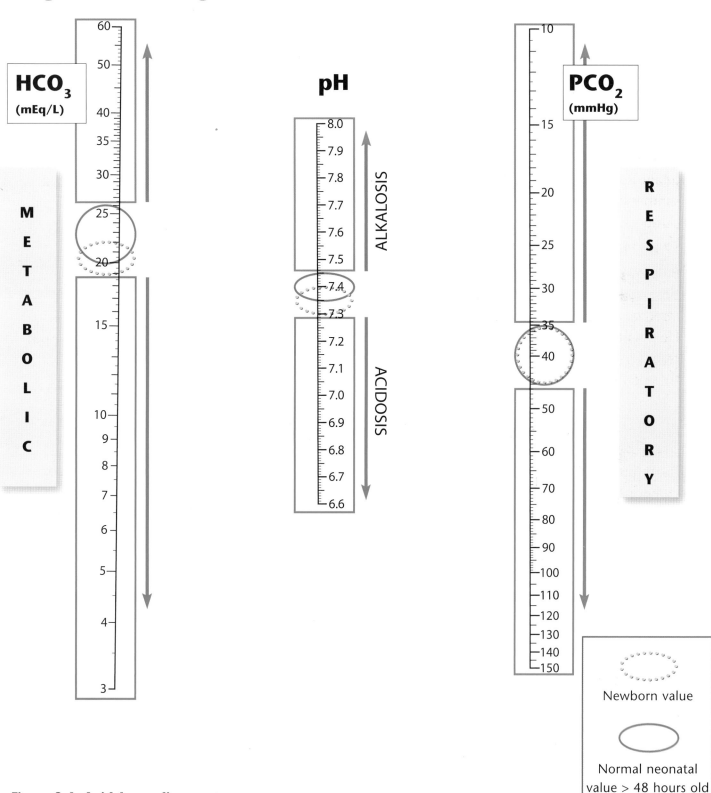

**Figure 3.4. Acid-base alignment nomogram.**

*Adapted with permission Taylor and Francis AS, from Andersen, S.O. (1963). Blood Acid-Base Alignment Nomogram. The Scandinavian Journal of Clinical and Laboratory Investigation. 15: 211-217.63*

## S.T.A.B.L.E. Blood Gas Rules[20,61,64,65]

Accurate interpretation of a blood gas is important because it guides appropriate treatment. The following steps explain how to use the nomogram found in Figure 3.4.

### Step 1.

a. Obtain the baby's pH, $PCO_2$ and $HCO_3$ values from a blood gas measurement.

b. Put a dot on the nomogram for each of these values. Notice the $HCO_3$ scale goes from high to low (top to bottom) and the $PCO_2$ scale goes from low to high (top to bottom).

c. Using a ruler, draw a straight line through the three dots.

• **If the line is not straight**, then something is wrong with the blood gas result. For example, if there is too much heparin in the sample, the sample pH will be decreased which will affect the calculations for base excess and $HCO_3$. In most cases, the test should be re-drawn and analyzed.

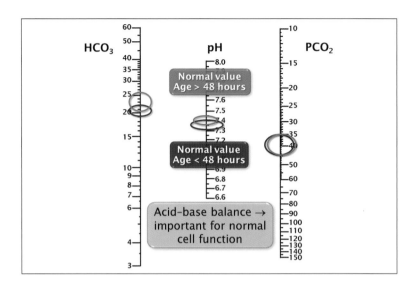

### Step 2. Interpret the blood gas.

Read rules 1 through 5 and decide into which category the blood gas falls. These rules apply to the very young infant and do not necessarily apply to older infants or children who have metabolic derangements from multiple other causes.

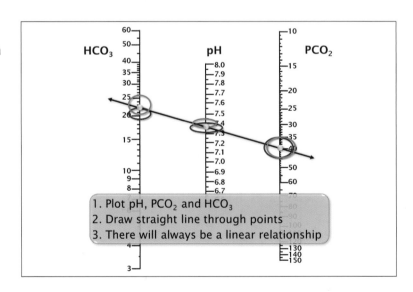

## RULE 1

Think of carbon dioxide ($CO_2$) as an **acid**. The only way to remove $CO_2$ is through the lung.

- $CO_2$ reflects the respiratory component of acid-base balance.

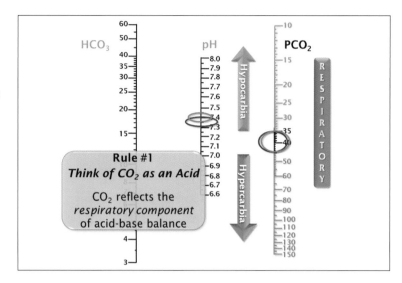

## RULE 2

Think of bicarbonate ($HCO_3$) as a **base** (a hydrogen ion acceptor).

- Changes in $HCO_3$ reflect the metabolic component of acid-base balance. To regulate acid-base balance, bicarbonate is retained or excreted by the kidney.

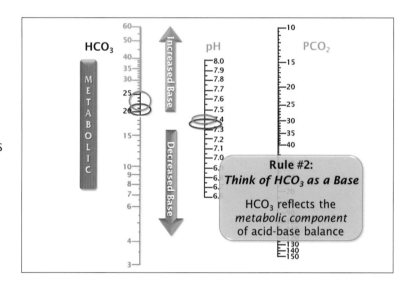

## RULE 3

That which happens on the acid side (loss of, or accumulation of, acid or $CO_2$) will be balanced by the base side ($HCO_3$), and vice versa.

- If the base side declines, the infant will try to blow off $CO_2$ to balance out or "compensate" for the change on the base side.

- The overall purpose of this balancing act is to maintain a normal pH value.

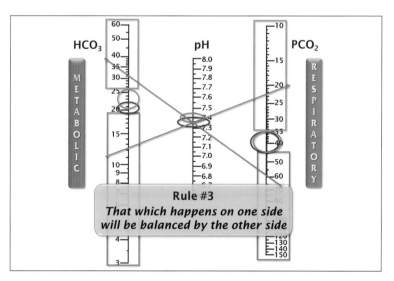

## The red zone.

If the blood gas dots are in the metabolic, respiratory, or both metabolic and respiratory red zones (the areas within the red boxes), then a **metabolic and/or respiratory abnormality** is the primary problem. For example, if a dot is in the metabolic red zone but not in the respiratory red zone, then the primary problem is metabolic.

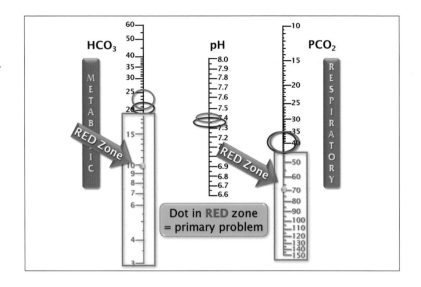

## The green zone.

The green zone is the area within the green boxes on the metabolic and respiratory scales. The green zone represents the **compensatory** area for both respiratory and metabolic components.

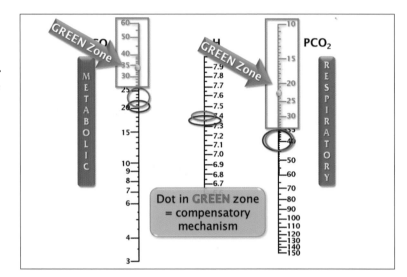

## Interpreting the pH.

If a dot is in the pH red zone then this would be considered "acidemia." If a dot is in the pH green zone, then this would be considered "alkalemia." Investigation into the underlying cause of the acidosis or alkalosis is important so that correct treatment may be initiated.

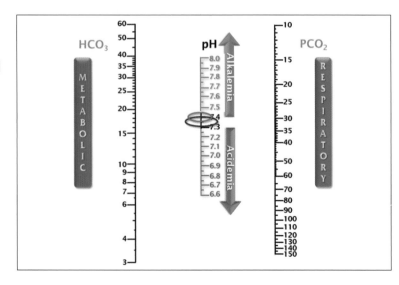

## RULE 4

If the pH is normal, the blood gas is normal *or* the blood gas is compensated.

- If the blood gas is **normal**, then all three dots will be within the three circles on the $HCO_3$, pH and $PCO_2$ scales. This does not necessarily mean the baby is normal, but the blood gas values are within a normal range.

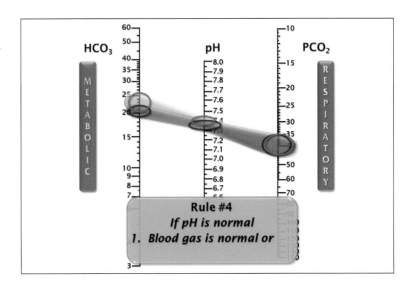

- If the blood gas is compensated, then the pH will be in the circle, but there will be a dot in the **red** zone on either the $HCO_3$ or $PCO_2$ scale.*

  *The focus of this discussion is on acidemia since acidosis is more often observed in sick newly born infants.

**Example of compensated metabolic acidosis:**

A dot is in the metabolic **red** zone

A dot is in the pH normal circle area

A dot is in the respiratory green zone

**Example of compensated respiratory acidosis:**

A dot is in the respiratory **red** zone

A dot is in the pH normal circle area

A dot is in the metabolic green zone

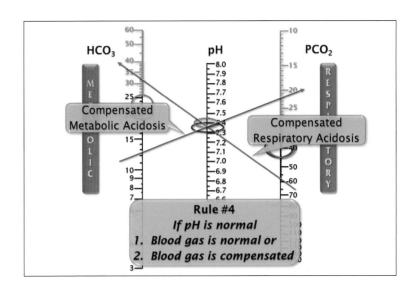

## RULE 5

**If the pH is low** then the blood gas is **uncompensated** secondary to metabolic and/ or respiratory acidosis.

- The pH dot will be in the **red** (acidosis) zone

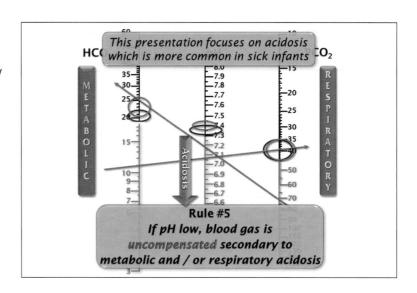

**Example of uncompensated metabolic acidosis:**

A dot is in the metabolic **red** zone

A dot is in the pH **red** zone

A dot is in the circle (normal area) on the respiratory side

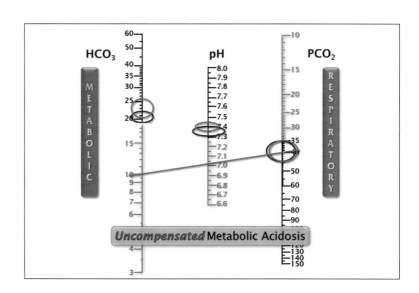

**Example of uncompensated respiratory acidosis:**

A dot is in the respiratory **red** zone

A dot is in the pH **red** zone

A dot is in the circle (normal area) on the metabolic side

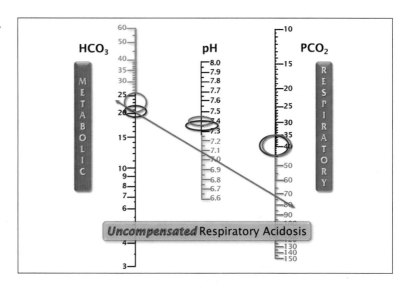

## Example of uncompensated mixed metabolic and respiratory acidosis:

A dot is in the metabolic red zone

A dot is in the respiratory red zone

A dot is in the pH red zone

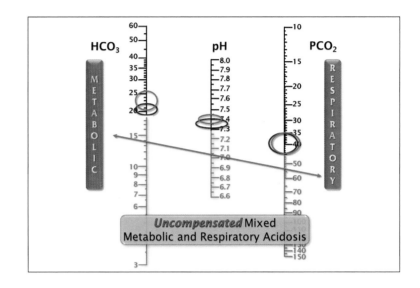

**If the pH is high,** then the blood gas is uncompensated secondary to metabolic and/or respiratory alkalosis*.

- The pH dot will be in the green (alkalosis) zone.

## Example of uncompensated respiratory alkalosis:

A dot is in the respiratory green zone

A dot is in the pH green zone

A dot is in the circle (normal area) on the metabolic (HCO$_3$) side

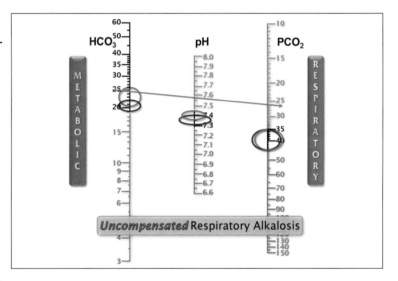

*The treatment of respiratory alkalosis starts with determining why the infant is alkalotic: too much ventilation (PCO$_2$ low) versus medication administration (consider a sodium bicarbonate overdose). In the example above, the infant was receiving more respiratory support than necessary. Reducing the ventilator rate allowed the PCO$_2$ to increase which in turn restored the pH to a normal value.

___

Notes

Venous blood pH values are usually 0.02 to 0.04 lower and PCO$_2$ 6 to 10 mmHg higher than the arterial sample results.[66] For capillary or venous samples, the PO$_2$ is not reflective of arterial PO$_2$. To assess oxygenation, evaluate the O$_2$ saturation by pulse oximetry.

## Causes of METABOLIC Acidosis

Increased lactic acid production can be secondary to:

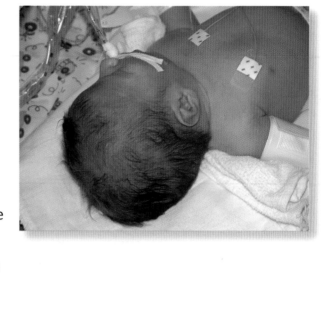

- Anaerobic metabolism secondary to:

  - Shock, poor tissue perfusion and oxygenation

  - Hypothermia (severe enough to result in anaerobic metabolism)

  - Hypoglycemia (severe enough to impair cardiac function and result in impaired oxygen and glucose delivery to the tissues)

  - Severe forms of congenital heart disease that cause severe hypoxemia or left outflow tract obstruction

- Sepsis

- Inborn errors of metabolism

  - Included in this list as an important reason for metabolic acidosis, but the problem is most often because of increased anion accumulation and infrequently lactic acid accumulation.

## Treatment of METABOLIC Acidosis

Identify and treat the underlying problems:

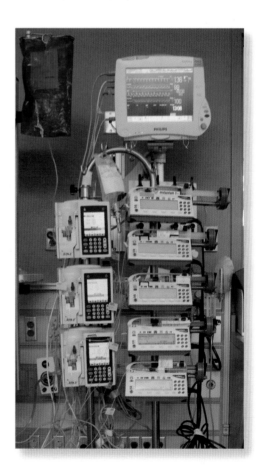

- Hypoxia is treated by improving oxygenation, ventilation and perfusion.

- It is not recommended that metabolic acidosis be treated with hyperventilation as this would be a temporary maneuver that does not effectively treat the underlying problem and could potentially cause other problems.

- Hypotension and shock are treated aggressively with volume infusions, blood pressure medications, and correction of anemia as necessary.

- Heart failure is treated once the primary cause has been identified (such as infection, structural heart disease, arrhythmias, hypoglycemia, and electrolyte disturbances).

- Inborn errors of metabolism require extensive workup and treatment to minimize acid production and reverse the effects of acids that accumulate in the bloodstream.

## Causes of RESPIRATORY Acidosis

$CO_2$ retention can result from inadequate ventilation due to:

### Loss of tidal volume

- Lung disease (pneumonia, aspiration, surfactant deficiency)

- Pneumothorax

- Airway obstruction

- Mechanical interference with ventilation as occurs with: chest wall deformities, hyperexpansion of the lungs in ventilated infants, and infants with abdominal distention

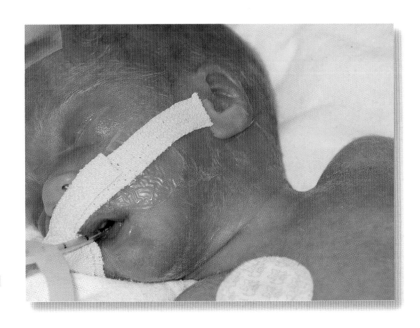

### Loss of respiratory drive

- Poor respiratory effort which occurs most often in preterm or very sick infants

- Neurologic injury: hypoxic ischemic encephalopathy, neonatal encephalopathy, structural brain abnormalities, and ischemic or hemorrhagic stroke, which can lead to respiratory depression

- Apnea

## Treatment of Respiratory Acidosis

- Renal compensation (retention of bicarbonate) for an elevated $PCO_2$ is a slow process. In most cases, providing continuous positive airway pressure (CPAP) or positive pressure ventilation by bag and mask or intubation will rapidly correct a respiratory acidosis. It is also important to continue to identify and treat the underlying cause of respiratory acidosis.

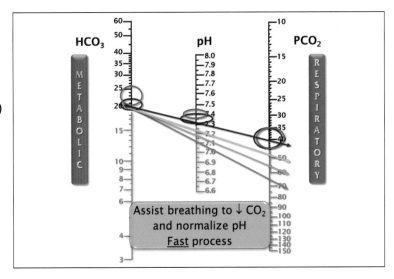

# Clinical Tip

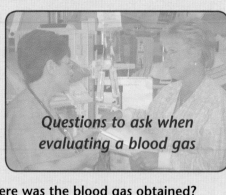

*Questions to ask when evaluating a blood gas*

**1. Where was the blood gas obtained?**

- ☐ Capillary (not useful for assessing oxygenation)
- ☐ Arterial
    - ☐ right radial artery (pre-ductal)
    - ☐ left radial artery (near ductus; juxta-ductal)
    - ☐ umbilical artery catheter (post-ductal)
    - ☐ posterior tibialis artery (post-ductal)
- ☐ Venous (UVC) (not useful for assessing oxygenation)

**2. Is the pH less than 7.30 and the $PCO_2$ greater than 50?**

If yes, this is respiratory acidosis and reflects difficulty exhaling $CO_2$.

- ☐ Re-evaluate the blood gas if the infant's distress worsens.
- ☐ Be prepared to assist ventilation with bag / mask ventilation, laryngeal mask airway placement, or endotracheal intubation and positive pressure ventilation.

**3. Is the pH less than 7.30 and the bicarbonate ($HCO_3$) less than 19?**

If yes, this is metabolic acidosis and means the infant is using bicarbonate as a buffer to neutralize the lactic acid. [Other causes of metabolic acidosis not related to lactic acidosis include renal tubular acidosis, excessive stool or stoma output, or inborn errors of metabolism].

- ☐ The lower the pH and $HCO_3$, the worse the situation.
- ☐ If the pH is less than 7.20, this is severely abnormal.

**4. Is the pH less than 7.30, the $PCO_2$ greater than 50, and the $HCO_3$ less than 19?**

If yes, this is a mixed respiratory and metabolic acidosis.

**5. Is the arterial $PO_2$ less than 50 when the infant is breathing 50% inspired oxygen?**

- ☐ Evaluate the $O_2$ saturation and if less than 85%, then the infant is hypoxemic.
- ☐ If drawn from an arterial location, evaluate whether the location was pre or post-ductal.
    - ☐ The right radial artery is the only pre-ductal site for blood gas sampling.
    - ☐ The left radial artery is close to the ductus (called juxta-ductal), and cannot be considered pre-ductal or post-ductal.
    - ☐ The umbilical or posterior tibialis arteries are the post-ductal arterial sites commonly used for blood gas sampling.
    - ☐ A blood gas drawn from a capillary or venous location cannot be used to assess oxygenation.
    - ☐ If the arterial PO2 in either a pre or post-ductal location is less than 50 on ≥ 50% inspired oxygen, try increasing the oxygen concentration.
    - ☐ Consider cyanotic congenital heart disease if unable to increase the arterial $PO_2$ to greater than 150 when the infant is breathing 100% oxygen. Unless indicated, the infant should **not** be left on 100% oxygen.
- ☐ Remain prepared to assist ventilation.

**6. What degree of respiratory distress was the baby in when the blood gas was drawn?**

☐ Mild  ☐ Moderate  ☐ Severe

- ☐ If the respiratory distress increased since the blood gas was drawn, then obtain another blood gas for comparison.
- ☐ Respiratory failure rapidly leads to $CO_2$ retention, hypoxemia and acidosis. If the infant was in severe distress when the blood gas was drawn, then the infant should receive full respiratory support, which includes laryngeal mask airway placement or intubation and assisted ventilation with a bag, t-piece resuscitator, or ventilator if available.
- ☐ Once intubated, the blood gas should be repeated to evaluate whether the degree of positive pressure support being provided is adequate to help normalize the blood gas.

# REVIEW

## Respiratory distress: what is important to evaluate and document?[1,2,8,10,11]

Evaluate respiratory rate, work of breathing, oxygenation, and ventilation by examining the infant, evaluating the $O_2$ saturation, blood gas and chest x-ray.

### Respiratory rate and effort

✧ Normal respiratory rate: 30 to 60 breaths per minute.

✧ Describe apneic episodes:

- Frequency per hour and length of apnea each time (in seconds) from start to resolution.

- How apnea was terminated: spontaneously versus with tactile stimulation and/or assisted ventilation.

- Heart rate and $O_2$ saturation during periods of apnea.

- Activity during episodes.

### Respiratory effort

Presence of:

✧ Nasal flaring.

✧ Audible grunting (heard without a stethoscope), including the infant's age when grunting started.

✧ Stridor (inspiratory or expiratory).

✧ Retractions, including location and severity.

✧ Quality of air entry on auscultation (equal, good entry, diminished, decreased on one side, extra sounds: moist rales/crackles, wheezes, grunting).

✧ Oxygen concentration being delivered (if any) and method of delivery

✧ $O_2$ saturation and location of the oximeter probe(s).

✧ Evaluation of the pre-and post-ductal $O_2$ saturation may be helpful if the infant has risk factors for pulmonary hypertension.

### Blood gas

✧ Arterial, capillary or venous blood gas to evaluate for respiratory and/or metabolic acidosis (or alkalosis).

### Chest x-ray

✧ To help identify any lung and/or cardiac pathology that may be present.

### Communication and documentation

✧ When communicating concerns to the infant's medical staff provider, it may be helpful to utilize a standardized communication tool called SBARR (http://teamstepps.ahrq.gov/) (see the Quality Improvement Module Appendix 7.1 for a detailed explanation).

- SBARR stands for Situation, Background, Assessment, and Recommendation. An additional "R" has been added by S.T.A.B.L.E. to represent Repeat back orders.

- The medical staff provider should be updated regarding the infant's condition, especially if the infant is deteriorating. Such communication and any additional orders received from the provider should be documented in the patient's chart.

✧ Remember to utilize the **Chain of Command or Chain of Communication** if your concerns are not being satisfactorily addressed.

# RESPIRATORY SUPPORT

→ **Continuous Positive Airway Pressure (CPAP)**
**Positive Pressure Ventilation with Bag and Mask or T-piece Resuscitator**
**Endotracheal Intubation**
**Assisting with Endotracheal Intubation**
**Securing the Endotracheal Tube**
**Location of the Endotracheal Tube on Chest X-ray**

If the infant is experiencing moderate to severe respiratory distress, then more aggressive levels of support, such as continuous positive airway pressure (CPAP) or endotracheal intubation may be indicated. Tables 3.4 and 3.5 identify infants who are and who are not candidates for CPAP.

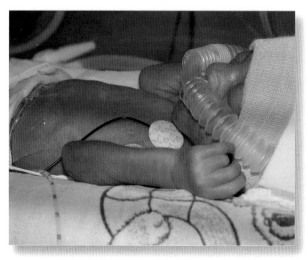

27-week gestation 5-day old infant

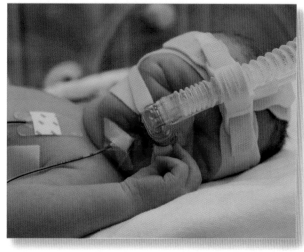

35-week gestation 1-day old infant

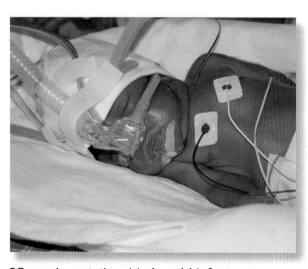

28-week gestation 11-day old infant

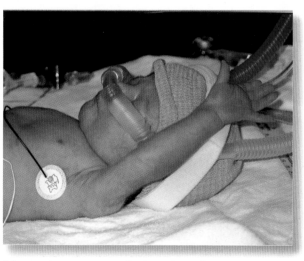

33-week gestation 2-day old infant

**Table 3.4.** Candidates for continuous positive airway pressure (CPAP).[64]

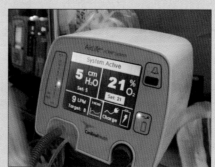

♢ Infant has adequate respiratory effort.

♢ An increased level of respiratory support is required, but infant does not yet meet clinical or blood gas criteria for endotracheal intubation and positive pressure ventilation.

  • Infant has increased work of breathing and / or increasing oxygen requirement.

  • Infant has mild $CO_2$ retention and mild acidosis.

  • CPAP may be helpful if the $PCO_2$ is less than 55 to 60 mmHg and the infant is requiring less than 40 to 70% supplemental oxygen to maintain an acceptable $O_2$ saturation (90 to 95%).[67]

  • A higher percent of supplemental oxygen may be required at higher elevations; however, amounts exceeding 60 to 70% should raise concern that an increased level of support (endotracheal intubation) may be required.

♢ Infant is experiencing increased frequency or severity of apnea, however episodes are not severe enough to warrant endotracheal intubation.

♢ Infant has atelectasis on chest x-ray.

♢ Infant has tracheobronchomalacia.

**Table 3.5.** Infants who are *not* candidates for CPAP.

♢ Infants with rapidly progressing respiratory failure.

  • Signs of respiratory failure include a rapidly increasing oxygen requirement, worsening retractions, tachypnea, worsening blood gas (hypercarbia and respiratory or mixed acidosis), or signs that the infant is becoming exhausted: slowing respiratory rate plus increased work of breathing, increased frequency and severity of apnea.[15,68]

♢ Infants with severe apnea with cyanosis and/or bradycardia or increased frequency and severity of apnea.[68]

♢ Infants who are gasping.

♢ Infants with any of the following conditions:

  • Poor respiratory drive
  • Diaphragmatic hernia
  • Tracheoesophageal fistula / esophageal atresia
  • Choanal atresia
  • Cleft palate
  • Cardiovascular instability and poor heart function

 Use CPAP with caution if the infant has a pneumothorax

## Continuous Positive Airway Pressure (CPAP)

→ **Positive Pressure Ventilation with Bag and Mask or T-piece Resuscitator**

## Endotracheal Intubation
## Assisting with Endotracheal Intubation
## Securing the Endotracheal Tube
## Location of the Endotracheal Tube on Chest X-ray

Positive pressure ventilation (PPV) using a bag and mask or T-piece resuscitator may be necessary to support the deteriorating infant. Indications for PPV include:[13,17]

- Apnea
- Inadequate breathing effort
- Bradycardia
- Hypoxemia not responsive to supplemental oxygen
- Gasping

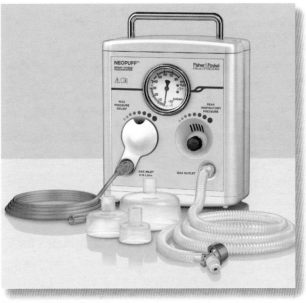

Neopuff™ Infant T-piece resuscitator
Photo courtesy of Fisher and Paykel, www.fphcare.com

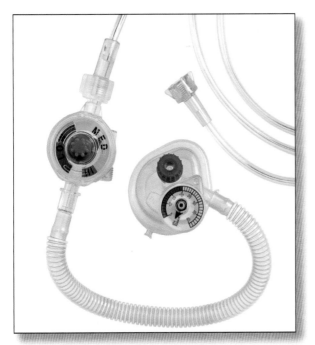
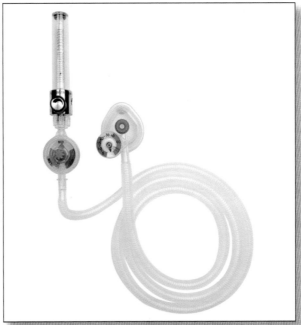

Neo-Tee® Infant T-piece resuscitator — Photos courtesy of Mercury Medical, mercurymed.com

!  Gasping respirations are a sign of impending cardiorespiratory arrest!

When an infant is gasping, ventilation and air exchange is ineffective. Positive pressure ventilation should be given immediately to reverse the hypoxic state.[13]

**If the infant is *not* already intubated,** effective positive pressure ventilation using a bag and mask or T-piece resuscitator should be started immediately.[13,14] If the infant's heart rate is low and not rising despite ***effective*** ventilation, insert a laryngeal mask airway or perform endotracheal intubation.[13,69] Cardiac stimulant medications may also be necessary.[13] Positive pressure ventilation should continue until the infant's heart rate is greater than 100 beats per minute and PPV may need to be continued even after the heart rate is greater than 100. Further evaluation for treatable causes of the respiratory deterioration (such as a pneumothorax), should be ongoing.

**If the infant *is* intubated,** the airway should be quickly assessed to determine whether the endotracheal tube is dislodged or obstructed. An acronym that is helpful for troubleshooting respiratory distress in the intubated infant is: **DOPE** – **D**isplaced, **O**bstructed, **P**neumothorax, **E**quipment failure (see Chameides, PALS reference, page 176[70] or Valente reference, page 7[71]).

!  Remember, when delivering positive pressure ventilation (PPV) with or without chest compressions, that all distractions should be minimized. The people performing PPV or compressions should stay focused on the important technical skill they are performing. If you are the team leader, then delegate the performance of PPV and chest compressions to others. Oftentimes the ventilation and/or compression rate becomes very erratic and uncoordinated when team members are distracted with questions and conversation.

## Proper positioning of the face mask.[13,17,71]

1. If not already done, apply a pulse oximeter so that oxygenation status and heart rate can be monitored continuously.

2. A well-fitting mask will help ensure a good seal. Position the cushioned, anatomically shaped face mask over the mouth and nose as shown. Cover the nose and mouth completely. The bottom rim of the mask should cover the edge of the chin and the eyes should not be covered by the top of the mask.

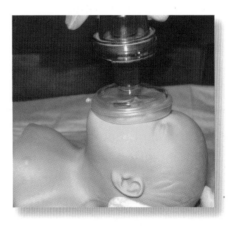 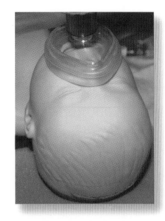

3. Hold the mask with your non-dominant hand and use your dominant hand for delivering the positive pressure ventilation.

4. Form a "C" with the thumb and index finger placed over the top of the mask and an "E" with the other three fingers. This method of holding the mask will allow for maintaining a good seal as well as good control over the chin position. Use the fingers forming the "E" to lift the jaw up to the mask rather than push the mask down onto the face which will be uncomfortable for the baby as well as may cause facial bruising.

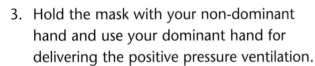

5. Precautions:

   • Be careful not to put pressure on the trachea with the fingers that are forming the "E".

   • Avoid pressure over the eyes.

   • Take care to not press the infant's head into the bed, which is especially possible when the infant is preterm.

   • If using a resuscitation bag, use a pressure gauge to monitor the amount of inflating pressure being given. If using a T-piece resuscitator, then the peak inspiratory pressure is set.

6. Watch for chest rise while squeezing the bag. **Avoid excessive chest rise!** If the heart rate is not increasing or the chest does not rise:

   • Recheck the mask seal and ensure the correct mask size is being used.

   • Reposition the head to open the airway.

   • Suction the mouth and nose to remove secretions that may be blocking the airway.

   • Ensure the mouth is open.

   • Increase the inflating pressure.

   • Consider an alternative airway – laryngeal mask airway or intubation.

7. If the infant was hypoxemic when bagging was initiated, look for improvement in $O_2$ saturation or color. If improvement is not seen, increase the oxygen concentration being delivered to the infant.

8. If the infant was bradycardic when bagging was initiated, look for improvement in the heart rate. If an improvement in heart rate is not seen, then check to be certain that oxygen is being delivered and that air entry can be heard in both lungs.

9. If the infant was newly born, remember the possibility of a congenital diaphragmatic hernia in any baby who deteriorates with bag/mask ventilation. Proceed with endotracheal intubation and positive pressure ventilation if this is suspected. A pneumothorax may also be the reason that an infant fails to improve. Be prepared to assess for pneumothorax (see page 162 for more details).

 If there is no improvement in heart rate or there is severe hypoxemia, consider endotracheal intubation or placement of a laryngeal mask airway (with positive pressure ventilation).

Table 3.6 identifies the warning signs of respiratory failure and when endotracheal intubation and assisted ventilation should be strongly considered. Table 3.7. reviews endotracheal tube (ET tube) sizes and insertion depth for orally intubated infants.

## Respiratory Failure Warning Signs

**Positive pressure ventilation via endotracheal tube or laryngeal mask airway should be considered for infants when:**

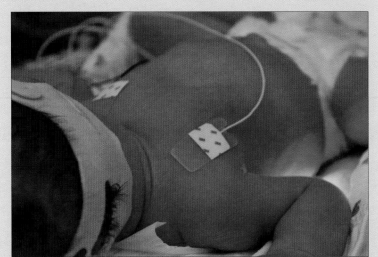

- The infant is gasping *(proceed with positive pressure ventilation immediately)*.

- The infant has periods of severe apnea and bradycardia.

- Persistent bradycardia despite properly performed positive pressure ventilation.

- Labored respiratory effort: moderate to severe retractions plus possibly grunting and nasal flaring.

- The infant is hypercarbic (elevated $PaCO_2$) with moderate to severe respiratory acidosis (low pH).

- Unable to ventilate and/or oxygenate adequately with PPV and the infant is not a candidate for nasal or mask continuous positive airway pressure (CPAP).

- Rapidly increasing $O_2$ concentration to maintain the $O_2$ saturation greater than 90%.

- Unable to maintain acceptable $O_2$ saturation for the infant's suspected disease process.

    *Note:* infants with some forms of cyanotic congenital heart disease may have $O_2$ saturation below 90%, however they may only have a mild degree of respiratory distress. Most often, these infants do not require intubation and positive pressure ventilation. Therefore, intubation should be at the direction of a neonatologist or pediatric cardiologist.

- The infant has a diaphragmatic hernia.

    *Note:* some infants with late onset diaphragmatic hernia are in minimal distress and they do not require endotracheal intubation.

**Consult the tertiary center neonatal physician if:**

1. Uncertain whether the infant should be placed on CPAP or intubated.

2. Unsure about the ventilatory support to provide once the infant is intubated.

3. Blood gases fail to improve after intubation.

4. Infant deteriorates after intubation.

**Table 3.6.** Respiratory failure warning signs and when endotracheal intubation and positive pressure ventilation should be strongly considered.[15,64,72]

Continuous Positive Airway Pressure (CPAP)

Positive Pressure Ventilation with Bag and Mask or T-piece Resuscitator

→ **Endotracheal Intubation**

Assisting with Endotracheal Intubation

Securing the Endotracheal Tube

Location of the Endotracheal Tube on Chest X-ray

## Supplies and Equipment[72-75]

The supplies and equipment necessary to perform endotracheal intubation should be kept together on either a resuscitation cart or intubation tray. Each delivery room, nursery, and emergency department should have a complete set of the items listed below.

- Laryngoscope with an extra set of batteries and extra bulb.

- Blades: (Straight rather than curved blades are preferred for optimal visualization).

  - No. 1 (term infant).

  - No. 0 (preterm infant).

  - No. 00 (very low birthweight infant).

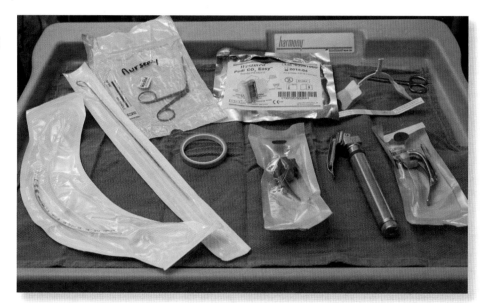

- McGill forceps (used for nasotracheal intubation).

- Uncuffed endotracheal (ET) tubes with an internal (inside) diameter of 2.5, 3.0, 3.5, and 4.0 mm.

- $CO_2$ detector (displays a color change when $CO_2$ is present when the infant exhales), or capnography equipment (displays the level of exhaled $CO_2$).

- Stylet (optional use, but should be available).

- Suctioning device, or suction setup with 8 and 10Fr suction catheters.

- Shoulder roll.

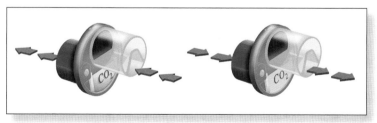

Mini StatCO$_2$ End Tidal $CO_2$ Detector

*Photo courtesy of Mercury Medical, mercurymed.com*

## Supplies and Equipment (continued)

- Roll of adhesive tape (½ or ¾ inch), or endotracheal tube stabilizer for securing the ET tube.

- Scissors.

- Extra thin hydrocolloid dressing.

- Oxygen source and blender (to permit administration of varying oxygen concentrations from 21% to 100%).

- Pulse oximeter (SpO$_2$).

- Resuscitation bag.

- T-piece resuscitator (if available).

- Appropriate sized masks for newborn and preterm infants.

- Stethoscope.

- Laryngeal mask airway – should be available in the event that intubation is not successful. Sizes vary depending upon the manufacturer and newer generation models may become available for smaller infants. Follow manufacturer instructions for appropriate size selection.

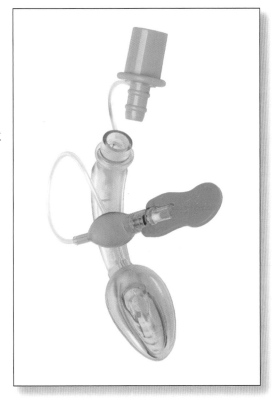

Size 1.0 airQ® Masked Laryngeal Airway

*Photo courtesy of Mercury Medical, mercurymed.com*

| Weight | Gestational Age (weeks) | ET tube size (mm ID) | Tube insertion depth at the lip (in centimeters) using the Lip-to-Tip Rule [b] (add 6 to the infant's weight in kilograms) |
|---|---|---|---|
| < 750 grams [a] (Below 750 grams) | < 28 | 2.5 [c] | 6 |
| < 1000 grams* (Below 1 Kg) | < 28 | 2.5 ~~3~~ | 7 |
| 1000-2000 grams (1 to 2 kg) | 28 – 34 | 3.0 | 8 |
| 2000-3000 grams (2 to 3 kg) | 34 – 38 | 3.5 | 9 |
| > 3000 grams (Greater than 3 kg) | > 38 | 3.5 – 4.0 | 10 |

**Table 3.7.** Endotracheal tube (ET tube) sizes and insertion depth for orally intubated infants according to weight and gestational age.[72-76] If the infant's weight is known, use the chart above to estimate the appropriate endotracheal tube size. If the weight is not known, use the gestational age to estimate correct size.

---

*Notes:

[a]  For extremely low-birth-weight infants, (less than 1000 grams), the ET tube insertion depth at the lip is usually between 5.5 cm and 7 cm (shorter distance with lower weights). At approximately 750 grams, the ET tube insertion depth is 6.5 cm.[76]

[b]  The ET tube tip should be positioned in the mid-trachea or halfway between the clavicles and the carina.[76] Confirm location by exam and chest x-ray. Tip location will vary with head position, therefore, take each x-ray with the head in the same position with the arms positioned along the side of the body and the chin in a neutral position. Flexing the head down (chin down) will advance the tube deeper and tipping the head back (chin up) will pull the tube upward.

[c]  A size 2.0 ET tube is so small that ventilation is impaired. By Poiseuille's Law, as the internal diameter of the tube is reduced, resistance is increased by the fourth power.[56] Because of this, a 2.0 ET tube has a 2.4-fold higher resistance than a 2.5 ET tube, therefore, insertion of a 2.0 ET tube should be avoided. Consult a tertiary center neonatologist to discuss individual circumstances and whether a 2.0 mm ET tube is necessary.

Continuous Positive Airway Pressure (CPAP)

Positive Pressure Ventilation with Bag and Mask or T-piece Resuscitator

Endotracheal Intubation

→ **Assisting with Endotracheal Intubation**

Securing the Endotracheal Tube

Location of the Endotracheal Tube on Chest X-ray

The performance of a successful intubation increases with opportunities to practice this skill and possibly through the level of support provided by those assisting with the procedure. It is best if two people are on hand to assist the person performing the intubation (the operator).

## Before intubation – prepare the patient and check equipment

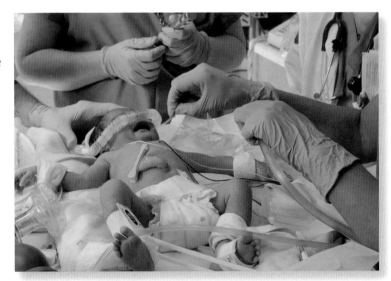

- Do a "time-out" to correctly identify the patient (if the patient condition allows).

- Provide protection from cold stress by using a radiant warmer or a heat lamp if no warmer is available. Limit the amount of time the infant will be exposed to a cooler environment. Do not block the heat output underneath the radiant warmer.

- Appropriate size endotracheal (ET) tube (see Table 3.7 for sizes).

- Do not leave the tube on the warmer surface or the tube will become too flexible. Keep the tube sterile when preparing it for use.

- Stylet: check with the operator before intubation to see if they want a stylet inserted into the ET tube.

- If a stylet is used, be sure the tip does not go beyond the end of the ET tube as this may injure the trachea upon insertion of the tube.

- Laryngoscope.

  - Check to make sure the bulb is bright and is screwed on tight.

  - Do not leave the bulb light on while waiting for the intubation to begin as this will heat up the blade and may burn the infant.

- Resuscitation bag or T-piece resuscitator and appropriate size face mask. A resuscitation bag should be available as back-up in the event it is needed.

- An anatomically correct shaped face mask should be used if available.

- Oxygen source and blender (to enable adjustment of inspired oxygen concentration).

- Suction equipment.

- Turn on and check to be sure the suction level is appropriate.

- Attach an 8 or 10Fr catheter to the suction tubing.

- Place the suction catheter close to the baby's head in the line of vision of the operator.

- Prepare tape or ET tube holder.

- If available, attach an $O_2$ saturation (pulse oximeter) monitor and cardiorespiratory monitor to the infant.

- If possible as outlined later in this module, provide analgesic medication before the intubation begins.

- Determine **before starting the procedure**, what the tube insertion depth will be (at the lip). For orotracheal intubation, refer to the Lip-to-Tip insertion depth guideline outlined Table 3.7.

## Assisting during intubation

- Stabilize the head and provide comfort to the infant.

- Hand equipment to the operator as they request: laryngoscope, suction catheter, ET tube.

- The goal is to provide equipment into the intubator's line of vision so that they do not have to take their eyes off the vocal cords.

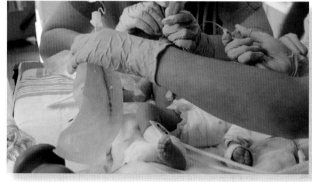

- If the infant is making a respiratory effort, provide free-flow oxygen. Remember this can be a source of cold stress to the infant so if not attached to a heated, humidified system, limit the amount of oxygen blown directly at the face and cheeks.

- If suction is requested, place the suction catheter into the operator's hand so that they do not have to take their eyes off the airway. Occlude the suction finger hole when requested.

- If asked by the operator for 'cricoid pressure', gently apply pressure on the cricoid cartilage of the trachea (just below the thyroid) and confirm with the operator that this is helping.

- Monitor the infant's heart rate and color (and $O_2$ saturation if this equipment was attached) during the procedure.

- When people have limited experience intubating small infants, it can be difficult for them to process a lot of information when they are performing the intubation. Therefore, the following is suggested:

  - If the infant is tolerating the procedure, offer reassuring but short statements to the operator such as: *"saturation is 94% (or color is pink)"*.

  - When the saturation begins to decline into the 80% range, or the heart rate drops below 100, notify the operator with short statements like: *"heart rate 90, saturation 80%"*.

  - If you think the operator should stop the procedure because the intubation time has exceeded 30 seconds[74] or the infant is not tolerating the procedure, then announce: *"We should stop now and bag/mask ventilate the baby"*.

- Assist as requested with bag and mask ventilation in between intubation attempts.

- Monitor the length of time spent on each intubation attempt. Follow established resuscitation guidelines for the length of time that an intubation should be attempted.[74]

## Assisting after intubation

## Using a $CO_2$ detector and assessing whether the infant is intubated

- Establish with the operator who will be responsible for holding the tube securely at all times (to prevent accidental dislodgment). Do not let the infant turn his or her head to either side.

- Immediately check the tube location at the upper lip. One of the most common mistakes when intubating is to insert the ET tube too deeply.

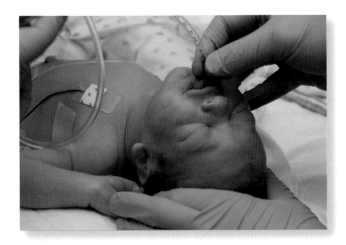

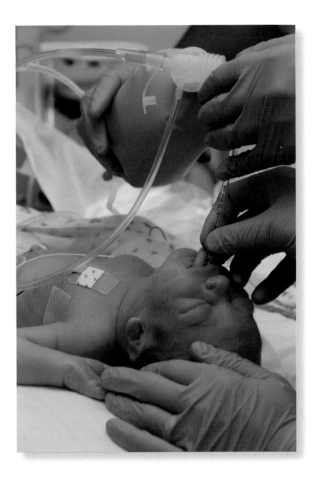

- Attach a $CO_2$ detector and confirm that you see the color change indicating the presence of $CO_2$ (this signifies the tube is in the trachea).

  - The $CO_2$ detector should be purple or blue initially. If it is a different color, then it should be discarded.

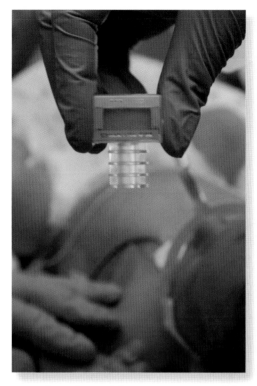

Purple or blue = negative $CO_2$

- A helpful reminder is that a **y**ellow color change signifies "**Y**es", or "yes for $CO_2$".

- The $CO_2$ color change may not occur until 6 or more breaths have been given to the infant.

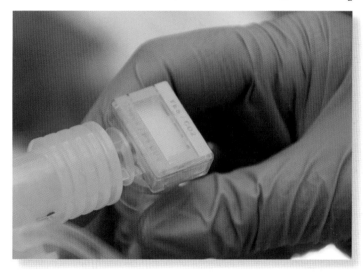

Yellow = positive $CO_2$

Notes:

1. If endotracheal epinephrine was given and the medication touches the $CO_2$ detector device, the color may change to yellow which will result in a false positive reading – the ET tube may not be in the trachea. Replace the contaminated $CO_2$ detector with a new one (and reassess for color change) and while giving PPV, assess breath sounds, chest rise and ascertain that the sounds over the stomach are diminished or absent compared to the sounds over the lungs. If the sounds are louder over the stomach, compared to the chest, the tube is most likely not in the trachea and should be removed.

2. $CO_2$ may not be detected if the infant has poor cardiac output and/or a low or no heart rate. The color may not change, yet the infant may be intubated. Examine the infant as explained above and remove the ET tube if not able to determine the infant is intubated.

3. $CO_2$ detector may also be used with a laryngeal mask airway and with a face mask.

## Assisting after intubation (continued)

- Watch for vapor condensation in the tube (this also signifies the tube is in the trachea).

- Attach a resuscitation bag or a T-piece resuscitator to the ET tube and provide breaths while someone listens with a stethoscope over both sides of the chest and stomach. Watch for gentle chest rise, an increase in heart rate, and an increase in $O_2$ saturation.

- Provide ventilation as required while the tube is being secured and after the tube is secured.

- Positive pressure ventilation must be provided once the infant is intubated.

> ⚠ Do not place an intubated infant into an oxygen hood as this will cause the infant to breathe with extreme difficulty. Airway resistance is higher once an ET tube is in place! The infant will not be able to effectively move air in and out of the lungs unless provided continuous positive airway pressure or positive pressure ventilation once intubated.

- Double check the tube location at the lip throughout the taping procedure.

- Insert a gastric tube if not done already and leave the tube open to air so air can escape from the stomach.

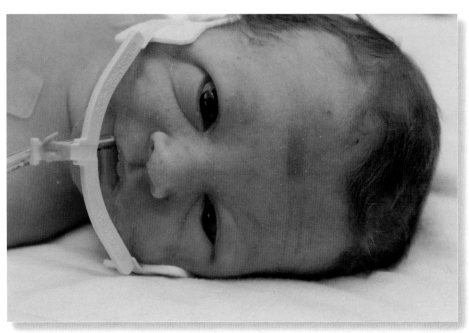

- Once the ET tube tip is in good position, **proceed with trimming the ET tube** so that the distance from the lip to the tube connector is approximately 4 centimeters. Cut the tube at a slight angle to make it easier to reattach the ET tube adapter. Since resistance is linearly proportional to the length of the tube, trimming the ET tube also offers the advantage of decreasing resistance, which will help improve ventilation.[56]

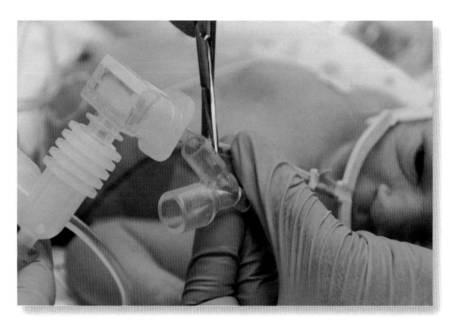

⚠ Accidental extubation while trimming the ET tube is a real risk! If not experienced in this procedure, it is advised that you leave the tube length alone and wait for the transport team or experienced NICU personnel to perform this procedure.

## Clinical Tip

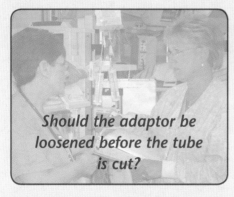

*Should the adaptor be loosened before the tube is cut?*

At times, especially with smaller ET tubes, it is helpful to loosen the adaptor before cutting the ET tube. That way, once the tube is cut, the adaptor can be placed quickly back on the cut ET tube. In addition, wiping the adaptor with an alcohol swab helps the adaptor to slip more easily into the tube.

Continuous Positive Airway Pressure (CPAP)

Positive Pressure Ventilation with Bag and Mask or T-piece Resuscitator

Endotracheal Intubation

Assisting with Endotracheal Intubation

→ **Securing the Endotracheal Tube**

Location of the Endotracheal Tube on Chest X-ray

## Securing the ET Tube with Tape:

The "X" and "V" method for taping an ET tube

There are various ways to secure the ET tube using tube holders (shown in the photos to the right) or with tape. If your facility does not already have an established way of securing the ET tube, then a taping method is shown on pages 145 to 147.

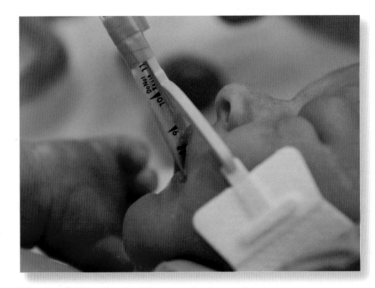

NeoBar® ET tube holder neotechproducts.com

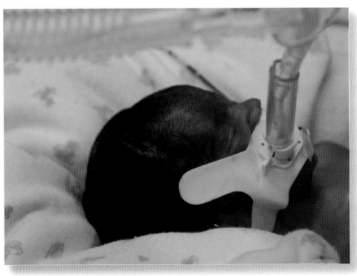

RSP® ET tube holder Smiths-Medical.com

1. If possible, prepare the cheeks and upper lip with a protective hydrocolloid base layer to protect the skin. This is especially important if the infant is preterm or it is expected that the infant will require prolonged intubation. Be sure the mouth area is clean and dry. Before applying the first piece of tape, confirm the ET tube location at the lip.

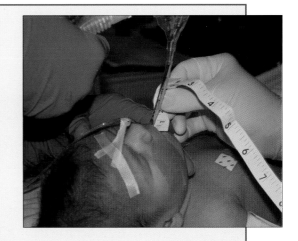

2. Cut adhesive tape into two pieces; a "V" and an "X."

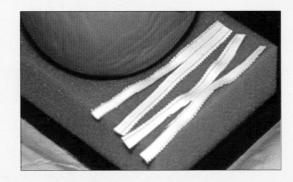

3. The assistant should hold the tube securely at all times. If possible, try to position the ET tube so it is slightly to the right of the center or, if re-taping the tube, in a different location against the upper gum than previously.

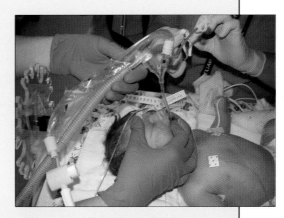

4. First, the "X" piece is applied firmly to the skin above the upper lip.

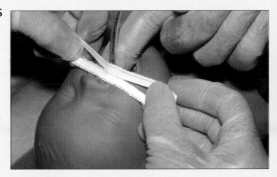

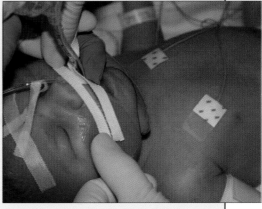

5. One arm of the lower tape is then wrapped around the tube. The other arm is then wrapped around the tube.

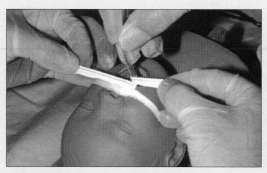
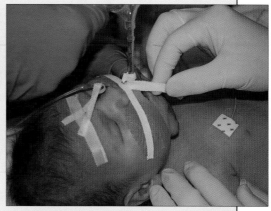

6. Move up slightly on the tube as you wrap but do not move up so much that the tape puts traction on the tube and pulls it into the mouth. Make a tab at the end of every piece so that it is easier to unwrap the tape if the tube needs to be repositioned. Be sure to check the tube markings at the lip throughout the procedure.

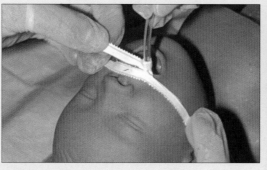
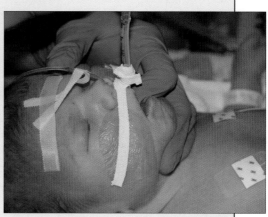

7. Next, apply the "V" shaped piece to help secure the underlying tape. The upper part of the "V" is applied first to the upper lip.

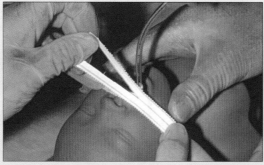
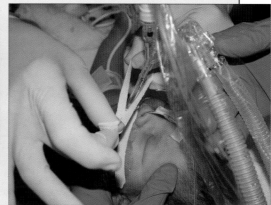

8. The lower piece wraps around the tube again. Continue to wrap the tape, moving up slightly until ½ inch of tape remains.

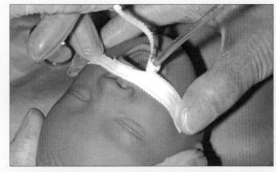

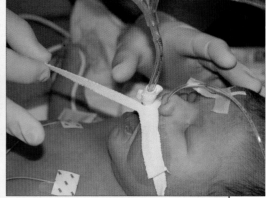

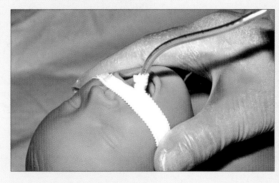

9. Fold the remaining ½ inch of tape to form a tab. This will allow for easier unfastening of the tape if the tube needs to be repositioned after the chest x-ray.

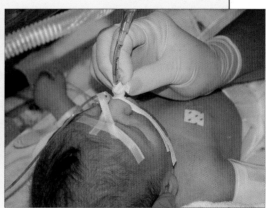

10. Once the ET tube has been secured, insert an orogastric or nasogastric tube to decompress the stomach.

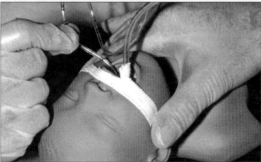

11. Confirm ET tube location on a chest x-ray.

Continuous Positive Airway Pressure (CPAP)
Positive Pressure Ventilation with Bag and Mask or T-piece Resuscitator
Endotracheal Intubation
Assisting with Endotracheal Intubation
Securing the Endotracheal Tube

→ **Location of the Endotracheal Tube on Chest X-ray**

Helpful advice for taking a chest x-ray

- Position the infant so that the infant's shoulders and hips lie flat on the bed or x-ray plate, with the arms in the same location on each side of the body (down by the sides rather than up over the head), and with the head turned slightly to the right or left (which is a more natural way for the infant to lie once the x-ray has been taken).

- Remember, the chin should be kept in a neutral position because, if the chin is down, (head flexed) the ET tube will move deeper. If the chin is up (head hyperextended), the ET tube will move upward.

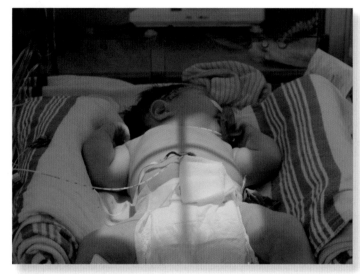

Infant positioned for an x-ray after placement of an umbilical venous catheter

- Use gonad protection whenever possible.

- If a chest x-ray must be repeated, position the infant in the same manner each time with the head turned in the same direction as the previous x-ray.

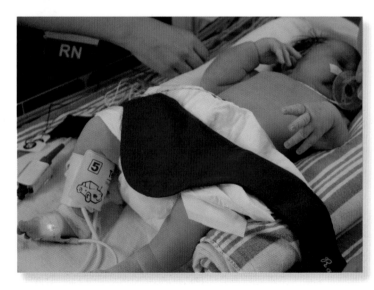

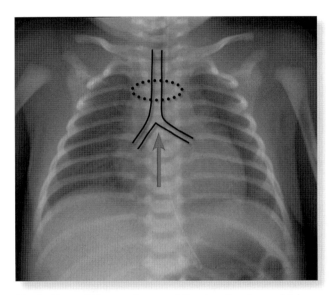

Illustration of the anatomy of the tracheobronchial tree. The dotted area represents the acceptable location for the ET tube tip (mid-trachea). The arrow points to the carina.

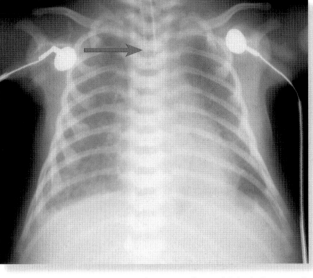

The arrow is pointing to the ET tube which is in good position in the mid-trachea.

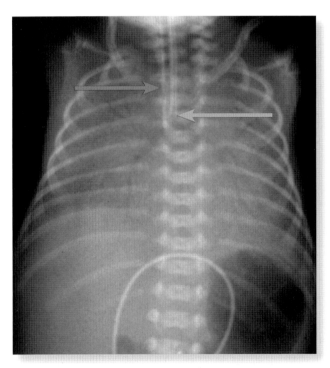

ET tube positioned too low and is at the carina or just slightly in the right mainstem bronchus. The arms are being held up along the sides of the head which might be causing head flexion. Flexing the head down (chin down) will advance the tube deeper and tipping the head back (chin up) will pull the tube upward. The blue arrow points to where the ET tube tip should be located. Both lungs are significantly atelectatic and air bronchograms are seen in this preterm infant with severe respiratory distress syndrome. Notice the large amount of gastric air in the absence of a gastric tube.

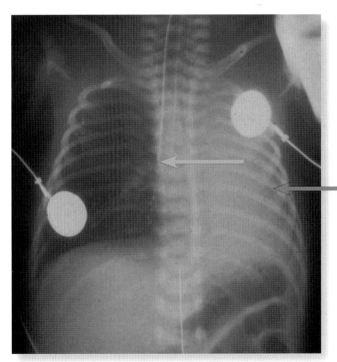

The ET tube is in the right mainstem bronchus and the left lung is completely atelectatic.

## Initial Ventilator Support

The infant's history, suspected disease process, response to ventilation, work of breathing, blood gas, and chest x-ray findings all need to be factored in when deciding which level of support to provide.[15] Figure 3.5 illustrates the settings that are adjusted when providing positive pressure ventilation (PPV) using a time-cycled mode.

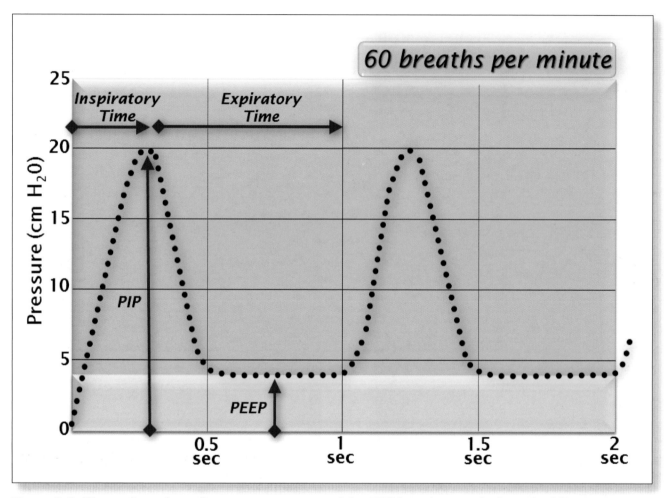

**Figure 3.5. Illustration of ventilator parameters used for PPV in a time-cycled mode.** PIP: positive inspiratory pressure, PEEP: positive end expiratory pressure, inspiratory time and expiratory time. Note, time is shown on the "X" axis and pressure (cmH$_2$O) is shown on the "Y" axis. In this example, each breath is delivered over one second to deliver a rate of 60 breaths per minute; the inspiratory time is 0.3 seconds and the expiratory time is 0.7 seconds.

Figure 3.6 provides suggestions for the **initial** ventilatory support of infants with varying weights. The goal is to provide adequate support of oxygenation and ventilation while trying to minimize lung injury.[15,77,78] **Therefore, it is advised to start with the lowest possible settings** and then increase if necessary. Aim for gentle chest rise; avoid excessive chest rise. If the infant is not improving on the selected ventilator support, then the ventilator settings should be adjusted (for additional information, see the Clinical Tip: How to approach the ventilated infant who is not oxygenating well).

**If unsure what level of support to provide, or the infant is not responding to the level of support you have chosen, call the tertiary center neonatologist or transport control physician for advice.**

| Settings | VLBW (< 1.5 kg) | LBW (1.5 to 2.5 kg) | Term (>2.5 kg) |
|---|---|---|---|
| **Rate (per minute)** | 30 to 45 | 20 to 40 | 20 to 40 |
| **Inspiratory Time (in seconds)** | 0.3 to 0.35 | 0.3 to 0.35 | 0.35 to 0.4 |
| **Positive Inspiratory pressure (PIP) [cmH$_2$O]** | 16 to 22 | 18 to 24 | 20 to 28 |
| **Positive End Expiratory Pressure (PEEP) [cmH$_2$O]** | 4 to 7 | 4 to 7 | 4 to 7 |

**Figure 3.6. Suggestions for initial ventilator support for infants of varying weights.** VLBW: very-low-birth weight, LBW: low-birth weight.

Notes:
1. PEEP
   a. The amount of PEEP selected will be based upon the infant's disease process and goals of therapy.
   b. A PEEP of 4 may be insufficient and may result in collapse of the alveoli.
   c. Excessive PEEP for the disease process and clinical situation may impair ventilation, lung perfusion, and/or venous return (return of deoxygenated blood to the right side of the heart).
2. The amount of pressure required (PIP) will also vary depending upon the infant's size, disease state and response to ventilation. Start with pressure in the lower end of the range and adjust up or down as needed based on the infant's response to treatment, chest x-ray, blood gas, and physical exam.
3. An inspiratory time greater than 0.5 seconds may result in air trapping and increase the risk for barotrauma and injury to the lung tissue.
4. A chest x-ray and blood gas may be helpful to assess response to changes.

# Clinical Tip

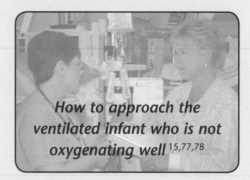

*How to approach the ventilated infant who is not oxygenating well* [15,77,78]

Several strategies may be used to improve oxygenation. The easiest thing to do initially is increase the inspired oxygen. If increasing the oxygen concentration does not improve oxygenation, or if the infant is already on a high percentage of oxygen, then the ventilator settings may be adjusted to increase Mean Airway Pressure (MAP). This can be achieved by increasing PEEP, PIP, or inspiratory time.[15] It is helpful to increase just one parameter at a time to see if oxygenation improves, in this order: PEEP first, then PIP (will also affect ventilation), and finally, inspiratory time.

**A few reminders regarding changes in ventilator settings:**[15,77]

- Increasing PIP will increase tidal volume so the $PCO_2$ may also go down.

- Increasing PEEP without increasing PIP may decrease tidal volume so although oxygenation improves, $PCO_2$ may actually go up.

- If the $PCO_2$ is already elevated, then PIP may be a better initial option.

- If the rate is kept the same, then increasing inspiratory time will decrease expiratory time, therefore $PCO_2$ may go up.

- An increase in inspiratory time reduces exhalation time.

- If the rate and inspiratory time are increased at the same time, the expiratory time may be significantly decreased, resulting in insufficient time to allow expiration and "breath stacking".

Notes:

1. These suggestions are for time-cycled pressure controlled ventilators. Other modes of ventilation, including volume ventilation and high frequency, require other adjustments than mentioned here. In addition, remember that air leak from pneumothorax, pulmonary interstitial emphysema, etc., and other severe forms of lung disease may preclude ventilator changes from being effective.

2. If not satisfied with the infants response to ventilation, repeat the chest x-ray as new information may be helpful to decide the next course of action.

# Neonatal Respiratory Illnesses

## Tachypnea and Low PCO$_2$

Fast breathing (tachypnea) with a low PCO$_2$ (less than 35) may be secondary to **NON-PULMONARY CAUSES** such as:

### Metabolic acidosis secondary to:

* Shock, poor tissue perfusion and oxygenation

  * To compensate for a metabolic acidosis, the infant will exhale CO$_2$ via the respiratory system. If the infant does not have concurrent pulmonary disease, then partial or complete compensation is possible.

* Congenital heart disease

  * The lungs can effectively ventilate, however the infant may be tachypneic secondary to shock or hypoxemia.

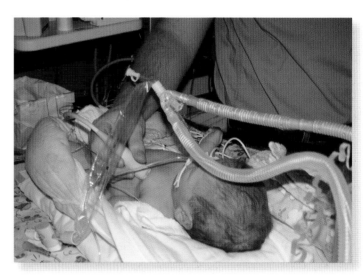

Echocardiogram being performed in a term infant with hypoplastic left heart syndrome

### Brain disorders

* The infant may be tachypneic because of brain irritation secondary to hemorrhage, meningitis, cerebral edema and/or brain injury secondary to perinatal or postnatal hypoxia.

## Tachypnea and Increased PCO$_2$

Fast breathing (tachypnea) or labored breathing plus an increased PCO$_2$ may be secondary to **PULMONARY CAUSES** such as:

* Transient tachypnea of the newborn (TTNB)
* Respiratory distress syndrome (RDS)
* Pneumonia
* Aspiration
* Pulmonary hemorrhage
* Tracheoesophageal fistula (TEF) / esophageal atresia (EA)
* Congenital diaphragmatic hernia (CDH)
* Airway obstruction
* Pneumothorax

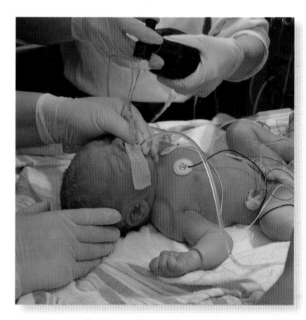

Resuscitation of an infant with congenital diaphragmatic hernia

As previously discussed in this module, in response to increased $CO_2$ in the bloodstream, the infant will breathe faster and use accessory muscles of respiration (e.g. will be retracting) to increase minute ventilation. A rising $PCO_2$ means the infant is no longer able to compensate despite the increased respiratory rate and work of breathing.

Other pulmonary causes of tachypnea with elevated $PCO_2$ (not included in this module) include chest or lung masses, chest wall deformity, and lung hypoplasia.

Infants with pulmonary and cardiac disease often both present with similar signs, including respiratory distress. Table 3.9 provides some guidance when differentiating between pulmonary and cardiac disease. It is important to remember that infants with cardiac disease may also have concurrent pulmonary conditions as further described in this section.

| | Pulmonary | Cardiac |
|---|---|---|
| **Cyanosis** | Yes | Yes or No |
| **Respiratory rate** | Tachypnea | Tachypnea – may be described as "comfortably tachypneic" |
| **Work of breathing** | Respiratory distress → flaring, grunting, retractions | Easy effort; but increased distress if congestive heart failure (CHF) has developed |
| **Acid / base** | Increased $PCO_2$ → Respiratory acidosis more common but may have mixed acidosis if shock also present | Decreased $PCO_2$ → Metabolic acidosis<br><br>Increased $PCO_2$ if CHF or concurrent pulmonary disease*<br><br>May have mixed acidosis |
| **Chest x-ray** | Asymmetric or symmetric pattern of infiltrates, pneumothorax, pleural effusion, retained fluid | Increased or decreased pulmonary vascular markings; pulmonary edema* |
| **Heart size, shape, heart location** | Normal or increased size | Normal or increased size; normal or abnormal shape |

*May have chest x-ray findings consistent with concurrent pulmonary disease*

**Table 3.9.** Differentiating between pulmonary and cardiac disease.[30]

## Transient Tachypnea of the Newborn (TTNB)[8,79-81]

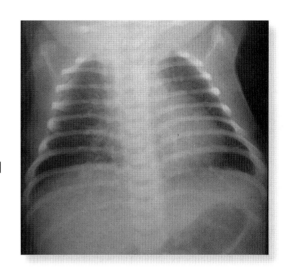

- Affects term or late preterm infants.

- TTNB is one of the most common causes of respiratory distress in the newborn period; estimated incidence is 5.7 per 1000 term births.

- Onset of respiratory distress is usually within 1 to 2 hours after birth and is a result of failure to adequately absorb fetal lung fluid into the pulmonary circulation and lymphatics.

- Risk factors include cesarean section birth (with or without labor), precipitous delivery, and preterm delivery.

- The infant may have mild to moderate respiratory distress, but usually the oxygen requirement remains less than 40%.

- Usually resolves within 2 to 3 days; sometimes within 24 hours.

- Chest x-ray typically shows fluid in the fissures and perihilar markings or opacity, and at times, lung overinflation and/or pleural effusion.

- Differentiate from pneumonia, sepsis, respiratory distress syndrome, aspiration, and pulmonary edema secondary to a cardiac cause.

## Respiratory distress syndrome (RDS)

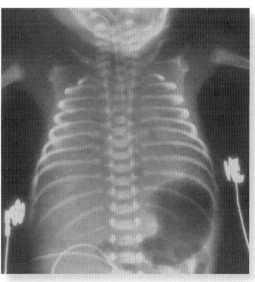

- Most commonly seen in preterm infants, including late preterm infants.[82]

- Immature lung anatomy and physiology and surfactant insufficiency.

- Infants of diabetic mothers (even if term gestation) have an increased incidence of RDS secondary to delayed surfactant production.[83]

- Onset of respiratory distress is usually at birth or shortly after birth.

- Chest x-ray shows uniform diffuse granular appearance with air bronchograms and low lung volumes.

## Pneumonia[79]

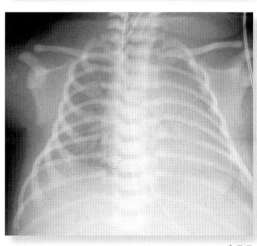

- Affects term or preterm infants.

- Onset of respiratory distress is at birth or with onset of the pulmonary infection.

- Differentiate pneumonia from sepsis, RDS, aspiration, and transient tachypnea of the newborn.

- Chest x-ray is variable and may show diffuse or focal infiltrates, hazy or opaque lung fields, or lobar consolidation.

## Aspiration of amniotic fluid, blood, or gastric contents[8,79,84]

- Affects term or preterm infants.

- Onset of respiratory distress is at birth or at the time of aspiration.

- The history should be carefully evaluated for clues that help differentiate aspiration from sepsis, pneumonia, or TTNB.

- Chest x-ray is variable and may show patchy infiltrates, areas of atelectasis, or hyperinflation.

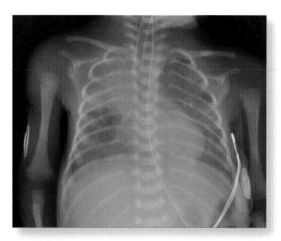

## Meconium aspiration syndrome (MAS)[79,85,86]

- Affects term and post-term infants predominantly.

- Common cause of hypoxemic respiratory failure.

- MAS is also associated with a several-fold increased risk for sepsis.

- *The problem begins in utero:*
  Poor placental blood flow and oxygenation causes the fetus to evacuate (pass) meconium ➔ gasping respirations move the meconium deep into the lungs ➔ after birth, obstruction of the airways leads to both atelectasis and hyperinflation ➔ this increases the risk for pneumothorax, impaired ventilation and oxygenation, surfactant inactivation, and pulmonary hypertension. At times, intrauterine infection is a predisposing factor in development of severe MAS.

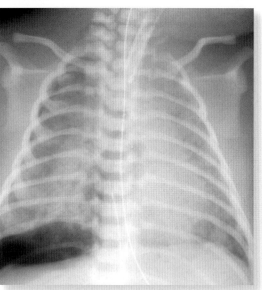

Subpulmonic pneumothorax also present on the right

- Chest x-ray typically shows coarse, nodular opacities (likely from meconium in the small airways), atelectasis, and overinflation.

## Pulmonary hemorrhage[79]

- Affects term or preterm infants.

- Onset of cardiorespiratory distress is sudden and is accompanied by blood in the trachea.

- Blood not only fills alveoli, but also inactivates surfactant.

- Etiologies include pulmonary edema, left-to-right ductal shunting through a patent ductus arteriosus (PDA), surfactant administration, sepsis, left ventricular failure, bleeding disorders.

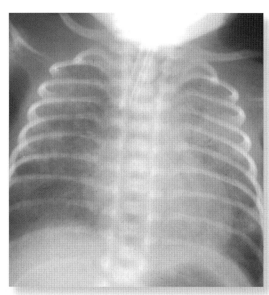

## Tracheoesophageal Fistula (TEF) / Esophageal Atresia (EA)[87,88]

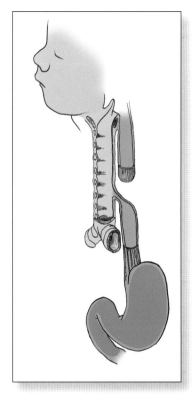

- Affects term or preterm infants.

- TEF and EA are rarely found alone; 85% of the time, both are present.

- Onset of respiratory distress is usually soon after birth. The infant often has excessive salivation and choking, coughing, and cyanosis with feeding.

*For more details, see Appendix 3.2. Neonatal Respiratory Diseases.*

## Congenital Diaphragmatic Hernia (CDH)[67,89,90]

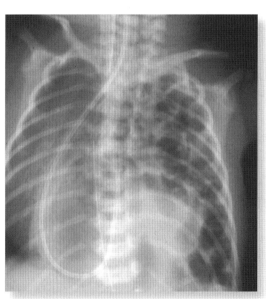

- Affects term or preterm infants.
- Onset of respiratory distress is at birth or very shortly thereafter. Infant will be cyanotic and have decreased breath sounds on the side with the hernia, which is usually the left. The abdomen may appear sunken (scaphoid) because the stomach and intestine are up in the chest.

- Immediately upon suspecting or diagnosing CDH, stop giving bag-and-mask or T-piece resuscitator PPV and prepare to intubate.

- Insert an orogastric or nasogastric tube and frequently remove air from the stomach to prevent the air from entering the bowel as this will further compromise lung expansion. Leave the tube open to air when not aspirating air with a syringe.

*For more details, see Appendix 3.2. Neonatal Respiratory Diseases.*

# Airway obstruction[2,89,91,92]

Obstruction may occur at the nose, mouth and jaw, larynx or trachea, bronchi. If the upper airway is narrowed or partially obstructed, in addition to respiratory distress (flaring, grunting, retractions), **stridor** may be heard.

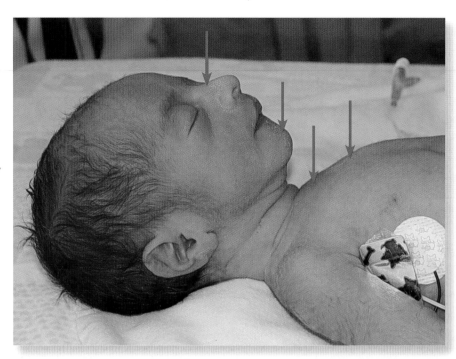

Stridor is a high-pitched sound heard with inspiration (usually associated with upper airway obstruction), expiration (usually associated with lower airway obstruction), or both. When the infant cries, is agitated, or breathes more forcefully, then stridor will sound louder. Figure 3.7 is a photo of swollen vocal cords taken during laryngoscopy in a former 3-month old preterm infant who subsequently required a tracheostomy.

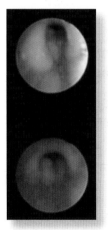
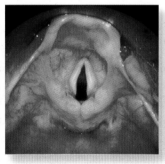

**Figure 3.7. Swollen vocal cords in a 3-month old former preterm infant.**

For comparison, a photo of a normal larynx is shown to the right;

Two obstructive airway conditions that present shortly after birth are **choanal atresia** and **Pierre-Robin syndrome.**

## Choanal atresia

- Affects term or preterm infants.

- Affects females more than males and the incidence is between 1 per 5000 and 1 per 9000 births. In more than half the cases there are other associated congenital anomalies.[89] The incidence of congenital heart disease is increased and therefore a cardiac evaluation should be strongly considered.[93]

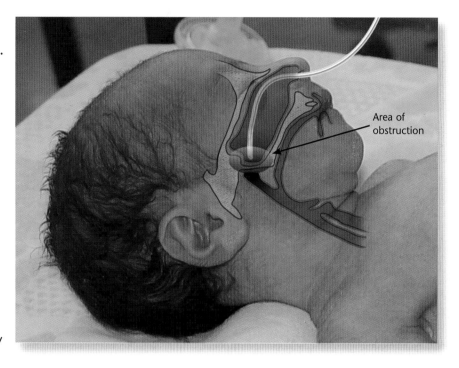

Area of obstruction

- One or both of the posterior nasal passages are blocked by a bony septum or soft tissue membrane. When both are blocked the infant may have significant difficulty breathing and may need an oral airway or endotracheal intubation.

- Infant may be cyanotic at rest (because the infant is a preferential nose breather and the nasal passages are blocked) but "pinks up" with crying because the infant breathes through the mouth.

- If bilateral choanal atresia is present, the infant may be severely cyanotic at rest, or even experience severe asphyxia.[80] In this case, an oral airway (neonatal airway size 00 for preterm or small infants and size 0 for term infants) may be necessary to provide a patent airway. If an oral airway cannot be located quickly, then ensure the mouth is open and the tongue is not obstructing the airway.

- If choanal atresia is suspected, gently try to pass a 6-French (water soluble lubricated) feeding tube through the nares.[80] Inability to pass this tube mandates further evaluation to rule out choanal atresia.

## Pierre Robin Syndrome[89,91,92]

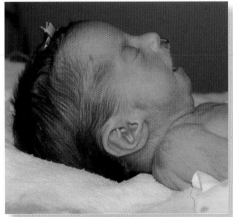
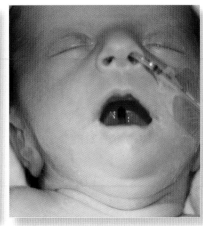

- Affects term or preterm infants.

- Infants with Pierre Robin syndrome have a very small jaw with a normal size tongue that obstructs the airway. As many as half of these infants also have a cleft palate.

- Respiratory distress may be mild to severe.

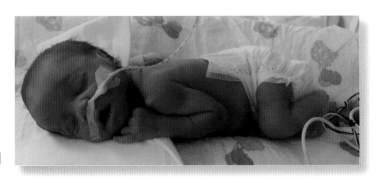

- To relieve airway obstruction, **turn the infant prone.** This will help the tongue fall forward by gravity.[92]

- **If the airway is still obstructed,** insert a nasopharyngeal (NP) tube as follows:

  - Coat the tip of a 2.5 mm endotracheal tube with water soluble gel (do **not** use oil based lubricant).

  - Gently pass the lubricated tube through one nostril until the tube is located at the end of the nasal passage.

    ⬦ Note: you are not attempting to place the endotracheal tube tip in the trachea and placement in the back of the throat often makes the baby gag.

    ⬦ Trimming the part of the tube that fits into the adaptor before inserting it in the nose can help prevent inserting the tube too deep.

  - Secure the tube with tape.

  - Once the NP tube is in place, support breathing and oxygenation by attaching the tube to a device which can provide continuous positive airway pressure (CPAP) at approximately 6 cm $H_2O$ pressure, or place the infant in a humidified oxygen hood with supplemental oxygen to maintain the $O_2$ saturation > 90%.

- Combined with prone positioning, a NP tube is often very effective for opening the airway. However, if the NP tube is not adequate to maintain an open airway, a **laryngeal mask airway** (LMA) is another alternative. Because of the infant's very small jaw, endotracheal intubation may be technically very difficult to perform.

## Persistent Pulmonary Hypertension of the Newborn (PPHN)[67,94,95]

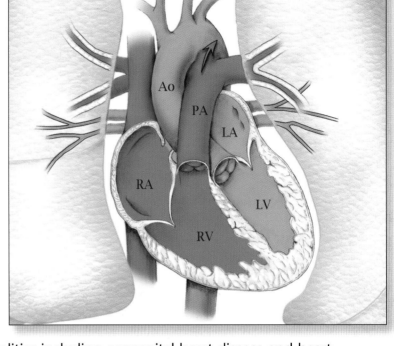

- Affects term infants predominantly, but may affect preterm infants at times.

- Elevated pulmonary vascular resistance causes right-to-left shunting of blood across the patent ductus arteriosus (PDA) and/or foramen ovale (FO) which leads to hypoxemia.

- Respiratory distress and cyanosis are usually apparent within hours of birth.

- PPHN may be associated with pulmonary diseases including meconium aspiration syndrome, pneumonia, respiratory distress syndrome, congenital diaphragmatic hernia or pulmonary hypoplasia; or with cardiovascular abnormalities including congenital heart disease and heart failure secondary to infection or asphyxia; associated with sepsis, and PPHN can be idiopathic (underlying cause undetermined).

- Investigate whether the mother took nonsteroidal antiinflammatory agents (aspirin, ibuprofen, indomethacin) during pregnancy, as these medications are prostaglandin synthetase inhibitors which may cause constriction of the ductus arteriosus and structural changes in the pulmonary vasculature leading to PPHN.

*For more details, see Appendix 3.2. Neonatal Respiratory Diseases.*

# Pneumothorax[18]

- Affects term or preterm infants.

- A pneumothorax occurs when air escapes from the air sacs in the lung and into the pleural space. The air can compress the lung, restrict ventilation, and in severe cases impair cardiac output.

- A pneumothorax can occur spontaneously in non-intubated infants with no history of assisted ventilation, or as a complication of positive pressure ventilation. Signs of a pneumothorax are described in Table 3.10.

**Table 3.10.** Signs of a pneumothorax.[18,47]

| Respiratory and cardiovascular deterioration | |
|---|---|
| ✧ Increased respiratory distress – cyanosis, tachypnea, nasal flaring, grunting, retractions | 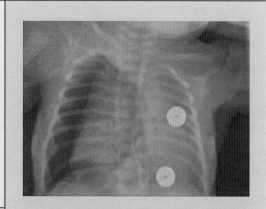 |
| ✧ Acute onset of bradycardia or tachycardia | |
| ✧ Irritability and restlessness | |
| ✧ Hypotension | |
| ✧ Blood gas may reveal a respiratory and/or metabolic acidosis, and hypoxemia | |
| **Evaluate for** | |
| ✧ Positive transillumination of the chest | 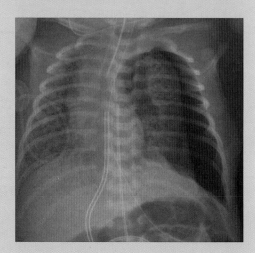 |
| ✧ Chest asymmetry (one side appears higher than the other) | |
| ✧ Asymmetric breath sounds (one side sounds quieter than the other) | |
| ✧ Shift in point of maximum impulse (PMI) | |
| ✧ Mottled appearance | |
| ✧ Poor peripheral pulses | |
| ✧ Hypotension | |
| ✧ Flattened or decreased QRS complex on ECG and if infant has an arterial line, dampened arterial waveform | |

## Chest x-ray for Pneumothorax Detection

Definitive diagnosis of a pneumothorax is by chest x-ray and one should be obtained if time allows (e.g., the infant is stable enough to tolerate the time it takes to complete the chest x-ray procedure). If the anteroposterior (AP) view is insufficient to determine whether a pneumothorax is present, then a lateral decubitus x-ray should be obtained.

### Preparing the infant for a lateral decubitus chest x-ray.

Turn the infant to his or her side for at least ten minutes (if the infant is stable) with the side of the suspected pneumothorax *up.* Keep the infant in this position by placing a roll behind the back. The lateral decubitus x-ray is taken with the infant in this position. When finished with the x-ray, turn the infant supine to allow optimal lung inflation.

 If the infant is severely compromised and a pneumothorax is strongly suspected, do not delay treatment by waiting for the chest x-ray result. Proceed with transillumination and if positive, evacuate the pneumothorax.

## Transillumination for Pneumothorax Detection

Rapid preliminary detection of a pneumothorax can often be accomplished by transillumination of the chest using a high-intensity fiberoptic light. Ideally a chest x-ray is also taken to provide important details about the pneumothorax size, location and for comparison when additional chest x-rays are taken (e.g., following evacuation of the pneumothorax).

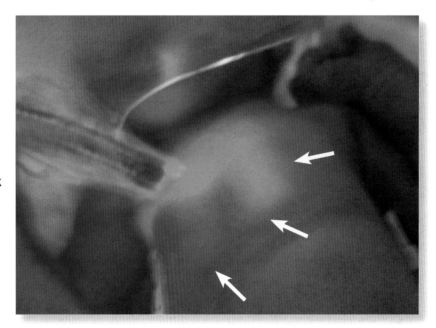

# Clinical Tip

*Transillumination: false positives, false negatives, and performing transillumination to evaluate for a pneumothorax*

## When transilluminating:

Darken the room as much as possible. Hold the light source perpendicular to the chest wall and compare each side by moving the light from right to left chest, under the midclavicular area bilaterally, in the axillae bilaterally, and under the subcostal regions bilaterally.

> ⚠ To prevent burns, use a cold light transilluminator. Be sure to clean the transilluminator between patients.

**A true positive transillumination** (meaning a pneumothorax appears to be present and in reality *is* present) is when the glow of light follows the shape of the chest cavity, not just the immediate region of the light source.

**A false *positive* transillumination** (meaning a pneumothorax appears to be present but in reality is *not* present) may be seen if the infant has chest wall edema, as occurs with hydrops fetalis, subcutaneous air in the chest wall, a pneumomediastinum, severe pulmonary interstitial emphysema, very preterm infants (small chest , thin skin and easily transmitted light), or if the light source is not held perpendicular to the chest wall.

**A false *negative* transillumination** (meaning a pneumothorax is present but is not detected by transillumination) may be seen if the infant has a thick chest wall or darkly pigmented skin, if the room is too light, or the transilluminator light source is weak.

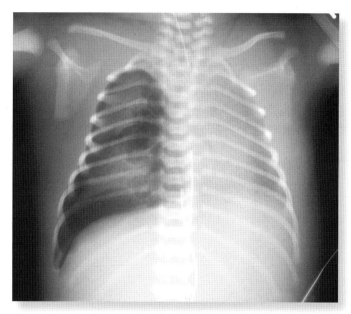

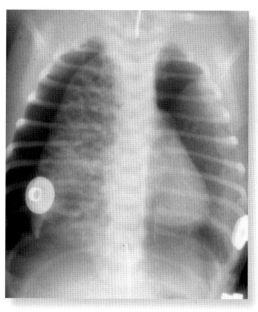

**Right-sided pneumothorax with mediastinal shift to the left and left lung atelectasis**

The ET tube is at T1, the UAC tip is at T6-T7 and the UVC tip is in good position at the IVC/RA junction or just in the right atrium.

**Bilateral pneumothoraces with significant collapse of both lungs and compression of the heart**

Very lordotic projection which makes the ET tube appear too high. With proper x-ray projection, the ET tube may be in satisfactory position. The UAC tip is malpositioned at T11.

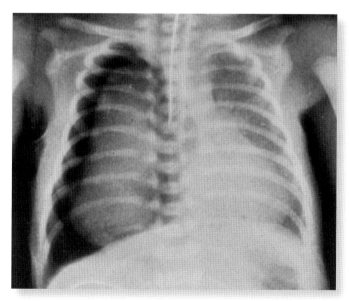

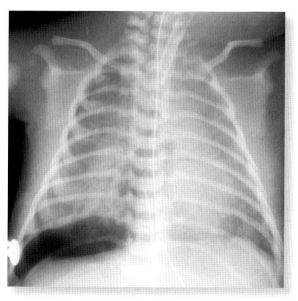

**Right-sided pneumothorax with mediastinal shift to the left**

The ET tube is in the right mainstem bronchus and there is significant collapse of the right lung.

**Subpulmonic pneumothorax**

The lung fields demonstrate severe atelectasis and / or infiltrates. The ET tube is in good position, the UAC tip is at T8 and the UVC tip is in the right atrium *(confirmed catheter types on abdominal films).*

**165**

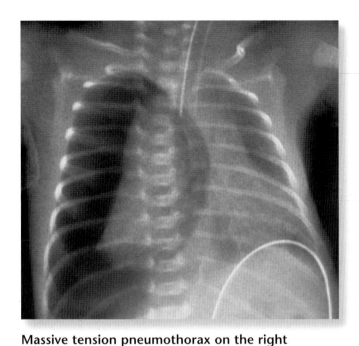

**Massive tension pneumothorax on the right**

The ET tube is in good position. Note complete collapse of the right lung, mediastinal shift and compression of the left lung.

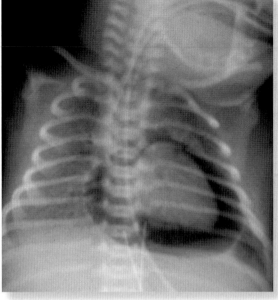

**Pneumopericardium**

Note the rim of air completely encircling and compressing the heart. The ET tube is in good position. Umbilical catheter tips are visible.

## Pneumopericardium[18,47]

A pneumopericardium rarely occurs in the absence of mechanical ventilation and usually occurs in association with other pulmonary air leaks. This complication can be an acute, life-threatening event. Air becomes trapped in the pericardial sac that surrounds the heart. As the air accumulates, it compresses the heart and impairs cardiac output. Most occurrences of pneumopericardium are symptomatic and require immediate detection and evacuation. Signs include sudden onset of severe cyanosis, muffled or inaudible heart sounds, and a flattened or decreased QRS complex (reduced cardiac voltage) on the ECG tracing. Other signs include initial tachycardia followed by bradycardia, poor or absent peripheral (brachial and femoral) pulses, and poor perfusion. If arterial monitoring is in progress, the waveform becomes acutely dampened as the pulse pressure narrows (pulse pressure is the difference between the diastolic blood pressure and the systolic blood pressure).

## Treatment of a Pneumothorax

If not experiencing respiratory distress or if only mildly symptomatic, then most infants can be observed closely while the pneumothorax resolves on its own. Infants with moderate to significant respiratory and/or cardiovascular compromise should have the pneumothorax evacuated. Needle aspiration may be attempted first and may be all that is necessary to resolve the pneumothorax. If however, air continually accumulates or the infant fails to improve to a satisfactory level following needle aspiration, a chest tube should be inserted. Figure 3.8 identifies the necessary equipment for performing needle aspiration. Needle aspiration of the chest and chest tube insertion are explained in more detail in the **Procedures Module** at the end of this manual.

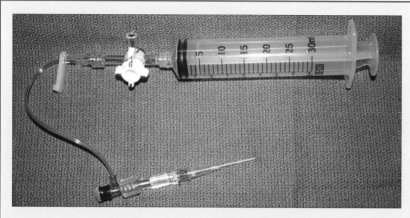

- 18, 20, or 22-gauge angiocatheter (use smaller sizes with smaller infants)

**Note:** using smaller gauge (22- and 24-gauge) angiocatheters may be problematic, as the thinner and more flexible catheter can collapse up the stylet needle when passing through the intercostal muscles.

- T-connector or other appropriate short IV extension tubing
- Three-way stopcock
- 20 – 30 mL syringe

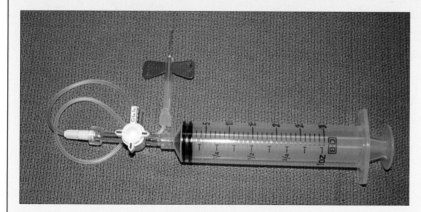

- 19, 21 or 23-gauge butterfly needle
- Three-way stopcock
- 20 – 30 mL syringe

**Figure 3.8. Pneumothorax (needle) aspiration kit assembly using an IV angiocatheter (preferred selection) or butterfly needle.** [92,96] For both set-ups, you will also need sterile gloves for the person performing the procedure and antiseptic cleanser to prepare the skin before the needle is inserted.

# Pain Control with Analgesics

Sick infants are exposed to numerous pain inflicting procedures including, but not limited to heel sticks and venipunctures for lab testing, IV insertion, arterial cannulation, endotracheal intubation and suctioning, lumbar puncture, needle aspiration of the chest, chest tube insertion, and surgery. In addition, they may experience varying degrees of pain as a result of their disease process.[97-100] Therefore, pain assessment and management is critically important for all sick and preterm infants.[101,102]

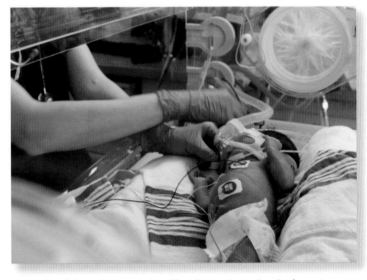

Whenever possible, offer non-pharmacologic comforting measures, which includes nonnutritive sucking, swaddling, facilitated tucking, kangaroo care, and music therapy, to reduce pain and stress the infant may be experiencing.[99,101,103-105] In addition, a major goal of everyday nursing and medical care should be to reduce the number of painful procedures and disruptions to the infant.

When analgesic medications are required for pain relief, morphine and fentanyl are the most commonly used opioids in neonates. Both of these medications block pain sensation at the level of the central nervous system.[106] Doses are titrated to clinical response and pain scores.[101] Indications for use include painful procedures such as intubation, chest tube insertion, and surgery. Infants who are mechanically ventilated and who become cyanotic with minimal stimulation or who are asynchronous with the ventilator may also benefit from opioid administration.[98] For more minor procedures such as heel stick or venipuncture, oral sucrose solution

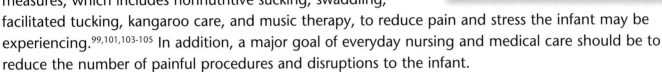

is effective.[104,105] Once an opioid is administered, monitor the blood pressure (for hypotension), heart rate (for tachycardia or bradycardia) and respiratory status (especially for apnea if not intubated). If unsure whether to use opioids, or how to use these medications, consult the transport control physician for guidance.

## Pre-medication before intubation.

Facilities capable of providing constant vital sign and $O_2$ saturation monitoring, as well as airway management, should strongly consider medicating the infant with an analgesic or a sedative prior to intubation, unless the intubation is done under emergency conditions. Recognize that sick infants who have not been medicated prior to intubation and who are experiencing pain, or who are air hungry, often become very agitated and difficult to manage once they are intubated. If the infant is air hungry, the agitation will most likely 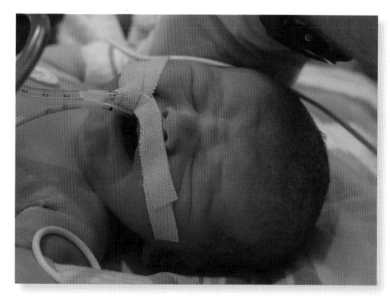 not diminish until oxygenation and ventilation are improved. Agitation and pain increase oxygen consumption and can worsen hypoxemia and pulmonary hypertension.

Provide optimal ventilatory and oxygen support and observe whether the agitation improves or whether analgesic medication is necessary. Some indications for analgesia include: if the patient is inconsolable, unable to tolerate necessary care (becomes cyanotic with minimal or necessary stimulation), or is breathing hard against ventilator breaths. If given slowly, most infants tolerate opioids without problems; however, blood pressure, heart rate, respiratory rate and $O_2$ saturation should be monitored closely during and after giving the medication. The goal is to provide pain control which allows for better tolerance of the care and procedures required.[100]

## Analgesic Medications

### Morphine[102,106,107]

**Dose:** 0.05 mg/kg (milligrams per kilogram) per dose every 4 to 8 hours.
**Route:** IV, IM, SubQ

- Dilute and give slowly, over at least 15 minutes.

- Start with a lower dose and repeat if there is insufficient response. Onset of action should be within 15 to 30 minutes.

- Causes respiratory depression and may lead to apnea.

- Be prepared to assist ventilation with bag and mask or endotracheal intubation.

- Most side effects are reversible with naloxone (Narcan).

> ⚠ Do not administer morphine to hypotensive preterm infants.

### Fentanyl[101,102,106]

**Dose:** 1 to 2 mcg/kg (micrograms per kilogram) per dose.
**Route:** IV

- Dilute to a 2 or 3 ml volume and give slowly, over at least 15 minutes.

- Fentanyl is a very potent opioid medication.

- Start with a lower dose and repeat if there is insufficient response. Onset of action is within minutes.

- Causes respiratory depression and may lead to apnea.

- Be prepared to assist ventilation with bag and mask or endotracheal intubation.

> ⚠ If given too rapidly, fentanyl may cause chest wall rigidity, which will block ventilation. Usually a paralytic medication may be necessary to treat chest wall rigidity. Fentanyl can be reversed with naloxone (Narcan); however, little response (if any) may be seen for chest wall rigidity. Contact the tertiary center neonatologist or transport control physician in the event of chest wall rigidity.

### Sucrose 24% solution[104,108,109]

**Dose:** Full-term infant: 0.5 to 2 mL
Preterm infant: 0.1 to 0.4 mL

**Route:** Place a few drops on the anterior portion of the tongue or into the buccal pocket two minutes before the painful stimulus. Duration of effect is 3 to 5 minutes.

- Provides short term analgesia for use during minor procedures.

- Sucking may be synergistic with sucrose in pain relief.

- Pacifier may be dipped in sucrose solution two minutes prior to the painful procedure.

- Do not give in a gastric tube as there is no effect when administered this way.

- Research is needed to establish safe use in very-low-birth-weight infants, therefore, use sucrose with extreme caution in preterm infants.

- The safest approach to using sucrose is to only administer it to infants who are able to protect their airway. Ensure there is an intact sucking reflex prior to administration.

# Appendix 3.1 **Practice Session: Blood Gas Interpretation**

This exercise is intended to be used with the blood gas practice session slides.

Refer to the **Acid-Base Alignment Nomogram on page 117** as a visual aid to help determine the primary problem (if any) and whether compensation has occurred.

**Remember the following tips:**

- If there is a "dot" in the red zone on the $HCO_3$ or $PCO_2$ scale, this is the primary problem. If there is a "dot" in the green zone for the $HCO_3$ or $PCO_2$ scale, this is the compensatory zone.

- If there is a "dot" in the red zone for pH, this is uncompensated acidosis, and if in the green zone for pH, this is uncompensated alkalosis.

- A "dot" in any of the circled areas represents a normal value for that parameter (pH, $HCO_3$ or $PCO_2$).

**Directions:**

1. For each of the following blood gases and clinical scenarios, determine whether:

2. The pH, $PCO_2$, $HCO_3$, and $PO_2$ are normal, high, or low.

3. The blood gas is compensated, uncompensated, or normal.

4. Identify the blood gas as normal versus respiratory, metabolic or mixed acidosis or alkalosis.

5. Answer the questions and when asked, identify your treatment plan!

## APPENDIX 3.1  **Practice Session: Blood Gas Interpretation**
(continued)

### Case One

A two day-old term infant is seen in the emergency room because of irritability and poor feeding. The mother reported that he only wet two diapers in the past 12 hours. The infant's perfusion is poor, brachial pulses are strong but femoral pulses are barely palpable. The infant has irregular breathing with periods of apnea and is sleepy but does cry when stimulated. The $O_2$ saturation is 93%.

The following blood gas was obtained from a right radial arterial stick while the infant was breathing room air.

| pH | $PCO_2$ | $PO_2$ | $HCO_3$ |
|-----|------|------|------|
| 7.1 | 38 | 58 | 11 |

pH is    ☐ normal    ☐ high    ☐ low

$PCO_2$ is    ☐ normal    ☐ high    ☐ low

$HCO_3$ is    ☐ normal    ☐ high    ☐ low

$PO_2$ is    ☐ normal    ☐ high    ☐ low

The blood gas is ☐ normal ☐ compensated ☐ uncompensated

If *uncompensated*, the blood gas reveals:

☐ Acidosis
☐ Respiratory ☐ Metabolic ☐ Mixed

☐ Alkalosis
☐ Respiratory ☐ Metabolic ☐ Mixed

If *compensated*, the blood gas reveals compensated:

☐ Acidosis
☐ Respiratory ☐ Metabolic

☐ Alkalosis
☐ Respiratory ☐ Metabolic

a) Identify two diagnoses that should be considered by the emergency physician:

_____

_____

b) Was the blood gas obtained from a pre-ductal, post-ductal, or juxta-ductal site?

_____

## Case Two

A six-hour old 37-week gestation, large for gestational age infant has required oxygen since birth. Currently he is on 70% oxygen by hood with an $O_2$ saturation of 70% (oximeter is on the left foot). The infant is tachypneic with intercostal and substernal retractions. Brachial and femoral pulses are equal but weak. He is intubated and placed on a ventilator.

The following blood gas was obtained from a right radial artery while the infant was breathing 70% oxygen.

| pH | PCO$_2$ | PO$_2$ | HCO$_3$ |
|------|------|------|------|
| 7.35 | 25 | 45 | 14 |

pH is     ☐ normal    ☐ high    ☐ low

PCO$_2$ is    ☐ normal    ☐ high    ☐ low

HCO$_3$ is    ☐ normal    ☐ high    ☐ low

PO$_2$ is     ☐ normal    ☐ high    ☐ low

The blood gas is ☐ normal ☐ compensated ☐ uncompensated

    If uncompensated, the blood gas reveals:

       ☐ Acidosis
       ☐ Respiratory ☐ Metabolic ☐ Mixed

       ☐ Alkalosis
       ☐ Respiratory ☐ Metabolic ☐ Mixed

    If compensated, the blood gas reveals compensated:

       ☐ Acidosis
       ☐ Respiratory ☐ Metabolic

       ☐ Alkalosis
       ☐ Respiratory ☐ Metabolic

a) A blood gas obtained from the right radial artery is (circle correct answer):

    pre-ductal         post-ductal         juxta-ductal

b) The physician orders pre and post-ductal saturation monitoring.

    The pre-ductal monitor should be placed on the: _____

    The post-ductal monitor probe should be placed on the: _____

# APPENDIX 3.1 **Practice Session: Blood Gas Interpretation**
(continued)

## Case Three

The same infant in Case Two is now 7-hours old. The transport team is en-route to the hospital and they are expected in the next hour. An umbilical artery catheter (UAC) was just inserted and the tip is at T7. The pre-ductal saturation is reading 92% and the post-ductal saturation is 80%.

The following blood gas was obtained from the UAC.

|  | pH | $PCO_2$ | $PO_2$ | $HCO_3$ |
|---|---|---|---|---|
|  | 7.0 | 55 | 38 | 13 |

pH is ☐ normal ☐ high ☐ low

$PCO_2$ is ☐ normal ☐ high ☐ low

$HCO_3$ is ☐ normal ☐ high ☐ low

$PO_2$ is ☐ normal ☐ high ☐ low

The blood gas is ☐ normal ☐ compensated ☐ uncompensated

If *uncompensated*, the blood gas reveals:

☐ Acidosis
☐ Respiratory ☐ Metabolic ☐ Mixed

☐ Alkalosis
☐ Respiratory ☐ Metabolic ☐ Mixed

If *compensated*, the blood gas reveals compensated:

☐ Acidosis
☐ Respiratory ☐ Metabolic

☐ Alkalosis
☐ Respiratory ☐ Metabolic

a) A blood gas obtained from a UAC is (circle correct answer):

pre-ductal        post-ductal            juxta-ductal

b) Explain the most likely reason there is a difference between the pre and post-ductal $O_2$ saturation readings: _____

## Case Four

A 15-year old mother does not reveal she is pregnant and delivers a 28-week gestation 950 gram infant unexpectedly at home. The paramedics transport the infant to the hospital. Upon arrival in the NICU, the infant is one hour old. Vital signs are: Axillary temperature 31.5°C (88.5°F), heart rate 100, spontaneous respiratory rate: 0 (bag / mask ventilation provided at 40 to 60 breaths per minute), blood pressure: will not register on the machine. The infant is immediately intubated.

The following blood gas was obtained from a left radial arterial stick.

| pH | $PCO_2$ | $PO_2$ | $HCO_3$ |
|----|---------|--------|---------|
| 6.9 | 80 | 28 | 15 |

pH is      ☐ normal    ☐ high    ☐ low

$PCO_2$ is    ☐ normal    ☐ high    ☐ low

$HCO_3$ is    ☐ normal    ☐ high    ☐ low

$PO_2$ is    ☐ normal    ☐ high    ☐ low

The blood gas is ☐ normal ☐ compensated ☐ uncompensated

    If uncompensated, the blood gas reveals:

        ☐ Acidosis
        ☐ Respiratory ☐ Metabolic ☐ Mixed

        ☐ Alkalosis
        ☐ Respiratory ☐ Metabolic ☐ Mixed

    If compensated, the blood gas reveals compensated:

        ☐ Acidosis
        ☐ Respiratory ☐ Metabolic

        ☐ Alkalosis
        ☐ Respiratory ☐ Metabolic

a) What size ET tube is appropriate for an infant this size? _____

b) What will be the insertion depth at the lip? _____

## APPENDIX 3.1 **Practice Session: Blood Gas Interpretation**
(continued)

**Case Five**

A 38-week gestation 2.4 kg infant with Pierre Robin syndrome is intubated because of severe airway obstruction. The initial ventilator settings are: PIP 24, PEEP 4, Rate 30, Inspiratory time 0.4, $FiO_2$ 0.3.

The first blood gas obtained after intubation is from a posterior tibial arterial stick, as follows:

| pH | $PCO_2$ | $PO_2$ | $HCO_3$ |
|------|------|------|------|
| 7.58 | 24 | 140 | 25 |

pH is ☐ normal ☐ high ☐ low

$PCO_2$ is ☐ normal ☐ high ☐ low

$HCO_3$ is ☐ normal ☐ high ☐ low

$PO_2$ is ☐ normal ☐ high ☐ low

The blood gas is ☐ normal ☐ compensated ☐ uncompensated

If *uncompensated*, the blood gas reveals:

☐ Acidosis
☐ Respiratory ☐ Metabolic ☐ Mixed

☐ Alkalosis
☐ Respiratory ☐ Metabolic ☐ Mixed

If *compensated*, the blood gas reveals compensated:

☐ Acidosis
☐ Respiratory ☐ Metabolic

☐ Alkalosis
☐ Respiratory ☐ Metabolic

a) Was the blood gas obtained from a pre-ductal, post-ductal, or juxta-ductal site? _____

b) What size ET tube is appropriate for an infant this size?_____

c) What will be the insertion depth at the lip? _____

d) What change in ventilator support will be most appropriate? _____

_____

## Case Six

A four day old 34-week gestation infant with Down syndrome (trisomy 21) is on a ventilator because of respiratory distress. Vital signs are: Axillary temperature 37°C (98.6°F), heart rate 140, spontaneous respiratory rate 40, blood pressure 60/38, mean 42. The ventilator settings are: PIP 18, PEEP 4, Rate 15, Inspiratory time 0.35, $FiO_2$ 0.28.

The following blood gas was obtained from an umbilical artery catheter:

| pH | $PCO_2$ | $PO_2$ | $HCO_3$ |
|------|------|------|------|
| 7.39 | 37 | 75 | 22 |

pH is     ☐ normal    ☐ high    ☐ low

$PCO_2$ is    ☐ normal    ☐ high    ☐ low

$HCO_3$ is    ☐ normal    ☐ high    ☐ low

$PO_2$ is     ☐ normal    ☐ high    ☐ low

The blood gas is ☐ normal ☐ compensated ☐ uncompensated

     If uncompensated, the blood gas reveals:

         ☐ Acidosis
         ☐ Respiratory ☐ Metabolic ☐ Mixed

         ☐ Alkalosis
         ☐ Respiratory ☐ Metabolic ☐ Mixed

     If *compensated*, the blood gas reveals compensated:

         ☐ Acidosis
         ☐ Respiratory ☐ Metabolic

         ☐ Alkalosis
         ☐ Respiratory ☐ Metabolic

a) The physician suggests the infant is ready for extubation. Do you agree that this infant would be a good candidate for extubation?

     If yes, explain why:_____

     If no, explain why: _____

# Appendix 3.2 **Neonatal Respiratory Diseases**: TEF/EA, CDH, PPHN

## Tracheoesophageal Fistula (TEF) / Esophageal Atresia (EA)[79,87,88]

The incidence of TEF / EA is estimated at 1 to 2 per 5000 live births. TEF and EA are rarely found alone; 85% of the time, both are present. Early in the first trimester, the esophagus and trachea form abnormally such that, in most cases of TEF/EA, the trachea communicates directly with the esophagus through a small hole, and the esophagus ends in a blind pouch.

There is a high association of other anomalies when an infant has TEF / EA. These are often grouped within the VACTERL association. VACTERL stands for **V**ertebral defects, **A**nal atresia (also called imperforate **a**nus or **a**norectal malformation), **C**ardiac defects, **T**racheo**E**sophageal fistula with esophageal atresia, **R**enal dysplasia, and **L**imb anomalies.

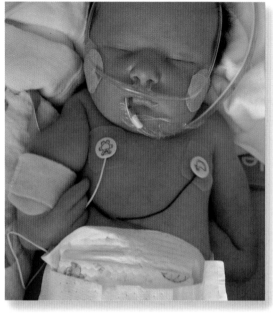

Late preterm infant with VACTERL association

## The Five Types of TEF

Note the following variations:

**Type C** is by far the most common.

**Type A** does not have a fistula from the esophagus to the trachea.

**If type A or B**, the x-ray will show absence of bowel gas.

**If type B or D**, the infant will aspirate directly into the lungs if given a feeding and all swallowed secretions will drain directly into the trachea.

**If types C or D**, air will be able to enter the stomach via the tracheal fistula, but there is no way to place a gastric tube to the stomach to remove air that collects. Significant gastric and abdominal distension may develop.

**Type E** (often called an "H-type" fistula) does not have esophageal atresia.

| Type A | Type B | Type C | Type D | Type E |
|--------|--------|--------|--------|--------|
| 8% | 1% | 86% | 1% | 4% |

## Signs of TEF / EA

Signs include choking, coughing, and cyanosis with feeding. The risk of aspiration and pneumonia is extremely high. There is usually excessive salivation because of the blind pouch esophagus. A history of **polyhydramnios** may indicate a problem of the fetus being unable to swallow amniotic fluid and should prompt suspicion of TEF / EA or bowel obstruction.

## Initial Stabilization

✧ **If TEF / EA is suspected,** attempt to pass a suction catheter or feeding tube into the stomach. Take a chest x-ray and be sure to include the abdomen, or obtain both a chest and abdominal x-ray.

- Evaluate whether the catheter is in the stomach or coiled in the esophageal pouch. Remember with some types of TEF, the gastric tube will pass all the way to the stomach, yet there is a fistula between the esophagus and trachea. Evaluate the abdomen for the presence or absence of bowel gas. In most cases, a contrast study is not indicated because the infant can aspirate the contrast material and develop a pneumonitis.

> ⚠ Any radiographic studies involving contrast material should be avoided. However, if necessary, they should be performed at a tertiary center by pediatric radiology staff skilled in these procedures.

✧ Establish IV access and withhold feedings.

✧ Insert a multiple end-hole suction tube (if available), or a vented gastric tube, into the proximal esophageal pouch or stomach if there is no blind pouch.

✧ Provide low continuous suction (between 20 and 30 cm $H_2O$ pressure) to remove secretions that collect in the pouch or stomach.

✧ Turn the infant prone with the head of the bed elevated 30 degrees to reduce reflux of stomach contents through the fistula and into the trachea and lungs.

✧ Support oxygenation and ventilation.

---

### EA / TEF

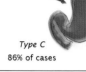

**Signs**

‣ Choking, coughing, cyanosis with feeding

‣ Excessive salivation → if esophageal atresia

‣ Respiratory distress secondary to aspiration

‣ Abdominal distension → fistula from trachea to stomach → air cannot escape stomach

**Maternal history**

‣ Polyhydramnios suggests esophageal atresia or bowel obstruction

Type C
86% of cases

---

### EA / TEF

**X-ray**

Esophageal pouch

‣ If esophageal atresia → oral gastric tube ends or curls in proximal esophageal pouch at T2 – 3

‣ If no esophageal pouch → may aspirate directly into trachea when fed

Gastric distension

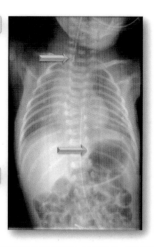

---

### EA / TEF

**Stabilization**

‣ Make NPO

‣ Assess oxygenation and ventilation

‣ Insert suction catheter into proximal esophageal pouch and connect to low intermittent suction to remove secretions

‣ Position prone → elevate head of bed to reduce reflux from stomach into trachea

⚠ If contrast study needed → perform at tertiary care center

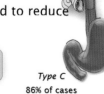

Type C
86% of cases

---

> ⚠ Continuous positive airway pressure (CPAP) is contraindicated as it may cause acute and severe gastric distension.

# Appendix 3.2 **Neonatal Respiratory Diseases** (continued)

## Congenital Diaphragmatic Hernia (CDH)[67,89,90]

The incidence of CDH is estimated at 1 in 2500 live births. At approximately the eighth week of gestation, the diaphragm develops and creates a barrier that separates the chest from the abdominal contents. Infants with congenital diaphragmatic hernia (CDH) have a disruption or hole in the diaphragm that allows the stomach and bowel to migrate up into the chest. Most often, diaphragmatic hernia occurs in the left chest. The lung on the side with the abdominal contents is compressed and therefore is hypoplastic. The lung on the contralateral side (the side without the abdominal contents) may be hypoplastic as well.

Following birth, when caring for an infant with CDH, several major challenges are commonly encountered. The first are the hypoplastic lungs, which makes oxygenation and ventilation very difficult. The second is the presence of **persistent pulmonary hypertension (PPHN)**, which is very common in infants with CDH. PPHN compounds the problem of oxygenation, as discussed later in this section. Infants with CDH may also have cardiac, renal, central nervous system, or gastrointestinal anomalies.

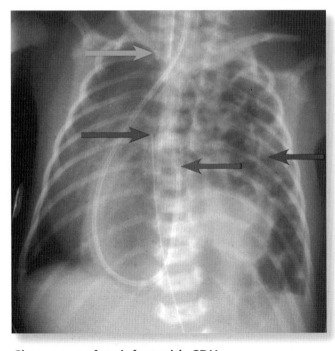

**Chest x-ray of an infant with CDH.**

→ ET tube in trachea, shifted to the right

→ UAC tip in aorta, shifted to the right

→ Intestine in chest

→ Gastric tube tip in stomach displaced in the chest

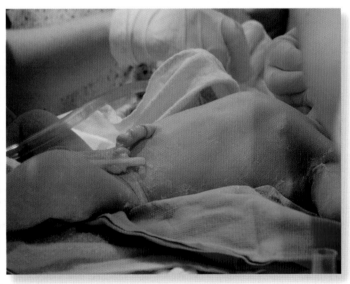

**Infant with left-sided congenital diaphragmatic hernia which was discovered after birth.** Physical exam findings included decreased breath sounds in the left chest (side with the hernia), bowel sounds in the left chest, and heart tones in the right chest (shifted mediastinum). Notice the sunken or scaphoid appearance of the abdomen which occurred because the bowel was in the chest. The chest became progressively barrel-shaped as the displaced stomach and bowel filled up with air in the left chest.

## Presentation of CDH

Infants with CDH usually present at birth or very shortly thereafter with profound cyanosis, respiratory distress, and scaphoid or sunken abdomen (because the abdominal contents are up in the chest).

If CDH was **not** diagnosed prenatally and birth healthcare providers respond to the infant's significant respiratory distress (appropriately so) by providing bag and mask positive pressure ventilation in the delivery room, the stomach and intestine fill up with air and expand in the chest. The dilated bowel and stomach compress the heart and lung and in turn, compress the contralateral lung (the lung on the side without the bowel herniation). This may significantly impair both circulation and ventilation. For this reason, it is very important, once a diaphragmatic hernia is suspected or diagnosed, bag and mask ventilation is not initiated, but the infant is quickly **intubated** and assisted ventilation is provided.

 Because the lung(s) are hypoplastic, an additional and significant risk is that a **pneumothorax** may develop. Therefore, one should achieve adequate inflation of the lungs, but be careful to avoid overinflation. The lowest pressure needed to move the chest should be used. If no ventilator is available, then provide gentle positive pressure ventilation by using a T-piece resuscitator or resuscitation bag connected to the ET tube.

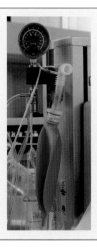

If using a resuscitation bag, use a pressure manometer to measure the delivered peak inspiratory pressure (PIP).

## Initial Stabilization

**Until the infant can be intubated:**

✧ Provide blow-by oxygen if $O_2$ saturation is not in the appropriate range.

✧ Insert a 10-French orogastric (or nasogastric) tube promptly.

✧ Attach a syringe and gently aspirate air from the tube every few minutes to prevent air from entering the intestines.

 • If a double-lumen (also called "vented") orogastric tube is placed, connect the tube to an intermittent suction device set at 30 to 40 mmHg suction pressure (if available).

✧ When the chest x-ray is taken, be sure the **gastric tube** is in place as this will help identify the stomach location.

✧ Ensure optimal oxygenation. This will help the pulmonary blood vessels to relax.

## Ongoing Stabilization

✧ Evaluate both **pre- and post-ductal $O_2$ saturation**. This will help detect whether right-to-left shunting through the ductus arteriosus secondary to PPHN is present. Remember, if a right-to-left shunt through the foramen ovale is also present, there may not be any difference in saturation for the pre- to post-ductal measurements.

✧ Evaluate the pulses, perfusion, and systolic, diastolic, and mean blood pressure and be prepared to provide a volume bolus if the infant appears **hypotensive**. If hypotension persists, consult the transport control physician or tertiary center for guidance regarding whether dopamine should be started.

✧ Watch closely for **pneumothorax** as the risk for air leak is increased with CDH.

✧ Provide analgesia to keep the infant calm and comfortable and to reduce oxygen consumption.

## Appendix 3.2 **Neonatal Respiratory Diseases** (continued)

### Persistent Pulmonary Hypertension of the Newborn (PPHN) [8,67,94,95,110,111]

### Understanding PPHN Starts with Understanding Fetal and Neonatal Circulation

#### Fetal circulation.

In utero, the placenta is responsible for the exchange of gases, nutrients, and metabolic waste products. The fetus receives blood from the placenta and returns it to the placenta via the following pathway:

> Blood flows from the **placenta** into the **umbilical vein**. This blood, which contains a $PO_2$ of approximately 35 mmHg, passes through the liver and fetal structure called the **ductus venosus**. From here blood drains into the inferior vena cava where a large amount streams in a path across the right atrium, through the **foramen ovale**, into the left atrium. Thus, blood entering the left atrium (oxygenated by the placenta) because of streaming across the foramen ovale, has a higher $PO_2$ than would be possible without this streaming effect.

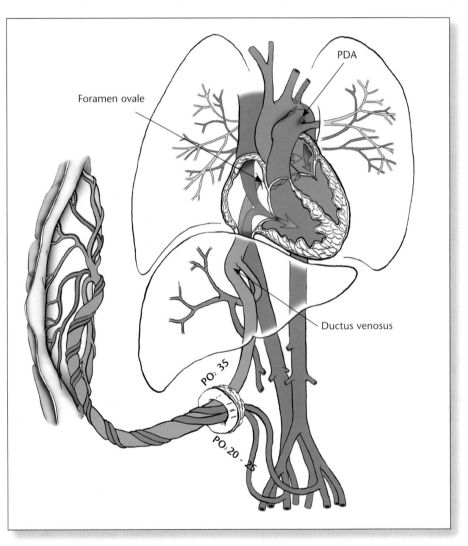

**Back on the right side of the heart**, the superior vena cava drains de-oxygenated blood from the brain to the right atrium. The right atrium then drains into the right ventricle. Approximately 90% of the right ventricular output is ejected into the pulmonary artery and then directly into the **ductus arteriosus** which connects to the aorta. This is called a *right-to-left shunt* (right ventricle ➔ ductus arteriosus ➔ aorta). The remaining 10% of the right ventricular output is ejected into the pulmonary artery and then into the lungs. The amount of blood entering the lungs is limited because of the high pulmonary vascular resistance present during fetal life and the fact that the lungs are not needed for gas exchange until after birth. The $PO_2$ in the right ventricular blood is somewhere between 19 and 21 mmHg. This is because of mixing that occurred in the right atrium when blood drained from the SVC and mixed with blood from the IVC.

**Back on the left side of the heart**, blood that streamed across the foramen ovale into the left atrium, plus the small amount of blood that returned from the lungs via the pulmonary veins, is drained into the left atrium, then left ventricle, where it is ejected into the aorta. This blood, which contains a $PO_2$ of approximately 28 mmHg, perfuses the coronary arteries, brain, and the rest of the body. Finally, blood in the aorta drains back to the placenta via the **two umbilical arteries**. The $PO_2$ of the blood entering the placenta is approximately 20 to 25 mmHg. The placenta has a low systemic vascular resistance and therefore, readily accepts the return of fetal arterial blood.

182

## Neonatal circulation.

After birth, the umbilical cord is cut which sets off a series of changes in blood pressure as follows:

The blood pressure in the aorta increases (increased systemic vascular resistance), while the blood pressure in the lungs decreases (decreased pulmonary vascular resistance). When the lungs expand and the infant begins to breathe, the $PO_2$ rises, and the pulmonary blood vessels begin to relax and dilate. As more blood enters the lungs, more blood is returned to the left atrium. The increased pressure in the left atrium helps to functionally close the right-to-left shunt through the foramen ovale. In addition, as the pulmonary blood vessels relax, more blood enters the lungs rather than shunt right-to-left through the ductus arteriosus. Because of the increased blood pressure in the aorta that occurred with clamping of the cord, the pathway of least resistance is no longer through the ductus arteriosus, but into the lungs. If the infant successfully makes the transition from fetal to neonatal life, blood that flows into the right ventricle should enter the lungs for appropriate gas exchange, and then return to the left heart. The left ventricle then ejects blood into the aorta and out to the body for organ perfusion.

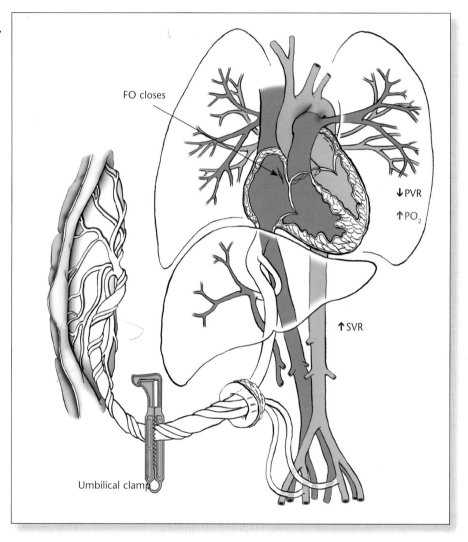

FO closes

↓PVR

↑PO₂

↑SVR

Umbilical clamp

# Appendix 3.2 **Neonatal Respiratory Diseases** (continued)

## Persistent Pulmonary Hypertension (PPHN)

At times however, the normal process of vessel relaxation is altered; the lung blood vessels fail to dilate properly and remain vasoconstricted in response to various causes, including hypoxemia, acidemia, (unintentional) hypothermia and sepsis. This presents as a clinical problem called persistent pulmonary hypertension of the newborn (PPHN), which is most often recognized in term or near term infants; however it can also occur in preterm infants. As shown in the following illustrations, with pulmonary vasoconstriction, blood shunts away from the lungs through the ductus arteriosus and / or the foramen ovale. This shunting interferes with the normal process of oxygenation and results in hypoxemia.

> Pulmonary blood vessels constrict ➔ ➔ increases resistance to blood flow into the lungs ➔ ➔ blood flows via pathway of least resistance ➔ ➔ right ventricle ➔ ➔ pulmonary artery ➔ ➔ ductus arteriosus ➔ ➔ aorta ➔ ➔ deoxygenated blood enters arterial circulation ➔ ➔ hypoxemia ➔ ➔ perpetuates pulmonary vasoconstriction and right-to-left shunting

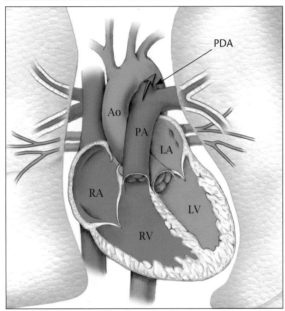

**Right-to-left shunting at the ductus arteriosus.** Deoxygenated blood enters the arterial circulation and results in hypoxemia. In this setting, the pre-ductal saturation would be higher than the post-ductal saturation.

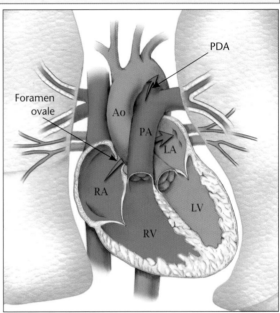

**Right-to-left shunting at the ductus arteriosus and foramen ovale.** Blood ejected into the aorta will have low arterial oxygen content because of the mixing at the atrial level. In this setting, there would be little, if any, difference between the pre and post-ductal saturation values. Yet the infant would still have pulmonary hypertension characterized by shunting of blood via the pathways of least resistance, which, in this case, are both the ductus arteriosus and the foramen ovale.

## Pathophysiology of PPHN

1. Increased, abnormal muscularization of the pulmonary arterioles prior to birth (also called remodeling). The presence of muscle in an area where there should be no muscle results in decreased diameter of the pulmonary arterioles. This, in turn, increases resistance to blood flow into the lungs, and encourages right-to-left shunting through the ductus arteriosus and away from the lungs. In addition, the extra muscle around the blood vessels means they can vasoconstrict with ease, thus compounding the problem.

2. Vasospasm and delayed relaxation of the pulmonary vasculature may be triggered or aggravated by hypoxemia, acidosis, sepsis, polycythemia, or possibly hypothermia. Associated lung diseases include meconium aspiration syndrome, pneumonia, congenital diaphragmatic hernia, and respiratory distress syndrome.

3. Underdeveloped (hypoplastic) pulmonary vasculature because of decreased lung size, such as occurs with pulmonary hypoplasia and congenital diaphragmatic hernia.

# References

1. Carlo WA, DiFiore JM. Assessment of Pulmonary Function. In: Martin RJ, Fanaroff AA, Walsh MC, eds. Fanaroff and Martin's Neonatal-Perinatal Medicine: Diseases of the Fetus and Infant. 9th ed. St. Louis: Elsevier Mosby; 2011:1092-106.

2. Smith JB. Initial Evaluation: History and Physical Examination of the Newborn. In: Gleason CA, Devaskar SU, eds. Avery's Diseases of the Newborn. 9th ed. Philadelphia: Elsevier Saunders; 2012.

3. Melton K, Pettett G. Transport of the ventilated infant. In: Goldsmith JP, Karotkin EH, Siede BL, eds. Assisted Ventilation of the Neonate. 5th ed. St. Louis: Elsevier Saunders; 2011:531-41.

4. Bhandari V. Nasal intermittent positive pressure ventilation in the newborn: review of literature and evidence-based guidelines. J Perinatol 2010;30:505-12.

5. Mahmoud RA, Roehr CC, Schmalisch G. Current methods of non-invasive ventilatory support for neonates. Paediatr Respir Rev 2011;12:196-205.

6. Wiswell TE, Courtney SE. Noninvasive Respiratory Support. In: Goldsmith JP, Karotkin EH, Siede BL, eds. Assisted Ventilation of the Neonate. 5th ed. St. Louis: Elsevier Saunders; 2011:140-62.

7. Sreenan C, Lemke RP, Hudson-Mason A, Osiovich H. High-flow nasal cannulae in the management of apnea of prematurity: a comparison with conventional nasal continuous positive airway pressure. Pediatrics 2001;107:1081-3.

8. Parker TA, Kinsella JP. Respiratory failure in the term newborn. In: Gleason CA, Devasker SU, eds. Avery's Diseases of the Newborn. 9th ed. Philadelphia: Elsevier Saunders; 2012.

9. Gardner SL, Enzman-Hines M, Dickey LA. Respiratory Diseases. In: Gardner SL, Carter BS, Enzman-Hines M, Hernandez JA, eds. Merenstein & Gardner's Handbook of Neonatal Intensive Care. 7th ed. St. Louis: Mosby Elsevier; 2011:581-677.

10. Askin DF. Chest and Lungs Assessment. In: Tappero EP, Honeyfield ME, eds. Physical Assessment of the Newborn: A Comprehensive Approach to the Art of Physical Examination. 4th ed. Santa Rosa: NICU Ink; 2009:75-103.

11. Sivieri EM, Abbasi S. Evaluation of Pulmonary Function in the Neonate. In: Polin RA, Fox WW, Abman SH, eds. Fetal and Neonatal Physiology. 4th ed. Philadelphia: Elsevier Saunders; 2011:1011-25.

12. Friedlich PS, Seri I. Regulation of Acid-Base Balance in the Fetus and Neonate. In: Polin RA, Fox WW, Abman SH, eds. Fetal and Neonatal Physiology. 4th ed. Philadelphia: Elsevier Saunders; 2011:1455-8.

13. Kattwinkel J, McGowan JE, Zaichkin J. Textbook of Neonatal Resuscitation. 6th ed. Elk Grove Village: American Academy of Pediatrics; 2011.

14. Wyllie J, Perlman JM, Kattwinkel J, et al. Part 11: Neonatal resuscitation: 2010 International Consensus on Cardiopulmonary Resuscitation and Emergency Cardiovascular Care Science with Treatment Recommendations. Resuscitation 2010;81 Suppl 1:e260-87.

15. Spitzer AR, Clark RH. Positive-pressure ventilation in the treatment of neonatal lung disease. In: Goldsmith JP, Karotkin EH, Siede BL, eds. Assisted Ventilation of the Neonate. 5th ed. St. Louis: Elsevier Saunders; 2011:163-85.

16. Yost GC, Young PC, Buchi KF. Significance of grunting respirations in infants admitted to a well-baby nursery. Arch Pediatr Adolesc Med 2001;155:372-5.

17. Chameides L. Part 5: Resources for Management of Respiratory Emergencies. In: Chameides L, Samson RA, Schexnayder SM, Hazinski MF, eds. Pediatric Advanced Life Support Provider Manual. Dallas: American Heart Association; 2011:61-7.

18. Bancalari E, Claure N. Principles of Respiratory Monitoring and Therapy. In: Gleason CA, Devaskar SU, eds. Avery's Diseases of the Newborn 9th ed. Philadelphia Elsevier Saunders 2012:612-32.

19. Levesque BM, Pollack P, Griffin BE, Nielsen HC. Pulse oximetry: what's normal in the newborn nursery? Pediatr Pulmonol 2000;30:406-12.

20. Durand DJ, Mickas NA. Blood Gases: Technical Aspects and Interpretation. In: Goldsmith JP, Karotkin EH, Siede BL, eds. Assisted Ventilation of the Neonate 5th ed. St. Louis Elsevier Saunders 2011:292-305.

21. Chock VY, Wong RJ, Hintz SR, Stevenson DK. Biomedical Engineering Aspects of Neonatal Monitoring. In: Martin RJ, Fanaroff AA, Walsh MC, eds. Fanaroff and Martin's Neonatal-Perinatal Medicine: Diseases of the Fetus and Infant. 9th ed. St. Louis: Elsevier Mosby; 2011:577-95.

22. Fernandes CJ. Neonatal Transport. In: Cloherty JP, Eichenwald EC, Hansen AR, Stark AR, eds. Manual of Neonatal Care. 7th ed. Philadelphia: Lippincott, Williams & Wilkins; 2012:192-202.

23. Ravert P, Detwiler TL, Dickinson JK. Mean oxygen saturation in well neonates at altitudes between 4498 and 8150 feet. Advances in neonatal care : official journal of the National Association of Neonatal Nurses 2011;11:412-7.

24. Bakr AF, Habib HS. Normal values of pulse oximetry in newborns at high altitude. J Trop Pediatr 2005;51:170-3.

25. Gonzales GF, Salirrosas A. Arterial oxygen saturation in healthy newborns delivered at term in Cerro de Pasco (4340 m) and Lima (150 m). Reprod Biol Endocrinol 2005;3:46.

26. O'Brien LM, Stebbens VA, Poets CF, Heycock EG, Southall DP. Oxygen saturation during the first 24 hours of life. Arch Dis Child Fetal Neonatal Ed 2000;83:F35-8.

27. Thangaratinam S, Brown K, Zamora J, Khan KS, Ewer AK. Pulse oximetry screening for critical congenital heart defects in asymptomatic newborn babies: a systematic review and meta-analysis. Lancet 2012;379:2459-64.

28. Thilo EH, Park-Moore B, Berman ER, Carson BS. Oxygen saturation by pulse oximetry in healthy infants at an altitude of 1610 m (5280 ft). What is normal? Am J Dis Child 1991;145:1137-40.

29. Kemper AR, Mahle WT, Martin GR, et al. Strategies for implementing screening for critical congenital heart disease. Pediatrics 2011;128:e1259-67.

30. Karlsen KA, Tani LY. S.T.A.B.L.E. Cardiac Module: Recognition and Stabilization of Neonates with Severe CHD. Salt Lake City: S.T.A.B.L.E., Inc.; 2003.

31. Wernovsky G. Transposition of the Great Arteries. In: Allen HD, Gutgesell HP, Clark EB, Driscoll DJ, eds. Moss and Adams Heart Disease in Infants, Children, and Adolescents. 6th ed. Philadelphia: Lippincott Williams & Wilkins; 2001:1027-84.

32. Park MT. Cyanotic Congenital Heart Defects. In: Park MK, Troxler RG, eds. Pediatric Cardiology for Practitioners. 4th ed. St. Louis: Mosby; 2002:174-240.

33. Ewer AK, Furmston AT, Middleton LJ, et al. Pulse oximetry as a screening test for congenital heart defects in newborn infants: a test accuracy study with evaluation of acceptability and cost-effectiveness. Health Technol Assess 2012;16:v-xiii, 1-184.

34. Smith AE, Vedder TG, Hunter PK, Carr MR, Studer MA. The use of newborn screening pulse oximetry to detect cyanotic congenital heart disease: a survey of current practice at Army, Navy, and Air Force hospitals. Mil Med 2011;176:343-6.

35. de-Wahl Granelli A, Wennergren M, Sandberg K, et al. Impact of pulse oximetry screening on the detection of duct dependent congenital heart disease: a Swedish prospective screening study in 39,821 newborns. BMJ 2009;338:a3037.

36. Mellander M, Sunnegardh J. Failure to diagnose critical heart malformations in newborns before discharge--an increasing problem? Acta Paediatr 2006;95:407-13.

37. Riede FT, Worner C, Dahnert I, Mockel A, Kostelka M, Schneider P. Effectiveness of neonatal pulse oximetry screening for detection of critical congenital heart disease in daily clinical routine--results from a prospective multicenter study. Eur J Pediatr 2010;169:975-81.

38. Mahle WT, Newburger JW, Matherne GP, et al. Role of pulse oximetry in examining newborns for congenital heart disease: a scientific statement from the American Heart Association and American Academy of Pediatrics. Circulation 2009;120:447-58.

39. Brown KL, Ridout DA, Hoskote A, Verhulst L, Ricci M, Bull C. Delayed diagnosis of congenital heart disease worsens preoperative condition and outcome of surgery in neonates. Heart 2006;92:1298-302.

40. Meberg A, Brugmann-Pieper S, Due R, Jr., et al. First day of life pulse oximetry screening to detect congenital heart defects. J Pediatr 2008;152:761-5.

41. Walsh W. Evaluation of pulse oximetry screening in Middle Tennessee: cases for consideration before universal screening. J Perinatol 2011;31:125-9.

42. Hall JE. Respiratory Insufficiency - Pathophysiology, Diagnosis, Oxygen Therapy. In: Hall JE, ed. Guyton and Hall Textbook of Medical Physiology. 12th ed. Philadelphia: Saunders Elsevier; 2011:515-23.

43. Johnson L, Cochran WD. Assessment of the Newborn History and Physical Examination of the Newborn. In: Cloherty JP, Eichenwald EC, Hansen AR, Stark AR, eds. Manual of Neonatal Care. 7th ed. Philadelphia: Lippincott, Williams & Wilkins; 2012:91-102.

44. Burns-Wechsler S, Wernovsky G. Cardiac Disorders. In: Cloherty JP, Eichenwald EC, Hansen AR, Stark AR, eds. Manual of Neonatal Care. 7th ed. Philadelphia: Lippincott, Williams & Wilkins; 2012:469-528.

45. O'Reilly D. Polycythemia. In: Cloherty JP, Eichenwald EC, Hansen AR, Stark AR, eds. Manual of Neonatal Care. 7th ed. Philadelphia: Lippincott, Williams & Wilkins; 2012:572-7.

46. Christou HA. Anemia. In: Cloherty JP, Eichenwald EC, Hansen AR, Stark AR, eds. Manual of Neonatal Care. 7th ed. Philadelphia: Lippincott, Williams & Wilkins; 2012:563-71.

47. Korones SB. Complications. In: Goldsmith JP, Karotkin EH, Siede BL, eds. Assisted Ventilation of the Neonate. 5th ed. St. Louis: Elsevier Saunders; 2012:389-425.

48. Phelps DL. Retinopathy of Prematurity. In: Martin RJ, Fanaroff AA, Walsh MC, eds. Fanaroff and Martin's Neonatal-Perinatal Medicine: Diseases of the Fetus and Infant. 9th ed. St. Louis: Elsevier Mosby; 2011:1764-9.

49. Mintz-Hittner HA. Retinal Development and the Pathophysiology of Retinopathy of Prematurity. In: Polin RA, Fox WW, Abman SH, eds. Fetal and Neonatal Physiology. 4th ed. Philadelphia: Elsevier Saunders; 2011:1875-81.

50. Wright KW, Sami D, Thompson L, Ramanathan R, Joseph R, Farzavandi S. A physiologic reduced oxygen protocol decreases the incidence of threshold retinopathy of prematurity. Trans Am Ophthalmol Soc 2006;104:78-84.

51. Carlo WA, Finer NN, Walsh MC, et al. Target ranges of oxygen saturation in extremely preterm infants. The New England journal of medicine 2010;362:1959-69.

52. Supplemental Therapeutic Oxygen for Prethreshold Retinopathy Of Prematurity (STOP-ROP), a randomized, controlled trial. I: primary outcomes. Pediatrics 2000;105:295-310.

53. Pirianov G, Mehmet H, Taylor DT. Apoptotic Cell Death. In: Polin RA, Fox WW, Abman SH, eds. Fetal and Neonatal Physiology. 4th ed. Philadelphia: Elsevier Saunders; 2011:93-101.

54. Auten RI. Mechanisms of Neonatal Lung Injury. In: Polin RA, Fox WW, Abman SH, eds. Fetal and Neonatal Physiology. 4th ed. Philadelphia: Elsevier Saunders; 2011:1034-9.

55. Vento M, Didrik-Saugstad O. Oxygen Therapy. In: Martin RJ, Fanaroff AA, Walsh MC, eds. Fanaroff and Martin's Neonatal-Perinatal Medicine: Diseases of the Fetus and Infant. St. Louis: Elsevier Mosby; 2011:468-74.

56. Keszler M, Abubakar MK. Physiologic Principles. In: Goldsmith JP, Karotkin EH, Siede BL, eds. Assisted Ventilation of the Neonate. 5th ed. St. Louis: Elsevier Saunders; 2012:19-46.

57. Chatburn RL, Carlo WA. Assessment of Neonatal Gas Exchange. In: Carlo WA, Chatburn RL, eds. Neonatal Respiratory Care. 2nd ed. Chicago: Year Book Medical Publishers, Inc.; 1988:40-60.

58. Hall JE. Transport of Oxygen and Carbon Dioxide in Blood and Tissue Fluids. In: Hall JE, ed. Guyton and Hall Textbook of Medical Physiology. 12th ed. Philadelphia: Saunders Elsevier; 2011:495-504.

59. Blackburn ST. Respiratory System. In: Blackburn ST, ed. Maternal, Fetal & Neonatal Physiology: A Clinical Perspective. 3rd ed. St. Louis: Saunders Elsevier; 2007:315-74.

60. Hall JE. Metabolism of Carbohydrates, and Formation of Adenosine Triphosphate. In: Hall JE, ed. Guyton and Hall textbook of medical physiology. 12th ed. Philadelphia: Saunders Elsevier; 2011:809-18.

61. Wood AM, Jones MD. Acid-base Homeostasis and Oxygenation. In: Gardner SL, Carter BS, Enzman-Hines M, Hernandez JA, eds. Merenstein & Gardner's Handbook of Neonatal Intensive Care. 7th ed. St. Louis: Mosby Elsevier; 2011:153-63.

62. Adams JM. Blood Gas and Pulmonary Function Monitoring. In: Cloherty JP, Eichenwald EC, Hansen AR, Stark AR, eds. Manual of Neonatal Care. 7th ed. Philadelphia: Lippincott, Williams & Wilkins; 2012:393-6.

63. Andersen OS. Blood acid-base alignment nomogram. Scales for pH, pCO2 base excess of whole blood of different hemoglobin concentrations, plasma bicarbonate, and plasma total-CO2. Scand J Clin Lab Invest 1963;15:211-7.

64. Donn SM, Sinha SK. Assisted Ventilation and Its Complications. In: Martin RJ, Fanaroff AA, Walsh MC, eds. Fanaroff and Martin's Neonatal-Perinatal Medicine: Diseases of the Fetus and Infant. 9th ed. St. Louis: Elsevier Mosby; 2011:1116-40.

65. Posencheg MA, Evans JR. Acid-Base, Fluid, and Electrolyte Management. In: Gleason CA, Devaskar SU, eds. Avery's Diseases of the Newborn. 9th ed. Philadelphia: Elsevier Saunders; 2012:367-89.

66. Kirk A. Pulmonology. In: Tschudy MM, Arcara KM, eds. The Harriet Lane Handbook. 19th ed. Philadelphia: Elsevier Mosby; 2012:584-605.

67. Ambalavanan N, Schelonka RI, Carlo WA. Ventilation strategies. In: Goldsmith JP, Karotkin EH, Siede BL, eds. Assisted Ventilation of the Neonate. 5th ed. St. Louis: Elsevier Saunders; 2011:265-76.

68. Goldsmith JP, Karotkin EH. Introduction to assisted ventilation. In: Goldsmith JP, Karotkin EH, Siede BL, eds. Assisted Ventilation of the Neonate. 5th ed. St. Louis: Elsevier Saunders; 2011:1-18.

69. Trevisanuto D, Micaglio M, Ferrarese P, Zanardo V. The laryngeal mask airway: potential applications in neonates. Arch Dis Child Fetal Neonatal Ed 2004;89:F485-9.

70. Chameides L. Part 11: Postresuscitation Management. In: Chameides L, Samson RA, Schexnayder SM, Hazinski MF, eds. Pediatric Advanced Life Support Provider Manual. Dallas: American Heart Association; 2011:171-97.

71. Valente C. Emergency Management. In: Tschudy MM, Arcara KM, eds. The Harriet Lane Handbook. 19th ed. Philadelphia: Elsevier Mosby; 2012:3-18.

72. Karlowicz MG, Karotkin EH, Goldsmith JP. Resuscitation. In: Goldsmith JP, Karotkin EH, Siede BL, eds. Assisted Ventilation of the Neonate. 5th ed. St. Louis: Elsevier Saunders; 2012:71-93.

73. MacKendrick W, Slotarski K, Casserly G, Hawkins HS, Hageman JR. Pulmonary Care. In: Goldsmith JP, Karotkin EH, Siede BL, eds. Assisted Ventilation of the Neonate. 5th ed. St. Louis: Elsevier Saunders; 2012:107-25.

74. Kattwinkel J. Endotracheal Intubation and Laryngeal Mask Airway Insertion. In: Kattwinkel J, McGowan JE, Zaichkin J, eds. Textbook of Neonatal Resuscitation. 6th ed. Elk Grove Village: American Academy of Pediatrics; 2011:159-210.

75. Rais-Bahrami K. Endotracheal Intubation. In: MacDonald MG, Ramasethu J, eds. Atlas of Procedures in Neonatology. 4th ed. Philadelphia: Lippincott Williams & Wilkins; 2007:241-55.

76. Peterson J, Johnson N, Deakins K, Wilson-Costello D, Jelovsek JE, Chatburn R. Accuracy of the 7-8-9 Rule for endotracheal tube placement in the neonate. J Perinatol 2006;26:333-6.

77. Eichenwald EC. Mechanical Ventilation. In: Cloherty JP, Eichenwald EC, Hansen AR, Stark AR, eds. Manual of Neonatal Care. 7th ed. Philadelphia: Lippincott, Williams & Wilkins; 2012:377-92.

78. Bhutani VK, Benitz WE. Pulmonary Function and Graphics. In: Goldsmith JP, Karotkin EH, Siede BL, eds. Assisted Ventilation of the Neonate. 5th ed. St. Louis: Elsevier Saunders; 2012:306-20.

79. Sivit CJ. Diagnostic Imaging. In: Martin RJ, Fanaroff AA, Walsh MC, eds. Fanaroff and Martin's Neonatal-Perinatal Medicine: Diseases of the Fetus and Infant. 9th ed. St. Louis: Elsevier Mosby; 2011:685-707.

80. Abu-Shaweesh JM. Respiratory Disorders in Preterm and Term Infants. In: Martin RJ, Fanaroff AA, Walsh MC, eds. Fanaroff and Martin's Neonatal-Perinatal Medicine: Diseases of the Fetus and Infant. 9th ed. St. Louis: Elsevier Mosby; 2011:1141-70.

81. Kienstra KA. Transient Tachypnea of the Newborn. In: Cloherty JP, Eichenwald EC, Hansen AR, Stark AR, eds. Manual of Neonatal Care. 7th ed. Philadelphia: Lippincott, Williams & Wilkins; 2012:403-5.

82. Yoder BA, Gordon MC, Barth WH, Jr. Late-preterm birth: does the changing obstetric paradigm alter the epidemiology of respiratory complications? Obstet Gynecol 2008;111:814-22.

83. Nold JL, Georgieff MK. Infants of diabetic mothers. Pediatr Clin North Am 2004;51:619-37, viii.

84. Burris HH. Meconium Aspiration. In: Cloherty JP, Eichenwald EC, Hansen AR, Stark AR, eds. Manual of Neonatal Care. 7th ed. Philadelphia: Lippincott, Williams & Wilkins; 2012:429-34.

85. Ghidini A, Spong CY. Severe meconium aspiration syndrome is not caused by aspiration of meconium. Am J Obstet Gynecol 2001;185:931-8.

86. Thureen PJ, Hall DM, Hoffenberg A, Tyson RW. Fatal meconium aspiration in spite of appropriate perinatal airway management: pulmonary and placental evidence of prenatal disease. Am J Obstet Gynecol 1997;176:967-75.

87. Ringer SA, Hansen AR. Surgical Emergencies in the Newborn. In: Cloherty JP, Eichenwald EC, Hansen AR, Stark AR, eds. Manual of Neonatal Care. 7th ed. Philadelphia: Lippincott, Williams & Wilkins; 2012:808-30.

88. Barksdale EM, Chwals WJ, Magnuson DK, Parry RL. Selected Gastrointestinal Anomalies. In: Martin RJ, Fanaroff AA, Walsh MC, eds. Fanaroff & Martin's Neonatal-Perinatal Medicine: Diseases of the Fetus and Infant. 9th ed. St. Louis: Elsevier Mosby; 2011:1400-31.

89. Keller RL, Guevara-Gallardo S, Farmer DL. Surgical Disorders of the Chest and Airways. In: Gleason CA, Devaskar SU, eds. Avery's Diseases of the Newborn. 9th ed. Philadelphia: Elsevier Saunders; 2012:672-97.

90. Stork EK. Therapy for Cardiorespiratory Failure. In: Martin RJ, Fanaroff AA, Walsh MC, eds. Fanaroff and Martin's Neonatal-Perinatal Medicine: Diseases of the Fetus and Infant. 9th ed. St. Louis: Elsevier Mosby; 2011:1192-206.

91. Arensman RM. Surgical Interventions for Respiratory Distress and Airway Management. In: Goldsmith JP, Karotkin EH, Siede BL, eds. Assisted Ventilation of the Neonate. 5th ed. St. Louis: Elsevier Saunders; 2012:435-51.

92. Kattwinkel J. Special Considerations. In: Kattwinkel J, McGowan JE, Zaichkin J, eds. Textbook of Neonatal Resuscitation. 6th ed. Elk Grove Village: American Academy of Pediatrics; 2011:237-66.

93. Blake KD, Prasad C. CHARGE syndrome. Orphanet J Rare Dis 2006;1:34.

94. Steinhorn RH, Abman SH. Persistent pulmonary hypertension. In: Gleason CA, Devaskar SU, eds. Avery's Diseases of the Newborn. 9th ed. Philadelphia: Elsevier Saunders; 2012.

95. Rabinovitch M. Developmental Biology of the Pulmonary Vasculature. In: Polin RA, Fox WW, Abman SH, eds. Fetal and Neonatal Physiology. 4th ed. Philadelphia: Elsevier Saunders; 2011:757-72.

96. Rais-Bahrami K, MacDonald M, G., Eichelberger MR. Thoracostomy tubes. In: MacDonald M, G., Ramasethu J, eds. Atlas of Procedures in Neonatology. 4th ed. Philadelphia: Wolters Kluwer / Lippincott Williams & Wilkins; 2007:261-84.

97. Anand KJ. Pharmacological approaches to the management of pain in the neonatal intensive care unit. J Perinatol 2007;27 Suppl 1:S4-S11.

98. Aranda JV, Carlo W, Hummel P, Thomas R, Lehr VT, Anand KJ. Analgesia and sedation during mechanical ventilation in neonates. Clin Ther 2005;27:877-99.

99. Cignacco EL, Sellam G, Stoffel L, et al. Oral sucrose and "facilitated tucking" for repeated pain relief in preterms: a randomized controlled trial. Pediatrics 2012;129:299-308.

100. Anand KJ, Johnston CC, Oberlander TF, Taddio A, Lehr VT, Walco GA. Analgesia and local anesthesia during invasive procedures in the neonate. Clin Ther 2005;27:844-76.

101. Batton DG, Barrington KJ, Wallman C. Prevention and management of pain in the neonate: an update. Pediatrics 2006;118:2231-41.

187

102. Anand KJ. Consensus statement for the prevention and management of pain in the newborn. Arch Pediatr Adolesc Med 2001;155:173-80.

103. Golianu B, Krane E, Seybold J, Almgren C, Anand KJ. Non-pharmacological techniques for pain management in neonates. Semin Perinatol 2007;31:318-22.

104. Stevens B, Yamada J, Ohlsson A. Sucrose for analgesia in newborn infants undergoing painful procedures. Cochrane Database Syst Rev 2010:CD001069.

105. Cignacco E, Axelin A, Stoffel L, Sellam G, Anand KJ, Engberg S. Facilitated tucking as a non-pharmacological intervention for neonatal pain relief: is it clinically feasible? Acta Paediatr 2010.

106. Taketomo CK, Hodding JH, Kraus DM. Pediatric & Neonatal Dosage Handook. 18th ed. Hudson: Lexicomp; 2011.

107. Anand KJ, Hall RW, Desai N, et al. Effects of morphine analgesia in ventilated preterm neonates: primary outcomes from the NEOPAIN randomised trial. Lancet 2004;363:1673-82.

108. Johnston CC, Filion F, Snider L, et al. Routine sucrose analgesia during the first week of life in neonates younger than 31 weeks' postconceptional age. Pediatrics 2002;110:523-8.

109. Walden M, Gibbins S. Pain Assessment and Management: Guideline for Practice. 2nd ed. Glenview: National Association of Neonatal Nurses; 2008.

110. Steinhorn RH. Pulmonary Vascular Development. In: Martin RJ, Fanaroff AA, Walsh MC, eds. Fanaroff and Martin's Neonatal-Perinatal Medicine: Diseases of the Fetus and Infant. 9th ed. St. Louis: Elsevier Mosby; 2011:1216-22.

111. Zahka KG. Cardiovascular Problems of the Neonate. In: Martin RJ, Fanaroff AA, Walsh MC, eds. Fanaroff and Martin's Neonatal-Perinatal Medicine: Diseases of the Fetus and Infant. 9th ed. St. Louis: Elsevier Mosby; 2011:1266-77.

**S**ugar and **S**afe Care

**T**emperature

**A**irway

**B**lood Pressure

**L**ab Work

**E**motional Support

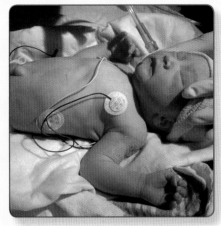

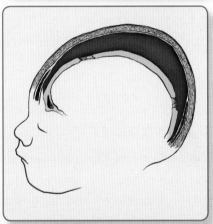

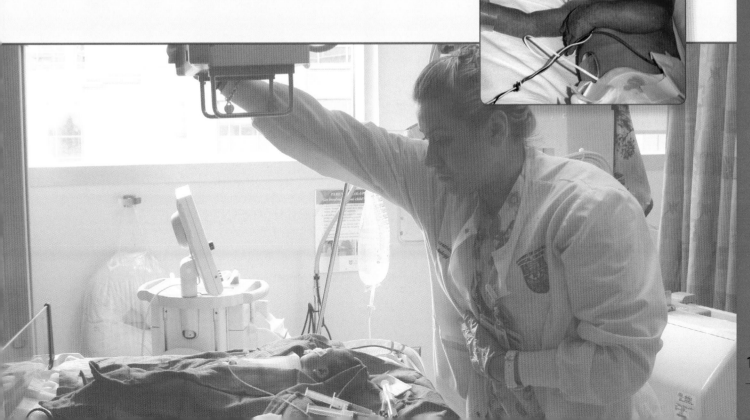

## Blood Pressure – Module Objectives

Upon completion of this module, participants will gain an increased understanding of:

1.  The difference between compensated and uncompensated shock.

2.  The principles of cardiac output and heart rate as they relate to shock and factors that can impair cardiac output.

3.  The physical examination to evaluate for shock.

4.  The causes and initial treatment of the three major types of shock seen in infants: hypovolemic, cardiogenic, and septic shock.

## What Is Shock?

For the cells to survive and function, they need oxygen. When tissue perfusion and oxygen delivery to vital organs becomes inadequate, a state of shock develops.[1-3] Two phases of shock are recognized: *compensated* and *uncompensated*.

### Compensated and Uncompensated Shock

In **compensated shock**, a complex series of responses are activated to maintain blood pressure and preserve blood flow to vital organs (e.g., brain, heart, and adrenal glands).[2,4] This response is not without consequence however, because blood is diverted away from non-vital organs, (e.g., skin, gastrointestinal tract, muscles, liver and kidneys), to preserve central blood pressure.[4,5] If shock is not quickly recognized and reversed, the oxygen debt worsens, metabolism converts from aerobic to anaerobic glycolysis, which produces large quantities of lactate, and metabolic acidemia develops. **Cardiac output** falls as the heart muscle weakens from lack of oxygen and the effects of acidemia. The body will compensate for as long as it can, but when hypotension develops, the phase of **uncompensated shock** has begun.[2,6]

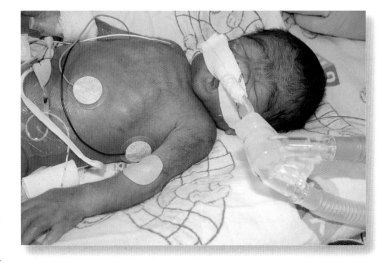

⚠ Hypotension is a late sign of cardiac decompensation,[5] therefore, it is very important to recognize that waiting for hypotension to develop may be deleterious to the infant's well-being. Failure to promptly recognize and treat shock may lead to cellular dysfunction, multiple organ failure (brain, heart, liver, kidneys, and gastrointestinal tract), and even death.[2,4,7] Therefore, treatment must be prompt and aggressive.

## Clinical Tip

**Are preterm infants experiencing uncompensated shock or are they simply "hypotensive?"**

Sick preterm infants (less than 1500 grams), with respiratory distress are commonly hypotensive, especially in the acute phase of their illness.[2,8,9] It is unclear what blood pressure value should be used for treatment and whether treating a low blood pressure value (primarily with a crystalloid volume infusion, dopamine and/or hydrocortisone), improves long-term neurodevelopmental outcomes.[9,10] Oftentimes, these very-low-birth weight preterm infants do not have other signs of shock, such as tachycardia or prolonged capillary filling time at the same time their blood pressure is low. Delaying treatment until these signs appear may result in worse outcomes.[11]

Commonly, mean blood pressure has been used as the parameter to assess when volume, dopamine, or hydrocortisone should be administered.[8,12,13] Until more research is done to determine the best approach to the hypotensive very-low-birth weight infant, it is recommended to discuss treatment with a neonatologist.

## Cardiac Output

A sustained heart rate greater than 180 beats per minute at rest, is called **tachycardia**.[5] Similar to why the infant breathes faster and deeper when trying to compensate for increased $CO_2$ levels, the heart rate will increase when the infant is trying to compensate for a low cardiac output. However, unlike the infant's ability to take a deeper breath when trying to compensate for increased $CO_2$ levels, the neonatal myocardium has poor capacity to increase the amount of blood that is ejected with each heart beat (stroke volume), unless augmented with a blood pressure medication and/or a volume infusion.

**The formula for cardiac output (CO) is: heart rate (HR) multiplied by stroke volume (SV)[2,4]**

$$HR \times SV = CO$$

**In addition to electrolyte, mineral, or energy imbalances, factors that can impair cardiac output include the following:[2,4]**

- Decreased volume of venous return to the heart *(preload)* – the heart has less to "pump" with each contraction (decreased stroke volume).

- Increased systemic vascular resistance *(afterload)* – the heart works harder to pump blood against the resistance.

- Decreased myocardial contractility – heart squeeze or contraction is poor so less blood is ejected with every beat.

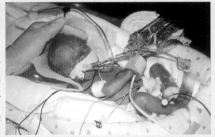

**Table 4.1.** Physical examination for shock.

## An infant in shock may exhibit the following signs:[2,14-17]

### Respiratory effort

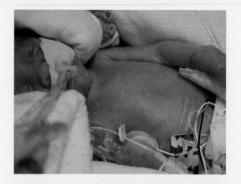

- ✧ Tachypnea (may be a sign that the infant is trying to compensate for a metabolic or mixed acidosis)

  - Evaluate the blood gas for respiratory, metabolic, or mixed acidosis

- ✧ Increased work of breathing (retractions, grunting, nasal flaring)

- ✧ Apnea

- ✧ *Gasping* (an ominous sign of impending cardiorespiratory arrest)

### Color

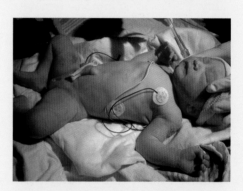

- ✧ Cyanosis, desaturation

  - Evaluate $O_2$ saturation

- ✧ Pale, white skin color

  - May indicate a very low hemoglobin secondary to hemorrhage

### Heart rate

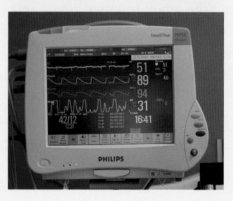

- ✧ A normal heart rate is between 120 and 160 beats per minute (bpm), but may range between 80 and 200 bpm depending upon the infant's activity level

- ✧ Bradycardia (< 100 bpm) with evidence of poor perfusion

  - Hypoxemia, hypotension, and acidosis all depress the conduction system and may cause bradycardia

  - Bradycardia combined with severe shock is an ominous sign of impending cardiorespiratory arrest

  - Other causes of bradycardia include hypothermia, increased intracranial pressure, abdominal distension, hypoglycemia, episodes of apnea (apnea of prematurity), and medications (digoxin and propranolol)[15]

  - Rule out complete heart block

- ✧ Tachycardia (sustained heart rate > 180 bpm at rest)

  - May indicate poor cardiac output and / or congestive heart failure

  - If the heart rate is above 220 bpm, consider supraventricular tachycardia (SVT), especially if the heart rate abruptly increases from a lower rate to a rate > 220 bpm[15]

  - Other causes of tachycardia include pain, fever, hypoxia, or medications (i.e., xanthine therapy, dopamine, epinephrine), and hyperthyroidism[15]

## Blood pressure

✧ Normal newborn blood pressure values are shown in Figure 4.2.

✧ May be normal or low

- The blood pressure reading may be within normal range because of vasoconstriction and centralization of blood pressure during the period of compensated shock

- The presence of hypotension signals uncompensated shock

## Pulses

✧ Weak peripheral pulses (the pulses feel decreased or the pulses are not palpable)

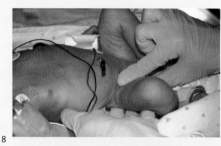

- If the brachial pulses are stronger than femoral pulses, consider coarctation of the aorta or interrupted aortic arch; if left outflow tract obstruction is present, with complete ductal closure, all pulses will be weak or absent[18]

## Peripheral perfusion

✧ Poor perfusion

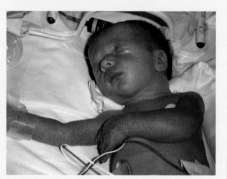

- Secondary to vasoconstriction and poor cardiac output

✧ Prolonged capillary refill time (CRT) (see Figure 4.1 for more information)

- Greater than 3 seconds in a sick infant is generally considered abnormal

✧ Cool skin

✧ Mottled skin

## Heart

✧ Enlarged heart size on chest x-ray (correlates with myocardial dysfunction and development of congestive heart failure)

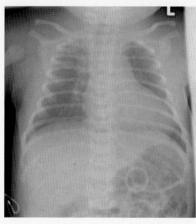

✧ Smaller than normal, or compressed heart on chest x-ray (may reflect poor filling or pre-load)

✧ Evaluate for the presence or absence of a heart murmur

- In shock, the most common reason for a loud systolic murmur is tricuspid regurgitation

- It is important to rule out other reasons for the heart murmur such as structural heart disease (usually valvular obstruction; a ventricular septal defect is typically silent in the first few weeks of life)

- Severe forms of congenital heart disease may be present even if there is no heart murmur

## Urine output

✧ Less than 1 mL/kg/hour or a declining urine output, especially if there are other signs of hypoperfusion

**Figure 4.1. Capillary Refill Time (CRT): How is the test done?**

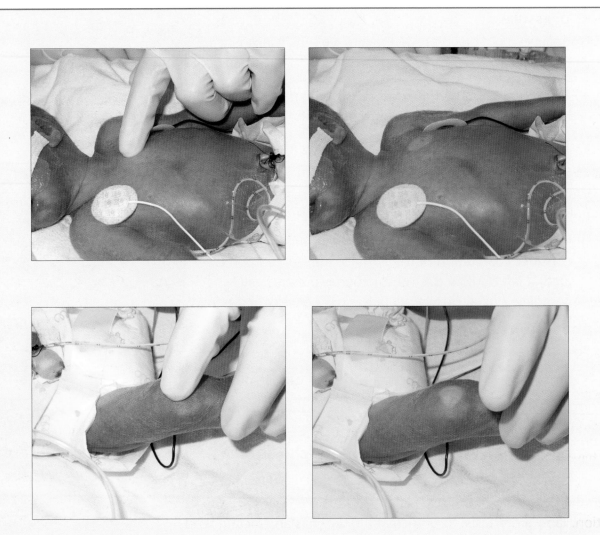

Evaluating CRT can be very subjective; therefore, try to perform the test using the same routine (location, time skin is pressed to blanch, method of counting) each time it is done. If the infant is hypothermic, the CRT will be prolonged; therefore, it is important to evaluate CRT when the infant is normothermic. Press firmly for 5 seconds and release. Count how many seconds it takes for the skin to re-fill. Compare the upper to lower body. If greater than 3 seconds on the upper or lower body, or if the lower body takes longer for the skin to refill compared to the upper body, report these findings to the infant's medical staff provider.

---

Notes:

1. Studies report variation in CRT because of gestational or postnatal age, skin temperature, ambient temperature, hydration status, polycythemia, duration of pressure applied to blanch the skin and location where CRT was assessed; therefore, it is important to realize that comparisons between studies are difficult to make.[2,19-25]

2. The Pediatric Advanced Life Support (PALS) course considers a CRT ≤ 2 seconds normal, unless there is clinical or historical evidence of hypotensive, vasodilated "warm" shock.[16,26]

## Blood Pressure

Defining a normal versus hypotensive blood pressure is a complicated issue.[6,9] In preterm infants, research is still lacking that identifies which preterm infants may benefit from interventions to raise blood pressure, which interventions improve outcomes and what is a "safe" blood pressure to allow (and not treat).[10,21]

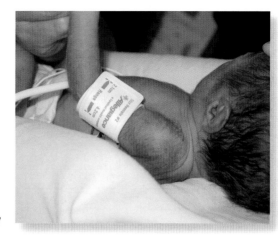

It is a common practice to use the mean arterial blood pressure to assess whether an infant is normotensive or not. Usually, when the mean blood pressure is equal to, or a few points above gestational age, neonatal caregivers conclude the blood pressure is in a normal range.[12,13] However, using mean blood pressure in this manner has not been empirically evaluated.[6] Until more data is available, it is advised that all three blood pressure parameters – systolic, diastolic, and mean – are assessed when evaluating blood pressure. Collectively all three parameters provide important information, including the information needed to calculate pulse pressure (see the Clinical Tip, How do I calculate and interpret pulse pressure?). Figure 4.2 contains normal arterial blood pressure values in healthy preterm and term infants.[27,28]

**Assessment of the infant's perfusion and overall well-being must accompany blood pressure measurement**. This is because an infant may have a blood pressure in the "normal range," but on exam, may have evidence of altered mental state and poor cardiac output: prolonged CRT, cool extremities, or mottled skin. Findings such as these would be consistent with a state of compensated shock. In addition, laboratory tests, in particular a blood gas and lactate level (see Table 4.2) may also provide useful information regarding the degree of shock an infant may be experiencing. However, if there is a clinical indication, treatment should not be delayed while awaiting laboratory results. Conversely, the blood pressure may be low, but there are no clinical signs of hypoperfusion. Report any concerns to the infant's medical staff provider. In addition, if using a blood pressure cuff, make sure the cuff is the correct size. See the Clinical Tip on taking blood pressures by the oscillometric method for more information.

> Assessment of the infant's perfusion and overall well-being must accompany blood pressure measurement

## Clinical Tip

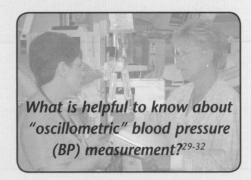

*What is helpful to know about "oscillometric" blood pressure (BP) measurement?*[29-32]

In nurseries and NICUs worldwide, noninvasive oscillometric measurement is the most common method for evaluating the infant's BP. A few important things to consider when assessing oscillometric BP results are:

• The BP will be higher when the infant is in an awake state compared with sleeping

• A second or third reading taken two minutes apart may be slightly lower than the initial reading

• Movement interferes with the accuracy of the reading

• Selecting the correct cuff size is very important[32]

To select the correct cuff, measure the arm circumference and then follow the manufacturer's recommendations for cuff size. For example, if using the Critikon® Neonatal Blood Pressure Cuff, a size 1 would be selected for a limb circumference of 3 to 6 centimeters, size 2 for 4 to 8 centimeters and size 3 for 6 to 11 centimeters, etc. A few important points about cuff size are:

• An undersized cuff will overestimate the BP, giving false reassurance that the infant has a normal blood pressure, when in fact it may be hypotensive.

• An oversized or loose cuff underestimates the BP, and will give a hypotensive reading, when in fact it may be normotensive.

To enable comparison of results, it is helpful to take the BP on the same limb (right upper arm if possible). Abnormal BP results should be repeated and always correlate findings with patient assessment.

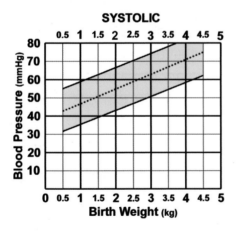 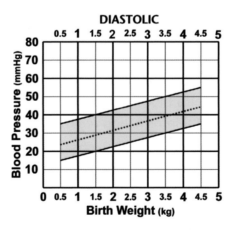 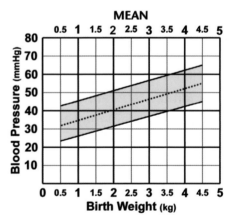

**The shaded yellow area is considered normal.**

**Figure 4.2. Average systolic, diastolic, and mean blood pressures during the first 12 hours of life in normal newborn infants according to birth weight.** Evaluation of blood pressure is an important component of patient evaluation, however, the decision to treat shock should be based on history, physical and laboratory exam, and patient condition, not just blood pressure.

*Graphs adapted with permission from Versmold, HT, et al. (1981). Aortic blood pressure during the first 12 hours of life in infants with birth weight 610 to 4,220 grams. Pediatrics, 67(5), 607-613.*[27,28]

Note:

The mean blood pressure values in Versmold's study were used for comparison in a recent study by Pejovic[32] who evaluated normal blood pressures in preterm and term infants using oscillometric (cuff) measurement. The mean blood pressures in the two studies were nearly identical.[27,32] Systolic and diastolic measurements were not compared, however visual inspection of graphs from both studies reveals the numbers are very comparable. For more information, see reference Pejovic.[32]

## Clinical Tip

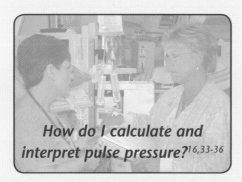

*How do I calculate and interpret pulse pressure?*[16,33-36]

| To calculate pulse pressure, subtract the diastolic pressure from the systolic pressure | |
|---|---|
| **Gestation** | **Normal pulse pressure (mmHg)[36]** |
| Term | 25 to 30 |
| Preterm | 15 to 25 |

| **Possible causes of a narrow or wide pulse pressure** | |
|---|---|
| Narrow | • Peripheral vasoconstriction<br><br>• Heart failure – low cardiac output, poor myocardial contractility<br><br>• Compression on the heart – low cardiac output secondary to pneumopericardium, pericardial effusion, tension pneumothorax<br><br>• Severe aortic valve stenosis |
| Wide | • Large aortic (diastolic) runoff lesion – patent ductus arteriosus, arteriovenous malformation, truncus arteriosus, aortopulmonary window, aortic regurgitation<br><br>• Sepsis with vasodilated (warm) shock |

⚠ A narrow or wide pulse pressure should be reported to the infant's medical staff provider.

## Exercise: A term, 3 kg infant has the following three blood pressures.

a) Mark the values on each blood pressure graph below.

b) Calculate the pulse pressure.

c) Evaluate whether the pulse pressure is narrow, normal or wide.

d) Use the information on page 197 to look at the various etiologies for abnormal results.

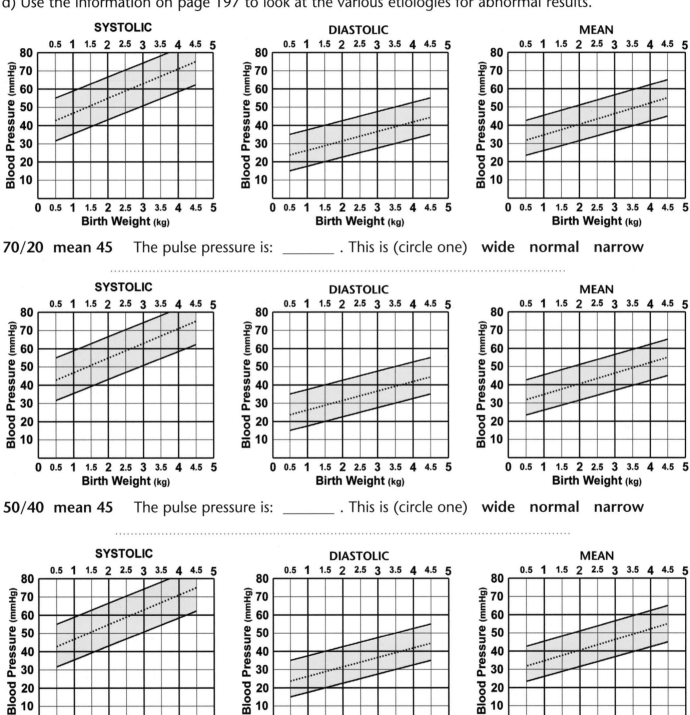

**70/20 mean 45** The pulse pressure is: _____ . This is (circle one) **wide   normal   narrow**

**50/40 mean 45** The pulse pressure is: _____ . This is (circle one) **wide   normal   narrow**

**60/30 mean 45** The pulse pressure is: _____ . This is (circle one) **wide   normal   narrow**

# The Three Types of Shock: Hypovolemic, Cardiogenic, Septic

## Hypovolemic Shock

Hypovolemic shock results from a low circulating blood volume.[4] Causes of hypovolemic shock include:[2,3,9,37-40]

## Acute blood loss during the intrapartum period

- Placental hemorrhage: placental abruption or placenta previa

- Umbilical cord injury

- Organ laceration (liver or spleen)

- Fetal-to-maternal hemorrhage

- Twin-to-twin transfusion syndrome (acute or chronic hemorrhage)

    - Criteria for diagnosis: single placenta, same-gender fetus, weight discordance of > 20%, amniotic fluid discordance[38]

    - The recipient twin may have signs of hydrops and heart failure (cardiomegaly, tricuspid regurgitation, and decreased left ventricular function) and the donor twin may be small in size, anemic and underperfused

## Postnatal hemorrhage

- Brain

- Lung

- Adrenal gland

- Scalp (of most concern is subgaleal hemorrhage; see Appendix 4.1 for more information on evaluation of scalp swelling)

## Obstructive etiology[41]

- Tension pneumothorax (decreases venous return and impairs cardiac output)

- Pneumopericardium (impairs cardiac output)

## Other non-hemorrhagic causes

- Umbilical cord accident (tight nuchal cord, cord prolapse, cord knot, cord entanglement, velamentous cord insertion, vasa previa) – blood flow to the fetus is interrupted and results in hypovolemic and cardiogenic shock[40]

- Severe capillary leak secondary to infection

- Dehydration

Some etiologies of postnatal hemorrhage may also occur prenatally or during the intrapartum period. As described in Table 4.1, infants in hypovolemic shock present with signs of poor cardiac output: tachycardia, weak pulses, prolonged capillary refill time, mottling, and cyanosis. If there is severe blood loss they will appear pale or white, and have acidosis and hypotension (a late sign of poor cardiac output).

Be aware of the very pale or 'white' appearing infant at delivery. Remember, 3 to 5 grams/dL of hemoglobin needs to be desaturated (not carrying any oxygen) for cyanosis to appear. If the infant has experienced a severe hemorrhage and only has 3 to 5 gm/dL of hemoglobin, then cyanosis will not be apparent. An emergency blood transfusion of O-negative packed red blood cells (PRBCs) may be lifesaving in this situation.

If the infant has experienced chronic anemia in utero, and/or is edematous at birth (hydrops fetalis), take care to give blood or volume infusions slowly. The infant may already be experiencing a degree of heart failure because of the anemia and chronic in-utero hypoxia. Giving blood or volume too quickly will worsen the situation.[39]

## Cardiogenic Shock

Cardiogenic shock (heart failure) results when the heart muscle functions poorly and may occur in infants with:[2,3,9]

- Intrapartum or postpartum asphyxia

- Hypoxia and/or metabolic acidosis

- Bacterial or viral infection

- Severe respiratory distress (requiring assisted ventilation)

- Severe hypoglycemia

- Severe metabolic and / or electrolyte disturbances

- Arrhythmias

- Congenital heart defects, especially those with severe hypoxemia or obstruction of blood flow into the systemic circulation

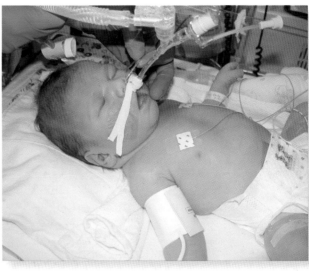

Term infant with hypoplastic left heart syndrome

## Septic (distributive) Shock

Severe infection may lead to a third type of shock known as septic or distributive shock. Infants in septic shock rapidly become critically ill. In the presence of bacterial infection, a host of complicated systemic reactions occur that result in circulatory insufficiency.[2,3] A hallmark of this type of shock is hypotension that responds poorly to fluid resuscitation.[9,41] Loss of vascular integrity allows fluid to leak out of the blood vessels and into the tissue spaces (also a cause of hypovolemic shock).[9] Poor myocardial contractility leads to poor tissue perfusion and oxygenation.[2] In addition to fluid resuscitation, these infants also often need blood pressure medication to treat the severe hypotension.[42] The risk for organ injury and death is very high.[17]

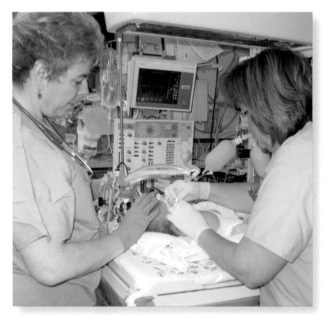

Not infrequently, infants may have a combination of the three types of shock.

**Table 4.2.** Laboratory evaluation for shock.[41,43] The following laboratory tests are useful to evaluate shock, and if abnormal, help determine appropriate corrective therapy.

## Blood gas

**Metabolic acidosis is present if the pH and bicarbonate are low.** If the infant is experiencing respiratory insufficiency, then the $PCO_2$ will also be elevated and the infant will have a mixed respiratory and metabolic acidosis.

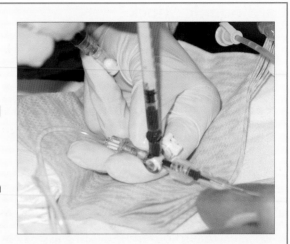

- ✧ pH < 7.30 is abnormal

- ✧ pH < 7.25 is concerning especially if in combination with poor perfusion, tachycardia, and/or low blood pressure

- ✧ pH < 7.20 is significantly abnormal

- ✧ pH < 7.10 indicates the infant is in severe crisis

## Other labs that are useful in the evaluation of shock

- ✧ Blood lactate

  - • Increased lactate level signifies anaerobic metabolism is occurring in the tissues

- ✧ CBC with differential

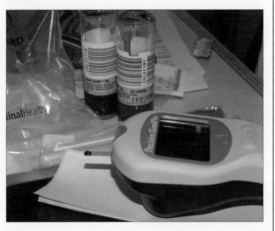

  - • Evaluate for sepsis, anemia, polycythemia, low platelet count

- ✧ Blood culture

  - • Evaluate for sepsis

- ✧ Coagulation studies (prothrombin time, partial thromboplastin time, fibrinogen, D-dimer)

- ✧ Liver function tests

- ✧ Glucose

  - • In response to stress, the infant may initially be hyperglycemic because of catecholamine release

  - • In the presence of shock, glucose utilization may be markedly increased which raises the risk for hypoglycemia

    - ◇ Anaerobic metabolism utilizes significantly more glucose than aerobic metabolism to produce adenosine triphosphate (ATP; energy for cell function)

  - • Evaluate the blood sugar frequently until a pattern of stability is demonstrated

- ✧ Electrolytes (hypo or hypernatremia, hypo or hyperkalemia)

  - • If metabolic acidosis present, calculate the anion gap

  - • For more information, see: **What's all the Phys about?** What is the Meaning of an Abnormal Anion Gap, low Ionized Calcium and Elevated Cardiac Enzymes

✧ Ionized calcium

  ● Calcium is needed for myocardial contractility

  ● If the calcium level is low, other inotropes will be significantly less effective

✧ Renal function tests (BUN, creatinine)

✧ Cardiac enzymes to look for myocardial tissue injury

  ● B-type Natriuretic Peptide (BNP), Troponin, Creatine phosphokinase-MB (CPK-MB)

**Other tests and observations**

✧ Echocardiogram to evaluate cardiac function and to rule out structural congenital heart disease

✧ Electrocardiogram (ECG) to assess for arrhythmias

✧ Evaluate urine output for oliguria or anuria

✧ If concerned about an inborn error of metabolism, many of the tests listed above will be useful (blood gas, serum lactate, coagulation profile and liver function tests, glucose, electrolytes, and renal function tests), but additional metabolic screening tests are also useful (state newborn screen, ammonia level, plasma amino acids, plasma acylcarnitine profile, and urine organic acids)

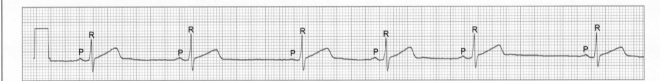

ECG of sinus bradycardia; the heart rate is 42 beats per minute.

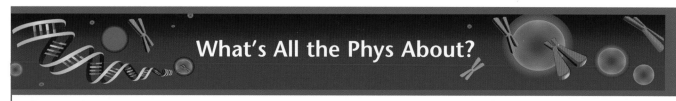

# What's All the Phys About?

## What is the Meaning of an Abnormal Anion Gap, Low Ionized Calcium and Elevated Cardiac Enzymes?

### If metabolic acidosis is present, calculate the anion gap as follows:

- $[(Na)] - [Cl + HCO_3)]$[44-46]

  - ⬥ Use the serum $CO_2$ on the electrolyte panel for the $HCO_3$.

- Normal values for the neonate are 5 to 15 mEq/L.[47,48]

  - ⬥ **High anion gap**[49,50]

    - ◇ Lactic acidosis – produced by anaerobic metabolism; shock, sepsis

    - ◇ Ketoacidosis – inborn error of organic acid or amino acid metabolism

    - ◇ Renal failure

    - ◇ Late metabolic acidosis

    - ◇ Toxins

  - ⬥ **Normal anion gap**

    - ◇ Loss of bicarbonate ($HCO_3-$), usually from gastrointestinal (small bowel drainage, diarrhea) or renal losses (bicarbonate wasting secondary to immaturity, renal tubular acidosis, diuretic treatment with carbonic anhydrase inhibitors)[44,47,49]

    - ◇ Excessive chloride in IV fluid

    - ◇ Aldosterone deficiency

    - ◇ Hyperchloremia is a compensatory mechanism[49]

  - ⬥ **Low anion gap**

    - ◇ Caused by hypoalbuminemia[47,51]

### Ionized calcium is the measure of 'free calcium' and the best indicator of physiologic blood calcium activity

- Hypocalcemia in term and late preterm infants is defined as an ionized calcium concentration < 4.4 mg/dL (1.1 mmol/L)[52,53]

- Calcium acts as a second messenger in myocardial contractility

- If there is insufficient calcium available for myocardial contraction, other inotropes will be significantly less effective

### Elevated Cardiac enzymes can be due to myocardial tissue injury

- *BNP – B-type natriuretic peptide* is synthesized and released by the ventricles of the heart in response to excessive stretching of cardiac myocytes or ventricular stress[54-57]

  - ⬥ Ranges Elevated in:[57-60]

    - ◇ Congestive heart failure

    - ◇ Pulmonary hypertension

    - ◇ Various congenital heart diseases

    - ◇ Septic shock

| Values in Preterm infants* | |
|---|---|
| Median values of 31 to 833[54] were obtained in 24- to 31-week gestation infants with patent ductus arteriosus (PDA) | Values increased as grade of PDA increased<br><br>If also intubated and ventilated, the BNP values were in the higher range[54] |
| **Values in Healthy Term Infants*** | |
| Mean BNP starts at 231.6 and declines to 48.4 in first week[57]<br><br>Values are highest in the first 3 days of life[61] | |

*Interpret in the context of clinical events and physical exam.*

- *Troponin I (cardiac Troponin)* is released in response to myocardial injury

  - ⬥ Newborns have slightly higher levels than adults and increase these levels when asphyxiated[62]

- Creatine phosphokinase (CPK) is an enzyme found mainly in the heart (MB fraction), brain (BB fraction), and skeletal muscle (BB fraction)

  - ⬥ CPK-MB rises 4 – 6 hours after myocardial injury and peaks at 24 hours

  - ⬥ Less reliable marker than Troponin I

*A special thank you to Dr. Howard Stein, neonatologist and pediatric cardiologist at Toledo Children's Hospital, Toledo, Ohio, for his assistance with preparing this information.*

# Treatment of Shock

The first step in the treatment of shock is to identify its cause or causes. The second step is to identify and correct any related or underlying problems that may impair heart function, such as poor cardiac filling because of hypovolemia, tamponade, excessive airway pressure, electrolyte disturbances, hypoglycemia, hypoxemia, or arrhythmias.[17] Figure 4.3 illustrates the principles underlying an improvement in blood pH.

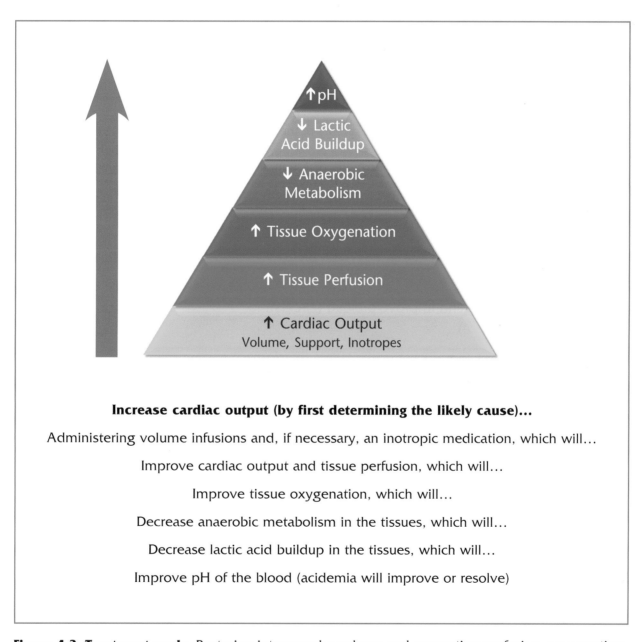

**Increase cardiac output (by first determining the likely cause)...**

Administering volume infusions and, if necessary, an inotropic medication, which will...

Improve cardiac output and tissue perfusion, which will...

Improve tissue oxygenation, which will...

Decrease anaerobic metabolism in the tissues, which will...

Decrease lactic acid buildup in the tissues, which will...

Improve pH of the blood (acidemia will improve or resolve)

**Figure 4.3. Treatment goals.** Restoring intravascular volume and supporting perfusion, oxygenation and ventilation is critically important when infants are in shock.[41] Oxygen delivery to the tissues must improve to reverse the effects of shock.[2]

# Treatment of Hypovolemic (low blood volume) Shock

The goal of treatment is to improve the circulating blood volume. This can be accomplished by administering the following crystalloids or blood products.

## IF THERE IS NO ACUTE BLOOD LOSS[3,41]

### Normal Saline (NS) 0.9%

**Indications:** Volume infusion, to improve preload (circulating blood volume)

**Dose:** 10 mL per kilogram per dose (10 mL/kg/dose)

**Route:** IV, UVC, intraosseous

**Time interval:** Administer over 15 to 30 minutes

Notes:

1. The administration time is dependent upon the severity of the situation and may need to be more rapid.

2. For treatment of severe shock, it may be necessary to provide two, three or more volume boluses. Evaluate the infant's response to treatment (changes in heart rate, perfusion, and blood pressure) following each bolus and decide if more volume is necessary.

## IF THERE IS ACUTE BLOOD LOSS

Give normal saline to begin volume resuscitation while awaiting Packed Red Blood Cells (PRBCs), or Whole Blood (usually reconstituted with PRBCs and Fresh Frozen Plasma)

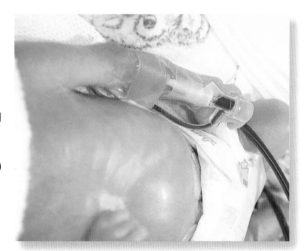

**Indications:** Treat anemia and improve preload (circulating blood volume)

**Dose:** 10 mL per kilogram per dose (10 mL/kg/dose)

**Route:** IV, UVC, intraosseous

**Time interval:** Administer over 30 minutes to 2 hours

Notes:

1. The administration time is dependent upon the severity of the situation, and may need to be more rapid than 30 minutes.

2. Remember to obtain the newborn screen whenever possible prior to any blood transfusions, but do not delay giving a transfusion if emergently needed.

> ⚠ If there is a history of chronic blood loss, some infants in severe shock may not tolerate volume boluses. Consultation with the tertiary center neonatologist is advised if in doubt about whether to administer volume or how much to give.

---

### *Example:* How to calculate the volume bolus

**Desired Dose:** 10 mL per kilogram per dose (10 mL/kg/dose)

**Weight:** 1800 grams or 1.8 kg

**Final Dose:** 10 (mL) X 1.8 (kg) = 18 mL

*Give 18 mL of volume over 15 to 30 minutes IV, UVC, or intraosseous (IO) route*

# Clinical Tip

*What packed red cell blood type can be administered during an emergency when there is not enough time to perform a type and cross-match?*[63,64]

**Type O-negative packed red blood cells may be provided during an emergency when time may not allow for cross matching of blood.**[41]

Very low birthweight neonates (<1200 grams) may benefit from special product modifications such as leukoreduction of cellular products for CMV safety and irradiation of cellular products to reduce the risk of transfusion-associated graft vs host disease (TA-GVHD). Cellular products are packed red blood cells and platelets.

## CMV Infection

- CMV infection is particularly problematic for very-low-birth weight infants, especially if the mother is sero-negative for CMV. This is because the infant would then lack any immunity to CMV.[65]

- The risk of acquiring cytomegalovirus (CMV) is proportional to the number of WBC's containing CMV virions in the blood (product).

- Packed red blood cells and platelets that are leukoreduced are considered to be 'CMV safe'. Packed red blood cells are **leukoreduced** (white blood cells removed) by filtration either soon after collection (before the PRBCs are stored – prestorage), after varying periods of storage in the laboratory, or at the bedside using a blood transfusion filter. Leukoreduction performed in the laboratory is subject to quality control, whereas leukoreduction at the bedside is not.

- The amount of leukocyte reduction that is achieved is a function of the filter system used. The American

Association of Blood Bank standard is that leukoreduced blood products must have a residual content of leukocytes less than $5 \times 10^6$.[66] Transfusion with **prestorage** leukoreduced red blood cells or platelets is preferred whenever possible.

- CMV transmission risk can also be decreased by the use of CMV sero-negative donors but leukoreduction provides additional benefits that CMV sero-negative cellular components do not.

## Who should receive filtered PRBCs?

All babies who receive a blood transfusion must receive filtered RBCs (and platelets).

## Transfusion-Associated Graft Vs Host Disease (TA-GVHD)

Irradiation is another process that may be performed on cellular components. Even after leukoreduction, there are enough residual T lymphocytes left in the PRBCs to potentially cause transfusion-associated graft versus host disease (TA-GVHD). The risk of TA-GVHD is especially concerning when viable donor lymphocytes are transfused into patients with severe cellular immunodeficiency, such as very-low-birth weight infants. Irradiation renders lymphocytes unable to proliferate, thereby reducing the risk that the blood product will cause transfusion-associated graft versus host disease.[66]

## Who should receive irradiated blood products?

The American Association of Blood Banks[66] recommends irradiation for preterm infants $\leq 1200$ grams. Irradiation is also recommended for fetal intrauterine transfusion, exchange transfusion, or if the infant has acquired or congenital immunodeficiency, such as DiGeorge syndrome.[63,64,67] There are additional candidates for irradiated blood products, however, that is beyond the scope of this discussion. Irradiation may not always be practical or possible in all hospital settings, especially if neonatal blood transfusions are infrequently required by the population served at that facility.

*(continued on next page)*

**Clinical Tip** (continued)

⚠ If an emergency blood transfusion is anticipated, (for example, if an emergency c-section for placental abruption is in progress), it is helpful to notify the blood bank ahead of time to request they prepare a unit of irradiated leukoreduced O-negative PRBCs in anticipation the infant may be severely anemic.

**However, do not withhold a life-saving transfusion if:**

a) There is not enough time to perform irradiation; or

b) Irradiation is not performed at that hospital.

Filtering of blood for the purpose of leuko-reduction should always be performed prior to administering blood to an infant.

## Staff Assignment

**Goal:** All staff members will know the process for rapidly accessing blood in an emergency.

Call the blood bank and inquire about the procedure to obtain O-negative packed red blood cells for emergencies in the delivery room or nursery (when cross-matching is not possible). This includes any paperwork that is necessary, whether a written order is required, and who may place the order for the blood (nurses, unit secretary, or physician). Ask whether this emergency supply of blood is available 24-hours per day, whether irradiated blood is available or not, whether the blood filter is sent with the packed red blood cells, and how long it will take to receive emergency blood once it is requested.

## Treatment of Cardiogenic (heart failure) Shock[3,41]

Evaluate the infant for tachycardia, bradycardia, hypotension, oliguria, hypoxemia, acidosis, and hypoglycemia, because these signs may be present when an infant is in cardiogenic shock. Treatment is aimed at correcting the underlying problems that may negatively affect heart function. These include (but are not limited to), hypoxia, hypoglycemia, hypothermia, hypotension, acidosis, arrhythmias, infection, and electrolyte or mineral imbalances.

## Treatment of Septic (distributive) Shock[3,17,41]

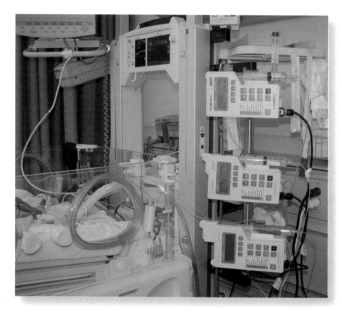

Treatment involves a combination of the therapies used to treat hypovolemic and cardiogenic shock. The septic infant may require more fluid boluses than in other types of shock given the movement of fluid from the intravascular compartment into the interstitial space, or extravascular compartment.[41] This is due to capillary injury as well as pooling of blood in the capillary bed. A continuous drip infusion of dopamine may be necessary to treat severe hypotension. Table 4.3 provides additional information about dopamine and page 212 provides a simple approach to mixing dopamine and selecting an infusion rate if a pharmacist is not available. It is critically important to optimize oxygenation and ventilation when treating septic shock.

## Clinical Tip

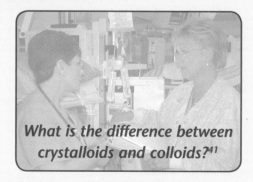

*What is the difference between crystalloids and colloids?*[41]

Crystalloid solutions, such as normal saline and Lactated Ringer's, are isotonic and contain water and electrolytes. They pass easily through semi-permeable membranes and therefore stay in the intravascular (circulating) compartment for shorter periods of time than colloids.

Advantages of crystalloid solutions are that they are readily available for the immediate treatment of shock, they require no special compatibility testing, they do not produce sensitivity reactions, they are inexpensive, and there are no religious objections to their use.

Colloid solutions have a large molecular weight and do not pass easily through semi-permeable membranes. Therefore, they stay in the intravascular (circulating) compartment longer than crystalloids. Colloid solutions include plasma protein, albumin, and synthetic colloid solutions such as Plasmanate®. The disadvantages of colloids include sensitivity reactions, their increased expense, and the need for compatibility testing (in some cases), before they can be administered.

# Medications Used to Treat Cardiogenic and Septic Shock

## Normal Saline (NS) 0.9%[41]

**Indications:** Volume infusion, to improve preload (circulating blood volume)

**Dose:** The dose recommendations are the same as for hypovolemic shock: 10 mL/kg per dose

**Route:** IV, UVC, Intraosseous

## Sodium Bicarbonate 4.2% solution (0.5 mEq/mL)

**Indications:** To treat severe metabolic acidosis (arterial pH is < 7.15)

**Contraindications:** Inadequate ventilation (see the caution below)

**Dose:** 1 to 2 milliequivalent per kilogram per dose (1 to 2 mEq/kg/dose)
When the 4.2% solution is used, this equals 2 to 4 mL/kg/dose

**Route:** Give over 30 to 60 minutes IV

---

Note:

The use of sodium bicarbonate to treat metabolic acidosis is controversial.[69,70] Research is lacking regarding the safety and efficacy of using this medication to treat infants with metabolic acidosis.[71] Therefore, it may be helpful to consult the transport control physician or tertiary center neonatologist to discuss whether sodium bicarbonate is indicated. Most important is to identify the potential causes of metabolic acidosis and institute appropriate corrective therapies.

 Sodium bicarbonate is a hypertonic solution and if given too rapidly may lead to intraventricular hemorrhage in preterm infants.[72] In addition, the infant must be adequately ventilated when sodium bicarbonate is administered or the acidosis will worsen because of an acute increase in $CO_2$ as the bicarbonate is metabolized.[73]

## Dopamine Hydrochloride[3,72,74]

**Indications:**      Poor cardiac contractility

**Dose:**      5 to 20 micrograms per kg per minute (mcg/kg/minute)

**Route:**      IV continuous infusion (IV pump)

 Do not give via any arterial route (umbilical or peripheral artery) or through an endotracheal tube.

**Table 4.3.** Dopamine dose and effect.[9]

| Dosage | Receptors | Effect |
|---|---|---|
| 0.5 to 2 mcg/kg/min | Dopaminergic (stimulation of dopaminergic receptors) | Renal and mesenteric vasodilatation; little effect on blood pressure |
| 2-10 mcg/kg/min | Beta-adrenergic (beta$_1$ receptors activated) | Increase in cardiac output and systolic blood pressure |
| Greater than 10 mcg/kg/min | Alpha-adrenergic (alpha receptors activated) | Vasoconstriction; increased systolic and diastolic blood pressure |

# Dopamine Dosing for Newborns

## How to Calculate a Final Standardized Concentration of 800 Micrograms per mL IV Fluid

In some practice settings, nurses and physicians may have limited experience in administering dopamine. In recognition of this, the S.T.A.B.L.E. Program recommends the use of a final dopamine infusion concentration that is relatively dilute. That dilution is explained in this section. More concentrated solutions are usually provided in the neonatal intensive care unit.

**Step 1:   Select the pre-mixed dopamine solution as described in** Option one, **or mix the solution as described in** Option two.

### Option One

Use this option when a commercially-prepared pre-mixed dopamine drip solution with a final concentration of 800 micrograms (mcg) per milliliter (mL) in $D_5W$ **IS** available.

- Please note, this solution is mixed in $D_5W$. Monitor the infant's blood glucose closely and adjust the maintenance dextrose infusion (concentration and/or rate) as necessary to maintain a normal blood sugar.

- To determine the appropriate rate, go to Step 2 on page 213. Rules for dopamine infusion may be found on page 214.

- Always administer dopamine using an infusion pump.

### Option Two

Use this option when a commercially prepared pre-mixed dopamine solution IS NOT available.

Mix the dopamine drip as follows:

1. Select a dopamine vial containing dopamine 40 milligrams (mg) per mL.

2. From this vial draw up 5 mL (or 200 mg) of dopamine.

3. Add this amount (5 mL or 200 mg of dopamine) to a 250 mL bag of $D_{10}W$.

4. This will provide a dopamine concentration of 800 mcg per mL of IV fluid (or 200 mg per 250 mL IV fluid).

5. Label the IV bag with the following: This 250 mL bag of $D_{10}W$ contains 800 mcg dopamine per mL IV fluid.

6. Always administer dopamine using an infusion pump.

## Step 2:   Using the graph, select the infusion rate.

1. Find the **patient's weight** in the first column marked **Weight in kg**. Round up or down as needed if the weight is in between the 0.5 kilogram increments.

2. Read across the row to the ordered infusion dose in mcg/kg/min.

3. Result = infusion pump setting in **mL/hr**.

> ⚠ Double check all calculations and reconstitution with another nurse or physician before administering dopamine to the infant.

| Weight In kg | 5 mcg/kg/min | 7.5 mcg/kg/min | 10 mcg/kg/min | 12.5 mcg/kg/min | 15 mcg/kg/min | 17.5 mcg/kg/min | 20 mcg/kg/min |
|---|---|---|---|---|---|---|---|
| **Ordered Dose  (mcg/kg/min)** — Using a dopamine solution containing 800 mcg per mL of IV fluid | | | | | | | |
| 0.5 kg | 0.2 mL/hr | 0.3 mL/hr | 0.4 mL/hr | 0.5 mL/hr | 0.6 mL/hr | 0.7 mL/hr | 0.8 mL/hr |
| 1 kg | 0.4 mL/hr | 0.6 mL/hr | 0.8 mL/hr | 1 mL/hr | 1.1 mL/hr | 1.3 mL/hr | 1.5 mL/hr |
| 1.5 kg | 0.6 mL/hr | 0.8 mL/hr | 1.1 mL/hr | 1.4 mL/hr | 1.7 mL/hr | 2 mL/hr | 2.3 mL/hr |
| 2 kg | 0.8 mL/hr | 1.1 mL/hr | 1.5 mL/hr | 1.9 mL/hr | 2.3 mL/hr | 2.6 mL/hr | 3 mL/hr |
| 2.5 kg | 1 mL/hr | 1.4 mL/hr | 1.9 mL/hr | 2.3 mL/hr | 2.8 mL/hr | 3.3 mL/hr | 3.8 mL/hr |
| 3 kg | 1.1 mL/hr | 1.7 mL/hr | 2.3 mL/hr | 2.8 mL/hr | 3.4 mL/hr | 3.9 mL/hr | 4.5 mL/hr |
| 3.5 kg | 1.3 mL/hr | 2 mL/hr | 2.6 mL/hr | 3.3 mL/hr | 3.9 mL/hr | 4.6 mL/hr | 5.3 mL/hr |
| 4 kg | 1.5 mL/hr | 2.3 mL/hr | 3 mL/hr | 3.8 mL/hr | 4.5 mL/hr | 5.3 mL/hr | 6 mL/hr |
| 4.5 kg | 1.7 mL/hr | 2.5 mL/hr | 3.4 mL/hr | 4.2 mL/hr | 5.1 mL/hr | 5.9 mL/hr | 6.8 mL/hr |
| 5 kg | 1.9 mL/hr | 2.8 mL/hr | 3.8 mL/hr | 4.7 mL/hr | 5.6 mL/hr | 6.6 mL/hr | 7.5 mL/hr |

Note: some rounding has occurred to simplify the infusion rate.

**If a pre-mixed dopamine solution is not available,** place the following items in a plastic bag or container and keep with emergency medications:

        250 mL bag of $D_{10}W$

        5 mL syringe

        Dopamine hydrochloride 40 mg/mL solution (5 ml vial  = 200 mg)

        This instructional information

# Rules for Dopamine Infusion

1. In most cases, volume boluses are administered before it is determined that dopamine is necessary.[41]

2. The starting dose for dopamine should be selected based on the infant's clinical status and reason for hypotension. Dopamine is usually started at 5 mcg/kg/minute and can be increased (or decreased) by 2.5 mcg/kg/minute as shown in the infusion graph on page 213.

   Note: In many neonatal intensive care units, dopamine is mixed to yield a more concentrated solution than presented in this module, and the rate of increase (or decrease) is usually limited to 1 mcg/kg/minute, each time the rate is changed.

3. Monitor the blood pressure and heart rate every 1 to 2 minutes for 15 minutes then every 2 to 5 minutes depending upon response to the medication. If an infant is failing to respond to a dose of 20 mcg/kg/minute, then increasing the dose further is not recommended.

- Never infuse dopamine, or any vasoconstrictor medication through any arterial site including the umbilical artery catheter or peripheral arterial line.

- Infuse dopamine on an infusion pump and to increase safety, use "smart pump" technology whenever possible.

- **Do not flush** dopamine or lines containing dopamine, as this will cause the blood pressure to surge up and the heart rate to abruptly slow down.

4. Since IV infiltration may lead to tissue sloughing and necrosis, it is recommended that dopamine be administered through a central venous line whenever possible.

- Administer via an umbilical venous catheter (UVC) if the catheter's position has been confirmed by chest x-ray and the tip is appropriately located above the liver at the inferior vena cava/right atrial junction; or, administer via a peripherally inserted central catheter (PICC).

- If no central venous access is available, infuse dopamine through a peripheral IV.

- If infused through a peripheral IV, monitor the infusion site closely. If infiltration occurs, and there is concern that dermal necrosis may develop, be prepared to treat the area with a subcutaneous injection of a saline solution containing phentolamine mesylate.[72,75]

## Practice Session: Dopamine rate

**A dopamine standardized concentration of 800 mcg per mL IV fluid has been prepared.**

Using the infusion graph on page 213 answer the follow questions:

1. A dose of 10 mcg/kg/minute of dopamine is ordered for a 3.8 kg infant.
   What infusion rate will this infant require? _____

2. A dose of 5 mcg/kg/minute of dopamine is ordered for a 1.4 kg infant.
   What infusion rate will this infant require? _____

# APPENDIX 4.1  Scalp Swellings: Caput Succedaneum, Cephalohematoma, Subgaleal Hemorrhage

Scalp swelling is a common finding in newborn infants. It is important to know the features of three types of swelling: caput succedaneum, cephalohematoma, and subgaleal hemorrhage, so that appropriate observation and management may be provided. In addition, parents may be concerned about the appearance of their infant's scalp. Being knowledgeable about the various types of swelling will allow you to offer words of reassurance as well as education about how long it will take for the swelling to resolve.

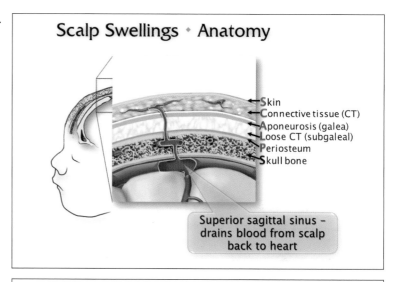

## Caput succedaneum

Following birth, molding of the head with concurrent swelling of the soft tissues of the scalp may be observed.[76] With caput succedaneum, swelling is superficial (extraperiosteal) and it recedes relatively quickly.[77] The swelling is composed of serosanguineous fluid that is usually limited to the region of the scalp that was the presenting part.[78] Because of its location, the edema may cross suture lines and it may be dependent. This means, as the infant's position changes, the swelling may shift. Bruising may be noted in the area of swelling and it is important to differentiate caput succedaneum from cephalohematoma, and from subgaleal hemorrhage, since all three may appear similarly at first. It is important to know however, that subgaleal hemorrhage, which is described further in this appendix, may extend rapidly, and lead to hypovolemic shock (hypotension, severe anemia, and altered level of consciousness). If subgaleal hemorrhage is not treated expeditiously, the risk of dying increases.[78]

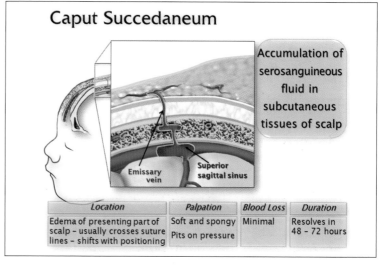

| Location | Palpation | Blood Loss | Duration |
|---|---|---|---|
| Edema of presenting part of scalp – usually crosses suture lines – shifts with positioning | Soft and spongy Pits on pressure | Minimal | Resolves in 48 - 72 hours |

# APPENDIX 4.1 Scalp Swellings: Caput Succedaneum, Cephalohematoma, Subgaleal Hemorrhage
(continued)

## Cephalohematoma

The periosteum is a membrane of fibrous connective tissue that wraps around bone. A hemorrhage that occurs under the periosteum of the skull (subperiosteal) is called a cephalohematoma.[77,79] The periosteum limits extension of the hemorrhage; therefore, the area of swelling will not cross suture lines. Often the hemorrhage feels firm and 85% of the time, the swelling is unilateral; 15% of the time bilateral cephalohematoma occurs. There is an occasional association of skull fracture, including depressed skull fracture, therefore additional testing such as a skull x-ray or CT scan may be indicated.[77] In rare cases, the bleeding can be severe enough to cause anemia. Usually a cephalohematoma will resolve within 2 to 12 weeks.[79]

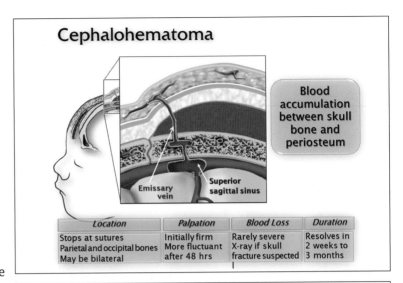

### Cephalohematoma

Blood accumulation between skull bone and periosteum

Emissary vein

Superior sagittal sinus

| Location | Palpation | Blood Loss | Duration |
| --- | --- | --- | --- |
| Stops at sutures Parietal and occipital bones May be bilateral | Initially firm More fluctuant after 48 hrs | Rarely severe X-ray if skull fracture suspected | Resolves in 2 weeks to 3 months |

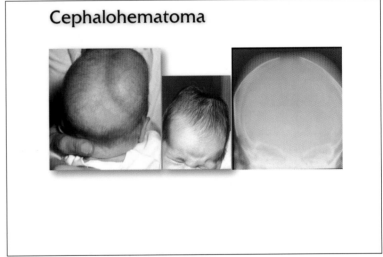

### Cephalohematoma

## Subgaleal hemorrhage

Venous return of blood from the scalp to the heart is via the scalp veins to the emissary veins to the dural sinuses, to the heart.[77] Rupture of the emissary veins can occur during a vacuum assist delivery secondary to the traction force applied, or as a consequence of pop-offs during vacuum assist delivery.[77] Subgaleal hemorrhage occurs when the emissary veins rupture and bleed into the subaponeurotic space which is located above the periosteum.[76,80,81] Unlike cephalohematoma, which has the periosteum to limit the spread of bleeding, there is no barrier to stop the bleeding, therefore, subgaleal hemorrhage can be massive.

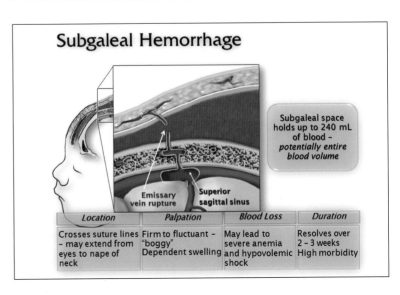

### Subgaleal Hemorrhage

Subgaleal space holds up to 240 mL of blood – potentially entire blood volume

Emissary vein rupture

Superior sagittal sinus

| Location | Palpation | Blood Loss | Duration |
| --- | --- | --- | --- |
| Crosses suture lines – may extend from eyes to nape of neck | Firm to fluctuant – "boggy" Dependent swelling | May lead to severe anemia and hypovolemic shock | Resolves over 2 – 3 weeks High morbidity |

APPENDIX 4.1 **Scalp Swellings: Caput Succedaneum, Cephalohematoma, Subgaleal Hemorrhage** (continued)

## Risk Factors for Subgaleal Hemorrhage

When a vaginal delivery is assisted by vacuum extraction or forceps, it is called an "operative vaginal delivery."[82,83] There are important specific indications for maternal and fetal candidacy for operative vaginal delivery, as well as guidelines for when it is safe to apply the vacuum or forceps, how to perform the procedure correctly, how many pop-offs should be permitted, how many minutes the procedure should be allowed to continue and importantly, when to abandon the attempt.[81] It should be noted that pop-offs are most often the result of an improperly placed cup and the more pop-offs there are, the risk for scalp injury is increased.[77,81,84] To prevent unplanned and unwanted injury to the mother and/or infant, it is important that obstetric caregivers observe standards of care regarding operative vaginal delivery.[84] When an operative vaginal delivery is performed, neonatal caregivers should be made aware so they may provide the appropriate assessment and monitoring for complications.[77] Especially if the procedure met with difficulty, the neonatal caregivers should be notified so that an appropriate monitoring guideline may be activated.[85]

Because there is no requirement for mandatory medical error reporting in the United States, the incidence of subgaleal hemorrhage is likely under-reported and under-appreciated. One estimate by the American College of Obstetricians and Gynecologists is that subgaleal hemorrhage occurs in 26 to 45 of every 1000 vacuum-assisted deliveries.[86] Another large study by Towner[87] reported subgaleal hemorrhage occurred in 1 in 860 vacuum-assisted deliveries compared with 1 in 1900 spontaneous vaginal deliveries. However, when vacuum and forceps were both used, the incidence was markedly increased; 1 in 280 deliveries.[87] Therefore, inspection of the scalp after a vacuum-assist delivery should include evidence of any apparent injury, lacerations, location and degree of swelling, bruising, and where the vacuum marks are located. An improperly applied cup increases the risk for scalp injury and/or subgaleal hemorrhage.[81,84,88,89] Following operative vaginal delivery, blood may also accumulate in other regions in the brain: subdural, subarachnoid, intraparenchymal, and intraventricular spaces.[77]

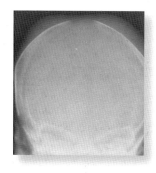
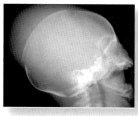
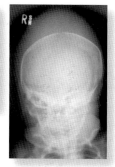

Skull x-ray of an infant with bilateral cephalohematoma (top) and subgaleal hemorrhage (bottom two x-rays). Notice the blood is limited to the subperiosteal space with cephalohematoma, but diffusely located in the scalp with subgaleal hemorrhage

# APPENDIX 4.1 **Scalp Swellings: Caput Succedaneum, Cephalohematoma, Subgaleal Hemorrhage**
(continued)

The subgaleal space is estimated to hold as much as 240 to 260 mL of blood. That amount of blood would be the entire blood volume of a 3 kilogram infant.[76,79] The scalp aponeurosis extends all the way from the orbits of the eyes to the nape of the neck. One characteristic finding of subgaleal hemorrhage is the lateral spreading of edema toward the ears, which may displace the ears anteriorly (shown in photo). Swelling around the eyes is also present in some cases.[78] A fluid wave may also be observed when pressing on the edematous scalp. Knowing this anatomy is helpful because inspection of the scalp that reveals swelling in these regions is significant.[79] Treatment of subgaleal hemorrhage may include any or all of the following to treat anemia, stop the bleeding and restore the blood pressure: PRBCs, fresh frozen plasma, platelets, cryoprecipitate, normal saline volume infusions, and dopamine.[78]

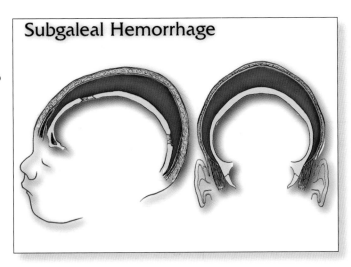
Subgaleal Hemorrhage

## Risk factors associated with development of SGH after vacuum-assisted delivery (VAD)[81,88,90-92] includes:

- Nulliparous mother

- Failed vacuum extraction

- Inadvertent cup release (pop-offs)

- Sequential use of vacuum and forceps

- Apgar score less than 8 at five minutes following vacuum assist delivery

- Deflexing cup application (edge of the cup application less than 3 cm from the anterior fontanel)

- Paramedian cup application (cup centered more than one centimeter lateral to the sagittal suture)

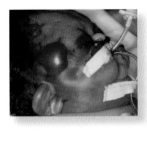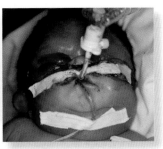

Infant with severe subgaleal hemorrhage. The infant required numerous blood product transfusions to stabilize. The infant's outcome is unknown.

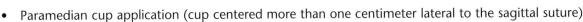

# Appendix 4.2 **It Isn't Just the Lungs: A Case Presentation**

## Case Study · Baby Boy Doe

- 15 year old, G1, P1 – 29 weeks gestation
- Double-footling breech presentation at Level I facility → unsafe to transport mother
- Fetal heart rate 140 – good variability
- SROM at delivery – normal volume, color, odor
- Precipitous delivery – 1200 gm male
- APGAR $1^1$, $7^5$
- Heart rate 60 despite tactile stimulation
  - Bag/mask ventilation with 100% $O_2$
  - Chest compressions
  - Intubated with 2.0 ET tube at 3 minutes of life → HR increased to 120

From Lynam L. (1992) *Neonatal Network, 11:3*

slide 1

## Case Study · Baby Boy Doe

- Umbilical venous catheter placed
  - $D_{10}W$ 80 mL/kg/day
- Blood cultures drawn
  - Ampicillin and gentamicin given IV
- 25 minutes of life → respiratory therapist providing ET – positive pressure ventilation (PPV) to keep $O_2$ saturation 90 – 100%
  - Rate, pressures not documented
- Chest X-ray
  - Severe respiratory distress syndrome
  - ET tube on carina → repositioned

From Lynam L. (1992) *Neonatal Network, 11:3*

slide 2

## Case Study · Baby Boy Doe

- 35 minutes of life → transport requested
- 2.5 hours of life → transport team arrived
- NNP – RN team configuration
- Nurse & respiratory therapist were with the baby
  - Physician had been called away to another emergency

From Lynam L. (1992) *Neonatal Network, 11:3*

slide 3

## Case Study · Baby Boy Doe

- Nurse reported no significant events prior to team arrival except physician unable to obtain arterial blood gas before being called away → acid base status undocumented
- Infant still in delivery room on radiant warmer, covered by sterile drape
  - Warmer on manual control → changed from servo because of 'frequent alarms'

From Lynam L. (1992) *Neonatal Network, 11:3*

slide 4

## Case Study · Baby Boy Doe

- ET tube – PPV given by respiratory therapist
- Vital signs last obtained 1 hour prior to team arrival
- Vital signs / blood sugar upon team arrival
  - Axillary temperature 31.5°C (88.7°F)
  - Heart rate "within normal limits"
  - Blood pressure – would not register
  - Bedside blood sugar by Dextrostix® 40 – 80

From Lynam L. (1992) *Neonatal Network, 11:3*

slide 5

## Case Study · Baby Boy Doe

***Transport team actions***
- Reviewed chest x-ray
- Replaced 2.0 ET tube with 3.0 mm ET tube
- Placed on transport ventilator → PIP 22, PEEP 5, rate 60, inspiratory time 0.4, 100% oxygen
  - Right radial blood gas 10 minutes later → pH 7.38, $PCO_2$ 19.7, $PO_2$ 151, $HCO_3$ 11.4
  - Actions: PIP ↓ 20, Rate ↓ 40, Oxygen ↓ 95%
- Administered surfactant
- Infant taken to see mother; infant's condition discussed

From Lynam L. (1992) *Neonatal Network, 11:3*

slide 6

# Appendix 4.2 **It Isn't Just the Lungs: A Case Presentation**
(continued)

## Case Study · Baby Boy Doe

- Team arrival to departure time = 40 minutes
- Vital signs and exam upon departure:
  - T 31.7°C (89°F), heart rate 136, RR 40, BP still would not register
  - Lethargic, mucous membranes pink, color pallid, PMI non-displaced, femoral pulses +1/4, brachial and radial pulses not palpable, extensive bruising lower extremities, capillary refill time 6 seconds
- Labs:
  - Plasma glucose 67 mg/dL
  - CBC: WBC 8,200, Hgb 14, Hct 39.6, platelets 218,000, neutrophils 22%, lymphocytes 64%

From Lynam L, (1992) *Neonatal Network, 11:3*

slide 7

## Case Study · Baby Boy Doe

- 16 minutes after departure from hospital, heart rate dropped to 60 bpm
- Breath sounds ↓ on left side (team concerned this could be a pneumothorax)
- Paramedic asked to turn around and return to referral community hospital
- Resuscitation enroute back to hospital:
  - 100% oxygen
  - Epinephrine x 3 via UVC
  - Needle aspiration chest → no air obtained
  - Chest compressions for 13 minutes until heart rate > 100 bpm

From Lynam L, (1992) *Neonatal Network, 11:3*

slide 8

## Case Study · Baby Boy Doe

- Arrived back in emergency room
- Chest x-ray → severe RDS, no pneumothorax
- Right radial ABG: pH 7.06, $PCO_2$ 42, $PO_2$ 99, $HCO_3$ 11.8
- Peripheral IV inserted → $NaHCO_3$ 2.4 mEq given
- UAC inserted
  - 20 minutes later, ABG: pH 7.00, $PCO_2$ 81, $PO_2$ 11, $HCO_3$ 20, $SaO_2$ 12%
- *Baby died shortly after blood gas obtained*

From Lynam L, (1992) *Neonatal Network, 11:3*

slide 9

## Case Study · Baby Boy Doe

*Discussion:*
- What other actions could have been taken by the transport team <u>before</u> departure?
- What was the source of hypotension and lethargy? Was it:
  - Fulminant sepsis?
  - Perinatal asphyxia?
  - Hypothermia?
- What was the cause of death?

From Lynam L, (1992) *Neonatal Network, 11:3*

slide 10

## Case Study · Baby Boy Doe

**Dr. Lynam's assessment:**

*"Closer inspection of both the initial arterial blood gas .....and subsequent blood gas results obtained after deterioration of the infant made it obvious that a profound primary metabolic acidosis was present"*

From Lynam L, (1992) *Neonatal Network, 11:3*

slide 11

# It Isn't Just the Lungs:
## A Case Presentation

*Lynn E. Lynam, RNC, MS, NNP*

CONTRIBUTING EDITOR

*When I began this column last year, I promised to try to use it as a forum to get back to the basics and present interesting case studies. This article represents my first attempt to combine those goals. The following true case occurred during the transport of a critically ill neonate to a Level III East Coast facility. The patient's name has been changed for legal protection of that facility.*

M s Long, a 15-year-old, gravida 1, para 0, black teen, delivered a 29-week 1,200-gm male fetus precipitously from a double-footling breech presentation shortly after her arrival at a Level I obstetrical facility. Just prior to delivery, the fetal heart rate had been assessed at 140 beats per minute with excellent variability. Amniotic membranes ruptured at delivery, and the fluid was noted to be normal in volume, color, and odor.

On initial physical assessment, the neonate's heart rate was auscultated at 60 beats per minute despite vigorous tactile stimulation and oropharyngeal suctioning. Hence, bag-mask ventilation with 100 percent oxygen and chest compressions were initiated, followed by successful endotracheal intubation with a 2.0 endotracheal tube by three minutes of life. The infant's heart rate increased to 120 almost immediately, and no further resuscitative efforts were necessary. Apgars were 1 and 7 at one and five minutes, respectively. A 10 percent dextrose infusion was started via an umbilical venous catheter at 80 cc/kg/day. After obtaining blood specimens for culture and hematologic analysis, ampicillin and gentamicin were administered intravenously.

By 25 minutes of life, the infant's oxygen saturation by pulse oximetry was consistently in the 90-100 percent range as long as a respiratory therapist delivered positive pressure ventilation to the endotracheal tube with an anesthesia bag. The initial chest x-ray film showed that the endotracheal tube was positioned at the carina and that the infant had severe respiratory distress syndrome. No other cardiorespiratory abnormalities were appreciated. After the endotracheal tube was repositioned at 35 minutes of life, a referral call was placed to the tertiary care facility requesting transport services.

When the transport team (neonatal nurse practitioner and nurse) arrived, the two and a half hour old premature infant was found lying in an open radiant warming bed located in the same room where he had been born, loosely covered by a sterile drape. The circulating nurse and respiratory therapist were present, but the referring pediatrician had been called away to another emergency.

They reported that no significant problems had occurred since the initial telephone call except for the attending physician being unsuccessful in obtaining an arterial blood gas before being called away. Hence, the infant's acid base status was undocumented. The transport nurse found that the circulating nurse had removed the bed's temperature sensor from skin contact because of "frequent alarms" and placed the bed on manual control mode.

Because almost an hour had elapsed since the last vital signs assessment, the transport nurse promptly obtained them. The infant's axillary temperature measured 88.7°F, and his blood pressure would not register on a noninvasive monitor. The Dextrostix measurement was 40-80. His other vital signs were within the expected normal range for his weight and gestational age.

After reviewing the chest x-ray examination, the transport team elected to replace the 2.0 endotracheal tube with a 3.0 and to administer exogenous surfactant. Baby Long was then placed on a transport ventilator set at the following parameters: PIP 22, PEEP 5, IMV 60, I-time 0.4 seconds, $FiO_2$ 100 percent.

The following blood gas values were obtained from a right radial artery specimen ten minutes later: pH 7.38, $PCO_2$ 19.7, $PO_2$ 151, bicarbonate 11.4, oxygen saturation 100 percent. Based on these values, the PIP was decreased to 20, the IMV was decreased to 40 breaths and the $FiO_2$ was decreased to 95 percent.

After visiting briefly with Ms. Long and discussing the infant's condition with her, the transport team left the referring hospital. Arrival time to departure time was 40 minutes. Vital signs and physical examination on departure from the referring hospital were recorded as follows:

Vital signs: Temperature 89°F, pulse rate 136, respiratory rate 40. Dextrostix had increased to 180; blood pressure continued to be nonrecordable.

Maternal medical history: No recollection of serious childhood illness. Denied personal drug or alcohol use, although the baby's father had been recently jailed for selling and dis-tributing cocaine. Ms. Long had had no contact with him for the last four months. There was no familial history of congenital anomalies, and the mother could not recall any exposure to communicable diseases during her pregnancy.

General: Length 39 cm, head circumference 27 cm, weight 1,200 gm. No obvious anomalies. Abundant lanugo. Skin turgor fair. Color pallid.

Head, eyes, ears, nose, throat: Normocephalic. Anterior fontanel open, flat, soft. Posterior fontanel not appreciated. Sutures overlapping. Pupils sluggishly reactive. Red reflex elicited. Pinna aligned above eye-occiput line with slow recoil. Nares patent without drainage. Palate intact. Mucous membranes pink. Neck supple without masses.

Chest: Clear to auscultation. Point of maximal impulse nondisplaced. Nipples visualized. No palpable areolar tissue.

Cardiovascular: Regular rate and rhythm without murmur. Femoral pulses +1/4. Brachial and radial puls-es not appreciated. Capillary refill 6 seconds.

Gastrointestinal: Soft, nontender, nondistended abdomen. No organomegaly. Absent bowel sounds. Anus grossly patent.

Extremities: All digits present. No sacral dimples or hair tufts. Hip check deferred. Full range of motion. Extensive bruising of lower extremities.

Neurological: Lethargic. Absent Moro reflex. Weak gag and palmar reflexes Intact plantar and Babinski reflexes.

Laboratory data: CBC: hemoglobin 14.1; hematocrit 39.6; WBC 8,200; platelets 218,000; neutrophils 22 percent; lymphocytes 64 percent; monocytes 12 percent; eosinophils 1 percent; basophils 1 percent. Glucose: 67 mg/dL.

Approximately 16 minutes after departing from the referring hospital, the infant's heart rate dropped precipitously to 60. The $FiO_2$ was immediately increased to 100 percent, and the infant's chest was auscultated. Decreased breath sounds were heard on the left side. Slight tension was placed on the endotracheal tube, and resusci-tation was initiated. The ambulance driver was instructed to return immed-iately to the referring hospital.

After 30 seconds, no improvement was observed, so 0.3 cc epinephrine 1:10,000 was given via the umbilical venous line. Because decreased breath sounds continued to be heard over the left chest, a 25-gauge butterfly needle was placed in the left, anterior second intercostal space at the midclavicular line. No air was obtained. Resuscitation continued, and two subsequent doses of epinephrine were given per AHA-AAP guidelines for neonatal resuscitation.

Chest compressions were halted 13 minutes into the code when the infant's

heart rate reached 100. A chest x-ray film in the referring hospital emergency room showed no evidence of pneumothorax and was essentially unchanged from the previous film—severe respiratory distress syndrome persisted. A right radial arterial blood gas specimen was profoundly acidotic: pH 7.06, $PCO_2$ 41.8, $PO_2$ 98.9, bicarbonate 11.8, oxygen saturation 97 percent.

A peripheral catheter was placed in the left antecubital vein, and 2.4 mEq sodium bicarbonate was infused while an umbilical artery catheter was inserted. The repeat arterial blood gas 20 minutes after the infusion demonstrated a worsening situation: pH 7.00, $PCO_2$ 80.5, $PO_2$ 11.5, bicarbonate 19.9, oxygen saturation 12 percent. Despite aggressive ventilatory and pharmacologic maneuvers, the neonate expired soon thereafter.

## What Is Your Assessment?

In a premature neonate with the history just presented, consideration must be given to the following possible clinical problems: (1) severe respiratory distress syndrome, (2) sepsis, (3) perinatal asphyxia, and (4) other.

Many clues were offered that lead to the conclusion that Baby Long had severe respiratory distress syndrome. Not only were several perinatal risk factors for the disease present, including prematurity and male gender, but factors likely to acutely impair surfactant production, release, or function (possible perinatal asphyxia and precipitous delivery) could also be identified.[1,2] Furthermore, in the postnatal period, the chest x-ray examination demonstrated the classic radiographic appearance of low-volume lungs with a reticulogranular pattern and air bronchograms.[3]

The keys to successful management of neonates with respiratory distress syndrome are (1) to prevent hypoxemia and acidemia in order to optimize endogenous surfactant production, (2) to reduce metabolic demands so as to minimize oxygen requirements and carbon dioxide production, (3) to improve lung function, and (4) to minimize barotrauma.[2,3] In this case, it seemed that early implementation of mechanical ventilation and appropriate use of an exogenous surfactant preparation were initially effective in accomplishing these goals, as evidenced by the first arterial blood gas results. However, the acute clinical deterioration that occurred during transport after surfactant administration, made it necessary for the team to look for other, concomitant problems.

Because decreased breath sounds were heard over the left chest and because some infants respond rapidly to surfactant replacement therapy with improved lung compliance and subsequent pneumothorax, the initial therapeutic goal was to rule out this possibility. As noted, neither direct needle aspiration nor radiograph supported this hypothesis. Closer inspection of both the initial arterial blood gas results obtained before surfactant administration and transport and subsequent blood gas results ob-tained after deterioration of the infant made it obvious that a profound primary metabolic acidosis was present. Respiratory compensation with mechanical ventilation had all but obscured it on the first blood gas results. What was the source? Why was the infant hypotensive and lethargic?

The possibility of fulminant septic shock should always be considered in the preterm infant who deteriorates suddenly with severe metabolic acidosis, signs of systemic hypoperfusion, unex-plained lethargy, and intractable hypotension.[4] Because initial clinical signs of septic shock are commonly sub-tle and nonspecific, a high index of sus-picion, a thorough investigation, and prompt initiation of appropriate treat-ment are essential to improve the outcome. Although not discounted at the time of clinical deterioration, maternal history suggested no clues, and the leukocyte or differential counts revealed no abnormalities. Blood cultures subsequently proved negative by 72 hours postmortem and discounted septic shock as the etiology of the metabolic acidosis.

Perinatal asphyxia should also be considered as a possible etiology of the metabolic acidosis and central nervous system depression, especially in the face of prematurity and a breech presentation.[5] However, because the fetal heart rate and beat-to-beat variability did not seem to be compromised prior to the birth and appropriate resuscitative mea-sures, including prompt assisted ventila-tion, were initiated at delivery, it was unlikely that perinatal asphyxia was the overriding problem for Baby Long. Additionally, although the infant did present in a breech manner, delivery occurred in an uncomplicated fashion, and the Apgar scores did not reflect ongoing perinatal depression.

FIGURE 1 • The effects of cooling

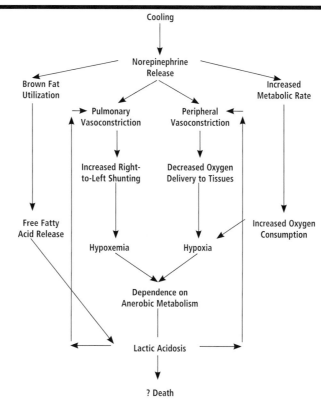

That leaves the dreaded "other" category to be considered. According to AHA-AAP guidelines, one of the cardinal initial steps after delivery involves preventing heat loss by placing the infant under a radiant heat source and drying off the amniotic fluid.[6] These steps become even more crucial for the premature neonate who is compromised by decreased amounts of subcutaneous fat to act as insulation against the cold, reduced amounts of mitochodria-enriched brown fat to serve as a heat source, increased surface area/body weight ratio from which to lose heat, and compromised oxygen resources due to immature lungs.[7]

The recommended interventions eliminate potential radiant and conductive losses of body heat and minimize evaporative losses.[8] Undoubtedly, the initial stabilization measures at the referring hospital included these cardinal steps. Retrospectively though, it became obvious that further heat losses were not or could not be prevented, as evidenced by the axillary temperature of 88.7°F at two and a half hours of life. As Figure 1 suggests, this cold stress had the potential to significantly complicate the infant's respiratory status by the time of the final blood gas results and probably was an important contributing factor leading to his demise.

Conclusion

It is a sad fact that in 1992, infants continue to die of hypothermia more than 30 years after Dr. W.A. Silverman and his colleagues described its effects on morbidity and mortality.[9] This case study represents one of two cases of documented intractable hypothermia encountered by the aforementioned transport team during the last year. Because it is not an uncommon problem, nurses must recognize the danger signs and symptoms of hypothermia, including pallid skin, cyanotic extremities, poor tissue perfusion, central nervous system depression, metabolic acidosis, alterations in glucose homeostasis, and compromised respiratory function.[7,8]

More important is preventing this complication by using common sense. Because heat loss cannot occur in the absence of a thermal gradient, it is essential to avoid exposing the baby to a cold environment by warming the environment (delivery room or nursery) to avoid radiant and conductive losses, by covering the baby with a clear plastic sheet or acrylic heat shield to minimize evaporative losses in a radiant bed, and by using equipment properly. A radiant warmer provides free access to infants who require frequent unimpeded procedures. It allows these procedures to be performed with minimal changes in an infant's skin temperature—as long as the temperature probe is firmly attached to the infant's skin and the heat source is not blocked by drapes or other unnecessary paraphernalia. Finally the value of frequent vital signs assessments in the first hours of life cannot be overemphasized.

## REFERENCES

1. Farrel PM, and ME Avery. 1975. Hyaline membrane disease. *American Review of Respiratory Diseases* 111: 657-688.
2. Liley HG, and AR Stark. 1991. Respiratory distress syndrome/hyaline membrane disease. In *Manual of Neonatal Care*, ed. JP Cloherty and AR Stark, 189-195. Boston: Little, Brown.
3. Martin RJ, MH Klaus, and AA Fanaroff. 1986. Respiratory problems. In *Care of the High Risk Neonate*, ed. MH Klaus and AA Fanaroff, 171-201. Philadelphia: WB Saunders.
4. Laurenti F. 1990. Granulocyte transfusion. In *Current Therapy in Neonatal-Perinatal Medicine*, ed. NM Nelson, 427-430. Philadelphia: BC Decker.
5. Phibbs R. 1990. Delivery room management of the newborn. In *Neonatology: Pathophysiology and Management of the Newborn*, ed. GB Avery, 212-231. Philadelphia: JB Lippincott.
6. Bloom RS, and C Cropley 1987. *Textbook of Neonatal Resuscitation.* Elk Grove: American Heart Association/ American Academy of Pediatrics.
7. Washington S. 1978. Temperature control of the neonate. *Nursing Clinics of North America* 13: 23-28.
8. Perlstein P. 1987. The thermal environment: Temperature and survival. In *Neonatal-Perinatal Medicine: Diseases of the Fetus and Infant,* ed. AA Fanaroff and RH Martin, 398-416. St. Louis: CV Mosby.
9. Silverman WA, JW Fertig, and AP Berger. 1958. The influence of thermal environment upon the survival of newly born premature infants. *Pediatrics* 22: 876.

## About the Author

*Lynn E. Lynam is currently employed as a neonatal nurse practitioner at the Medical Center of Delaware in Newark. She received her masters degree in maternal-child nursing from the University of Delaware and her neonatal nurse practitioner certificate from Georgetown University Hospital. She is a member of NAACOG and is president of NANN's Special Interest Group for Advanced Practice in Neonatal Nursing.*

# References

1. Corneli HM. Evaluation, treatment, and transport of pediatric patients with shock. Pediatr Clin North Am 1993;40:303-19.

2. Seri I, Markovitz B. Cardiovascular Compromise in the Newborn Infant. In: Gleason CA, Devaskar SU, eds. Avery's Diseases of the Newborn. 9th ed. Philadelphia: Elsevier Saunders; 2012:714-31.

3. Agrawal PB. Shock. In: Cloherty JP, Eichenwald EC, Hansen AR, Stark AR, eds. Manual of Neonatal Care. 7th ed. Philadelphia: Lippincott, Williams & Wilkins; 2012:463-8.

4. Noori S, Friedlich PS, Seri I. Pathophysiology of Shock in the Fetus and Neonate. In: Polin RA, Fox WW, Abman SH, eds. Fetal and Neonatal Physiology. 4th ed. Philadelphia: Elsevier Saunders; 2011:853-63.

5. Turner DA, Cheifetz IM. Shock. In: Kliegman RM, Stanton BF, St. Geme JW, Schor NF, Behrman RE, eds. Nelson Textbook of Pediatrics. 19th ed. Philadelphia: Elsevier Saunders; 2011:305-14.

6. Dempsey EM, Barrington KJ. Evaluation and treatment of hypotension in the preterm infant. Clin Perinatol 2009;36:75-85.

7. Carcillo JA, Kuch BA, Han YY, et al. Mortality and functional morbidity after use of PALS/APLS by community physicians. Pediatrics 2009;124:500-8.

8. Ng PC, Lee CH, Bnur FL, et al. A double-blind, randomized, controlled study of a "stress dose" of hydrocortisone for rescue treatment of refractory hypotension in preterm infants. Pediatrics 2006;117:367-75.

9. Osborn D, Evans N, Kluckow M. Diagnosis and treatment of low systemic blood flow in preterm infants. NeoReviews 2004;5:e109-e21.

10. Dempsey EM, Barrington KJ. Treating hypotension in the preterm infant: when and with what: a critical and systematic review. J Perinatol 2007;27:469-78.

11. Kluckow M, Evans N. Low superior vena cava flow and intraventricular haemorrhage in preterm infants. Arch Dis Child Fetal Neonatal Ed 2000;82:F188-94.

12. Pellicer A, Valverde E, Elorza MD, et al. Cardiovascular support for low birth weight infants and cerebral hemodynamics: a randomized, blinded, clinical trial. Pediatrics 2005;115:1501-12.

13. Cunningham S, Symon AG, Elton RA, Zhu C, McIntosh N. Intra-arterial blood pressure reference ranges, death and morbidity in very low birthweight infants during the first seven days of life. Early Hum Dev 1999;56:151-65.

14. Allen HD, Phillips JR, Chan DP. History and Physical Examination. In: Allen HD, Clark EB, Gutgesell HP, Driscoll DJ, eds. Moss and Adams' Heart Disease in Infants, Children, and Adolescents. 6th ed. Philadelphia: Lippincott, Williams & Wilkins; 2001:143-52.

15. Van Hare GF. Neonatal Arrhythmias. In: Martin RJ, Fanaroff AA, Walsh MC, eds. Fanaroff and Martin's Neonatal-Perinatal Medicine: Diseases of the Fetus and Infant. 9th ed. St. Louis: Elsevier Mosby; 2011:1277-89.

16. Chameides L. Part 6: Recognition of Shock. In: Chameides L, Samson RA, Schexnayder SM, Hazinski MF, eds. Pediatric Advanced Life Support Provider Manual. Dallas: American Heart Association; 2011:69-83.

17. Brierley J, Carcillo JA, Choong K, et al. Clinical practice parameters for hemodynamic support of pediatric and neonatal septic shock: 2007 update from the American College of Critical Care Medicine. Crit Care Med 2009;37:666-88.

18. Karlsen KA, Tani LY. S.T.A.B.L.E. Cardiac Module: Recognition and Stabilization of Neonates with Severe CHD. Salt Lake City: S.T.A.B.L.E., Inc.; 2003.

19. Raju NV, Maisels MJ, Kring E, Schwarz-Warner L. Capillary refill time in the hands and feet of normal newborn infants. Clin Pediatr (Phila) 1999;38:139-44.

20. LeFlore JL, Engle WD. Capillary refill time is an unreliable indicator of cardiovascular status in term neonates. Adv Neonatal Care 2005;5:147-54.

21. Miletin J, Pichova K, Dempsey EM. Bedside detection of low systemic flow in the very low birth weight infant on day 1 of life. Eur J Pediatr 2009;168:809-13.

22. Lobos AT, Lee S, Menon K. Capillary refill time and cardiac output in children undergoing cardiac catheterization. Pediatr Crit Care Med 2012;13:136-40.

23. Strozik KS, Pieper CH, Roller J. Capillary refilling time in newborn babies: normal values. Arch Dis Child Fetal Neonatal Ed 1997;76:F193-6.

24. Wodey E, Pladys P, Betremieux P, Kerebel C, Ecoffey C. Capillary refilling time and hemodynamics in neonates: a Doppler echocardiographic evaluation. Crit Care Med 1998;26:1437-40.

25. Gale C. Question 2. Is capillary refill time a useful marker of haemodynamic status in neonates? Arch Dis Child 2010;95:395-7.

26. Chameides L. Part 2: Systematic Approach to the Seriously Ill or Injured Child. In: Chameides L, Samson RA, Schexnayder SM, Hazinski MF, eds. Pediatric Advanced Life Support Provider Manual. Dallas: American Heart Association; 2011:7-29.

27. Versmold HT, Kitterman JA, Phibbs RH, Gregory GA, Tooley WH. Aortic blood pressure during the first 12 hours of life in infants with birth weight 610 to 4,220 grams. Pediatrics 1981;67:607-13.

28. Kitterman JA, Phibbs RH, Tooley WH. Aortic blood pressure in normal newborn infants during the first 12 hours of life. Pediatrics 1969;44:959-68.

29. Chock VY, Wong RJ, Hintz SR, Stevenson DK. Biomedical Engineering Aspects of Neonatal Monitoring. In: Martin RJ, Fanaroff AA, Walsh MC, eds. Fanaroff and Martin's Neonatal-Perinatal Medicine: Diseases of the Fetus and Infant. 9th ed. St. Louis: Elsevier Mosby; 2011:577-95.

30. Nuntnarumit P, Yang W, Bada-Ellzey HS. Blood pressure measurements in the newborn. Clin Perinatol 1999;26:981-96, x.

31. Arafat M, Mattoo TK. Measurement of blood pressure in children: recommendations and perceptions on cuff selection. Pediatrics 1999;104:e30.

32. Pejovic B, Peco-Antic A, Marinkovic-Eric J. Blood pressure in non-critically ill preterm and full-term neonates. Pediatr Nephrol 2007;22:249-57.

33. Bernstein D. Acyanotic Congenital Heart Disease: The Left-to-Right Shunt Lesions. In: Kliegman RM, Stanton BF, St. Geme JW, Schor NF, Behrman RE, eds. Nelson Textbook of Pediatrics. 19th ed. Philadelphia: Elsevier Saunders; 2011:1551-61.

34. Park MK. Physical Examination. In: Park MK, Troxler RG, eds. Pediatric Cardiology for Practitoners. St. Louis: Mosby; 2002:10-33.

35. Johnson WH. Diagnostic Methods. In: Johnson WH, Moller JH, eds. Pediatr Cardiol. Philadelphia: Lippincott, Williams, & Wilkins; 2001:1-55.

36. Johnson GL. Clinical Examination. In: Long WA, Tooley WH, McNamara DG, eds. Fetal and Neonatal Cardiology. Philadelphia: W.B. Saunders Company; 1990:223-35.

37. Janjua HS, Batisky DL. Renal Vascular Disease in the Newborn. In: Gleason CA, Devaskar SU, eds. Avery's Diseases of the Newborn. 9th ed. Philadelphia: Elsevier Saunders; 2012:1235-44.

38. Cleary-Goldman J, D'Alton ME. Physiologic Effects of Multiple Pregnancy on Mother and Fetus. In: Polin RA, Fox WW, Abman SH, eds. Fetal and Neonatal Physiology. 4th ed. Philadelphia: Elsevier Saunders; 2011:197-210.

39. Kattwinkel J. Medications. In: Kattwinkel J, McGowan JE, Zaichkin J, eds. Textbook of Neonatal Resuscitation. 6th ed. Elk Grove Village: American Academy of Pediatrics; 2011:211-36.

40. Kalkunte S, Padbury JF, Sharma S. Immunologic Basis of Placental Function and Diseases: The Placenta, Fetal Membranes, and Umbilical Cord. In: Gleason CA, Devaskar SU, eds. Avery's Diseases of the Newborn. 9th ed. Philadelphia: Elsevier Saunders; 2012:37-50.

41. Chameides L. Part 7: Management of Shock. In: Chameides L, Samson RA, Schexnayder SM, Hazinski MF, eds. Pediatric Advanced Life Support Provider Manual. Dallas: American Heart Association; 2011:85-108.

42. Han YY, Carcillo JA, Dragotta MA, et al. Early reversal of pediatric-neonatal septic shock by community physicians is associated with improved outcome. Pediatrics 2003;112:793-9.

43. Losek JD. Hypoglycemia and the ABC'S (sugar) of pediatric resuscitation. Ann Emerg Med 2000;35:43-6.

44. Greenbaum LA. Acid-Base Balance. In: Kliegman RM, Stanton BF, St. Geme JW, Schor NF, Behrman RE, eds. Nelson Textbook of Pediatrics. 19th ed. Philadelphia: Elsevier Saunders; 2011:229-42.

45. Kraut JA, Madias NE. Serum anion gap: its uses and limitations in clinical medicine. Clin J Am Soc Nephrol 2007;2:162-74.

46. Hines EQ. Fluids and Electrolytes. In: Tschudy MM, Arcara KM, eds. The Harriet Lane Handbook. 19th ed. Philadelphia: Elsevier Mosby; 2012:271-92.

47. Doherty EG. Fluid and Electrolyte Management. In: Cloherty JP, Eichenwald EC, Hansen AR, Stark AR, eds. Manual of neonatal care. 7th ed. Philadelphia: Wolters Kluwer / Lippincott Williams & Wilkins; 2012:269-83.

48. Gomella TL. Body Water, Fluid, and Electrolytes. In: Gomella TL, Cunningham MD, Eyal FG, Tuttle D, eds. Neonatology Management, Procedures, On-Call Problems, Diseases, and Drugs. 6th ed. New York: McGraw Hill Medical; 2009:68-76.

49. Posencheg MA, Evans JR. Acid-Base Fluid, and Electrolyte Management. In: Gleason CA, Devaskar SU, eds. Avery's Diseases of the Newborn 9th ed. Philadelphia: Elsevier Saunders; 2012:367-89.

50. Dell KM. Acid-Base Management. In: Martin RJ, Fanaroff AA, Walsh MC, eds. Fanaroff and Martin's Neonatal-Perinatal Medicine: Diseases of the Fetus and Infant. 9th ed. St. Louis: Elsevier Mosby; 2011:677-84.

51. Feldman M, Soni N, Dickson B. Influence of hypoalbuminemia or hyperalbuminemia on the serum anion gap. J Lab Clin Med 2005;146:317-20.

52. Abrams SA. Abnormalities of Serum Calcium and Magnesium. In: Cloherty JP, Eichenwald EC, Hansen AR, Stark AR, eds. Manual of Neonatal Care. 7th ed. Philadelphia: Lippincott, Williams & Wilkins; 2012:297-303.

53. Rigo J, Mohamed MW, De Curtis M. Disorders of Calcium, Phosphorus, and Magnesium Metabolism. In: Martin RJ, Fanaroff AA, Walsh MC, eds. Fanaroff and Martin's Neonatal-Perinatal Medicine: Diseases of the Fetus and Infant. 9th ed. St. Louis: Elsevier Mosby; 2011:1523-56.

54. da Graca RL, Hassinger DC, Flynn PA, Sison CP, Nesin M, Auld PA. Longitudinal changes of brain-type natriuretic peptide in preterm neonates. Pediatrics 2006;117:2183-9.

55. El-Khuffash A, Molloy EJ. Are B-type natriuretic peptide (BNP) and N-terminal-pro-BNP useful in neonates? Arch Dis Child Fetal Neonatal Ed 2007;92:F320-4.

56. Farombi-Oghuvbu I, Matthews T, Mayne PD, Guerin H, Corcoran JD. N-terminal pro-B-type natriuretic peptide: a measure of significant patent ductus arteriosus. Arch Dis Child Fetal Neonatal Ed 2008;93:F257-60.

57. Koch A, Singer H. Normal values of B type natriuretic peptide in infants, children, and adolescents. Heart 2003;89:875-8.

58. Davlouros PA, Karatza AA, Xanthopoulou I, et al. Diagnostic role of plasma BNP levels in neonates with signs of congenital heart disease. Int J Cardiol 2011;147:42-6.

59. Maisel A. B-type natriuretic peptide levels: diagnostic and prognostic in congestive heart failure: what's next? Circulation 2002;105:2328-31.

60. Maisel A. Algorithms for using B-type natriuretic peptide levels in the diagnosis and management of congestive heart failure. Crit Pathw Cardiol 2002;1:67-73.

61. Cantinotti M, Passino C, Storti S, Ripoli A, Zyw L, Clerico A. Clinical relevance of time course of BNP levels in neonates with congenital heart diseases. Clin Chim Acta 2011;412:2300-4.

62. Trevisanuto D, Picco G, Golin R, et al. Cardiac troponin I in asphyxiated neonates. Biol Neonate 2006;89:190-3.

63. Galel SA. Therapeutic techniques: Selection of blood components for neonatal transfusion. NeoReviews 2005;6:e351-e5.

64. Sloan SR. Blood Products Used in the Newborn. In: Cloherty JP, Eichenwald EC, Hansen AR, Stark AR, eds. Manual of Neonatal Care. 7th ed. Philadelphia: Lippincott, Williams & Wilkins; 2012:529-37.

65. Matthews DC, Glader B. Erythrocyte Disorders in Infancy. In: Gleason CA, Devaskar SU, eds. Avery's Diseases of the Newborn 9th ed. Philadelphia: Elsevier Saunders; 2012:1080-107.

66. Roback JD, Grossman BJ, Harris T, Hillyer CD. Technical Manual. 17th ed. Bethesda: American Association of Blood Banks; 2011.

67. Manco-Johnson M, Rodden DJ, Hays T. Newborn Hematology. In: Gardner SL, Carter BS, Enzman-Hines M, Hernandez JA, eds. Merenstein & Gardner's Handbook of Neonatal Intensive Care. 7th ed. St. Louis: Mosby Elsevier; 2011:503-30.

68. Axsom KM, Friedman DF, Manno CS. Transfusion Therapy. In: Spitzer AR, ed. Intensive Care of the Fetus & Neonate. 2nd ed. Philadelphia: Elsevier Mosby; 2005:1333-49.

69. Aschner JL, Poland RL. Sodium bicarbonate: basically useless therapy. Pediatrics 2008;122:831-5.

70. Ammari AN, Schulze KF. Uses and abuses of sodium bicarbonate in the neonatal intensive care unit. Curr Opin Pediatr 2002;14:151-6.

71. Lawn CJ, Weir FJ, McGuire W. Base administration or fluid bolus for preventing morbidity and mortality in preterm infants with metabolic acidosis. Cochrane Database Syst Rev 2005:CD003215.

72. Thomson Reuters Editorial Staff. NeoFax. 24th ed. Montvale: Thomson Reuters; 2011.

73. Goldsmith JP. Chest Compressions, Medications, and Special Problems. In: Martin RJ, Fanaroff AA, Walsh MC, eds. Fanaroff and Martin's Neonatal-Perinatal Medicine: Diseases of the Fetus and Infant. 9th ed. St. Louis: Elsevier Mosby; 2011:474-84.

74. Taketomo CK, Hodding JH, Kraus DM. Pediatric & Neonatal Dosage Handook. 18th ed. Hudson: Lexicomp; 2011.

75. Subhani M, Sridhar S, DeCristofaro JD. Phentolamine use in a neonate for the prevention of dermal necrosis caused by dopamine: a case report. J Perinatol 2001;21:324-6.

76. Waller SA, Gopalani S, Benedetti tJ. Complicated Deliveries: Overview. In: Gleason CA, Devaskar SU, eds. Avery's Diseases of the Newborn 9th ed. Philadelphia: Elsevier Saunders; 2012:146-58.

77. Doumouchtsis SK, Arulkumaran S. Head trauma after instrumental births. Clin Perinatol 2008;35:69-83, viii.

78. Mangurten HH, Puppala BL. Birth Injuries. In: Martin RJ, Fanaroff AA, Walsh MC, eds. Fanaroff and Martin's Neonatal-Perinatal Medicine: Diseases of the Fetus and Infant. 9th ed. St. Louis: Elsevier Mosby; 2011:501-30.

79. Bonifacio SL, Gonzalez FF, Ferriero DM. Central Nervous System Injury and Neuroprotection. In: Gleason CA, Devaskar SU, eds. Avery's Diseases of the Newborn 9th ed. Philadelphia: Elsevier Saunders; 2012:869-91.

80. Uchil D, Arulkumaran S. Neonatal subgaleal hemorrhage and its relationship to delivery by vacuum extraction. Obstet Gynecol Surv 2003;58:687-93.

81. McQuivey RW. Vacuum-assisted delivery: a review. J Matern Fetal Neonatal Med 2004;16:171-80.

82. Hoyt MR. Anesthetic Options for Labor and Delivery. In: Martin RJ, Fanaroff AA, Walsh MC, eds. Fanaroff and Martin's Neonatal-Perinatal Medicine: Diseases of the Fetus and Infant. 9th ed. St. Louis: Elsevier Mosby 2011:433-48.

83. Prapas N, Kalogiannidis I, Masoura S, et al. Operative vaginal delivery in singleton term pregnancies: short-term maternal and neonatal outcomes. Hippokratia 2009;13:41-5.

84. Hook CD, Damos JR. Vacuum-assisted vaginal delivery. Am Fam Physician 2008;78:953-60.

85. Davis DJ. Neonatal subgaleal hemorrhage: diagnosis and management. Cmaj 2001;164:1452-3.

86. Ali UA, Norwitz ER. Vacuum-assisted vaginal delivery. Rev Obstet Gynecol 2009;2:5-17.

87. Towner D, Castro MA, Eby-Wilkens E, Gilbert WM. Effect of mode of delivery in nulliparous women on neonatal intracranial injury. N Engl J Med 1999;341:1709-14.

88. Vacca A. Vacuum-Assisted Delivery. OBG Management Supplement 2004:S1-S12.

89. Boo NY, Foong KW, Mahdy ZA, Yong SC, Jaafar R. Risk factors associated with subaponeurotic haemorrhage in full-term infants exposed to vacuum extraction. Bjog 2005;112:1516-21.

90. Boo NY, Ng SF, Lim VK. A case-control study of risk factors associated with rectal colonization of extended-spectrum beta-lactamase producing Klebsiella sp. in newborn infants. J Hosp Infect 2005;61:68-74.

91. Castro MA, Hoey SD, Towner D. Controversies in the use of the vacuum extractor. Semin Perinatol 2003;27:46-53.

92. Gardella C, Taylor M, Benedetti T, Hitti J, Critchlow C. The effect of sequential use of vacuum and forceps for assisted vaginal delivery on neonatal and maternal outcomes. Am J Obstet Gynecol 2001;185:896-902.

**S**ugar and **S**afe Care

**T**emperature

**A**irway

**B**lood Pressure

**L**ab Work

**E**motional Support

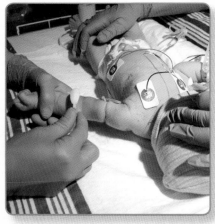

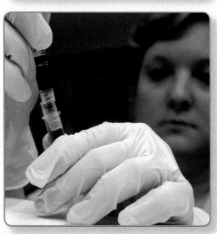

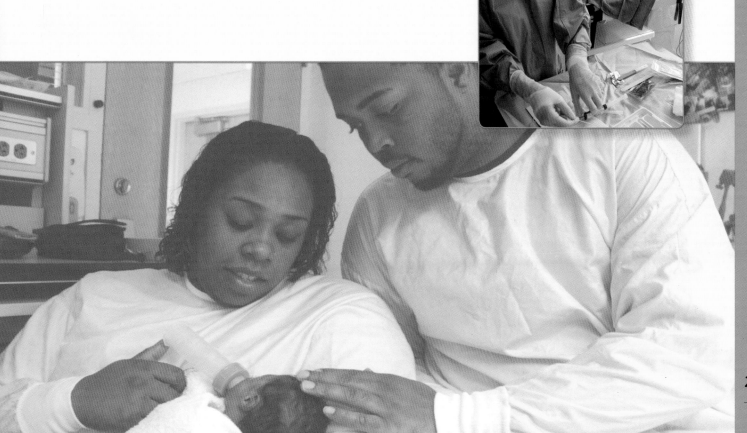

## Lab Work – Module Objectives

Upon completion of this module, participants will gain an increased understanding of:

1. Perinatal and postnatal risk factors that predispose infants to infection.
2. The clinical signs of neonatal sepsis.
3. Bacterial and viral organisms that may cause infection.
4. Laboratory tests to obtain in the pre-transport / post-resuscitation period.
5. White blood cell (WBC) development, how to calculate and interpret the absolute neutrophil count and immature to total ratio.
6. The initial antibiotic treatment of an infant with suspected sepsis.

## Lab Work – General Guidelines

### I. Neonatal infection can be devastating for the immunologically immature infant.

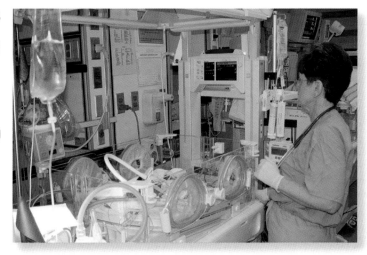

**The neonate's immune system is immature, which places them at increased risk for acquiring and succumbing to infection.**[1,2] They also have an impaired ability to effectively eliminate invading organisms.[3] Preterm infants are at an even greater disadvantage than term infants.[1,4] Mortality rates for preterm infants with early-onset infection may be as high as 40%.[5] Evaluation for, and treatment of suspected sepsis* when the infant is critically ill should be a top priority in the pre-transport / post-resuscitation period.[6] Table 5.1 lists risk factors that predispose an infant to infection.

### II. Signs of sepsis may range from subtle and non-specific to unmistakably apparent.

It is best practice to administer antibiotics to any neonate who has any signs that could indicate infection. Keep in mind that early signs of infection can be subtle and non-specific, and include respiratory distress, apnea, unexplained tachypnea, tachycardia or poor cutaneous perfusion. Broad spectrum antibiotic coverage is discussed on page 250. In addition, Appendices 5.1, 5.2, and 5.3 contain algorithms that may be useful when determining treatment options for **asymptomatic infants** with risk factors for sepsis.[6]

*The term sepsis is used interchangeably with infection in this module.*

**Table 5.1.** Risk factors for neonatal infection.[1,2,4,7]

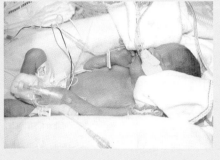

- ◇ Preterm premature rupture of membranes (PPROM)

- ◇ Premature onset of labor

- ◇ Rupture of membranes longer than 18 hours

- ◇ Chorioamnionitis (infection of the amniotic fluid, membranes, umbilical cord of the placenta, and/or decidua)[6,8]

  - Signs include maternal temperature > 100.4°F (38°C), maternal tachycardia > 100 beats per minute (BPM), fetal tachycardia > 160 BPM, uterine fundal tenderness, foul smelling amniotic fluid or vaginal discharge, purulent appearing amniotic fluid

- ◇ Recent maternal infection or illness

- ◇ Maternal fever in the peripartum period

- ◇ Maternal genitourinary tract infection, including urinary tract infection and sexually transmitted diseases

- ◇ Perinatal asphyxia, especially in conjunction with prolonged rupture of membranes

  - During an asphyxial event, the fetus or newborn may gasp and deeply inhale infected amniotic fluid

- ◇ Procedures

  - **Prior to delivery** that interfere with the integrity of the amniotic cavity: amniocentesis, chorionic villous sampling[8]

  - **Instrumentation at delivery** – vacuum assist, placement of a fetal scalp electrode[6]

  - **After delivery** – inserting intravenous lines, placing central lines, endotracheal intubation, other invasive procedures

Notes:

1. Appendix 5.4 contains guidance from the Centers for Disease Control on which newborns require full diagnostic evaluations, limited diagnostic evaluations, antibiotic therapy, and observation for the purpose of secondary prevention of early-onset Group B Streptococcal (GBS) infection. The recommended management depends on whether the newborn shows signs of neonatal sepsis or was exposed to maternal chorioamnionitis, whether the mother had an indication for GBS intrapartum antibiotic prophylaxis and received adequate GBS intrapartum antibiotic prophylaxis, the duration of the mother's rupture of membranes, and the newborn's gestational age.[7]

2. Appendix 5.5 contains information on the indications and nonindications for intrapartum antibiotic prophylaxis (IAP) to prevent early-onset GBS.[7]

3. Appendices 5.6 through 5.8 are algorithms for GBS screening and use of intrapartum antibiotic prophylaxis (IAP) for women with preterm labor, preterm premature rupture of membranes, and recommended regimens for IAP for prevention of early-onset GBS.[7]

Preterm infant with bacterial sepsis

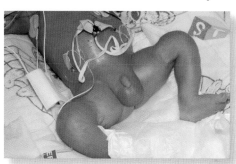

## Neonatal Infection

Infants may become infected with bacteria, virus, fungi, or other pathogens. Infection can begin prior to birth (in-utero, called *congenital* infection), during the birth process, or within the first 72 hours of life, called *early-onset sepsis*, or after the first 72 hours of life, called *late-onset sepsis*.[9,10] Infection that begins in utero, may be a result of the fetus swallowing or inhaling infected amniotic fluid, therefore a history of birth asphyxia with the possibility of in-utero gasping is important to recognize.[4] Most infants with early-onset sepsis have signs of infection within the first 24 to 48 hours of life.[11,12] Signs of infection are summarized in Table 5.2.

### Bacterial organisms that may infect the fetus or infant

Group B Streptococcus (a Gram-positive organism) and Escherichia coli (a Gram-negative organism) are the two most common organisms that cause early-onset bacterial infection.[13] Other organisms that cause early-onset and late-onset bacterial infection include:[4,9,13-15]

- Gram-positive organisms
  - Coagulase-negative Staphylococcus
  - Staphylococcus aureus
  - Listeria monocytogenes
  - Streptococcus pneumoniae
  - Group A Streptococcus

- Gram-negative organisms
  - Neisseria meningitides
  - Haemophilus influenzae
  - Klebsiella pneumoniae
  - Pseudomonas aeruginosa
  - Acinetobacter species
  - Citrobacter species
  - Enterobacter species
  - Serratia marcescens
  - Proteus species

## Clinical Tip

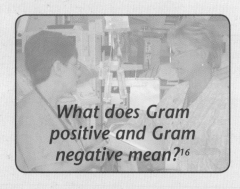

*What does Gram positive and Gram negative mean?*[16]

Gram staining refers to a bacterial staining procedure that was developed by a Danish bacteriologist, Hans Christian Gram in 1884. Gram staining is the first step in identifying an organism. The procedure allows differentiation of bacteria into one of two categories – positive or negative. The determination is based on color change. Organisms that stain a blue/purple color (because they retain the stain applied to them) are Gram-positive bacteria. Organisms that stain a pink/reddish color (because they lose their color when the destaining step is performed) are Gram-negative bacteria.

## Viral organisms that may infect the fetus or infant

Viruses that cause infection in the fetus or infant include, but are not limited to, **herpes simplex virus (HSV), human immunodeficiency virus (HIV), hepatitis, cytomegalovirus (CMV), parvovirus, and rubella.**[9,10] It is important to carefully evaluate the maternal history for viral exposure during any of the trimesters. Infection during the first trimester may result in severe consequences for both fetal growth and organ development. The fetus with viral exposure in early gestation is at greatly increased risk for intrauterine growth restriction (small for gestational age) and visual, hearing, brain, cardiac and/or liver damage. Late pregnancy, intrapartum, or post-partum viral exposure may result from maternal or family illness that presents with diarrhea and/or vomiting. It is important when taking the maternal medical history to ask about early gestation viral exposure, as well as recent viral illness in siblings, other family members and the mother.[17]

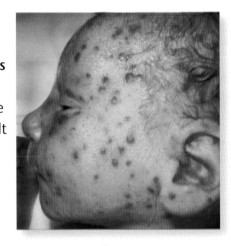

"Blueberry muffin" lesions secondary to extramedullary hematopoiesis in an infant with congenital CMV. These lesions may also observed with congenital rubella syndrome and other viral infections.
Photo courtesy Dr. David A. Clark

**Herpes simplex virus** (HSV) type 1 or 2 may be present in the maternal genital tract without the mother even knowing she has this infection.[10] Therefore, when taking a maternal history, this fact should serve as a reminder that HSV infection may still be possible even if the mother denies symptoms present or past for HSV.[17,18] It is also very important to interview the mother about her sexual partner(s) history of infection, since the mother may not think to introduce this information if not specifically asked. **Severe neonatal infection** is much more likely if the mother contracted a primary (first episode) HSV infection in late gestation than if she had a HSV infection before or early in pregnancy, or with recurrent infection.[10]

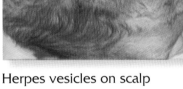

Herpes vesicles on scalp
Photo courtesy Dr. David A. Clark

- Infants exposed to HSV during delivery may not have symptoms for 3 to 7 days and even as late as 10 to 14 days.[10]

- Signs may include skin vesicles (which are not always present), poor feeding, lethargy, fever, shock, and if the infection is in the central nervous system, seizures.[17]

- If the history and/or presentation suggest HSV infection, treatment with acyclovir should be strongly considered while awaiting culture or Polymerase Chain Reaction (PCR) testing. Acyclovir can be stopped if the cultures or tests are negative. If the mother has active genital and/or buttock herpes lesions, acyclovir should be administered to the infant.[17]

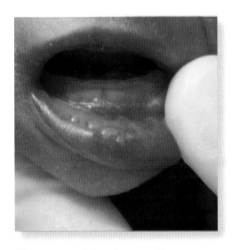

Herpes vesicles in mouth
Photo courtesy Dr. David A. Clark

233

**Table 5.2. Clinical signs of sepsis.** Infected infants most commonly present with some degree of respiratory distress. Additional signs that may be present are summarized in the table.[1,2,4,11]

Many of these signs may also be present with other concurrent illnesses, if the infant is in shock from other causes than infection, or if the infant has a metabolic condition, such as, is hypoglycemic.

### Respiratory distress
- Tachypnea, nasal flaring, grunting, retractions
- Apnea
- Cyanosis
  - Development of an oxygen requirement or an increase in oxygen requirement and/or ventilator support

### Temperature instability
- Hypothermia (more common) and hyperthermia (less common)
- Persistent hyperthermia (temperature remains elevated beyond a single temperature measurement) is especially concerning as a presenting sign for neonatal sepsis[4]

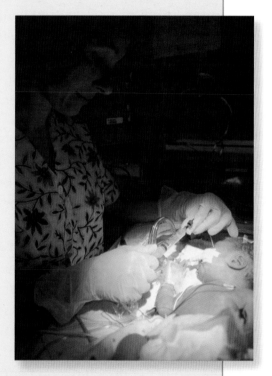

### Feeding intolerance
- Increased gastric pre-feeding residuals
- Poor feeding pattern
- Vomiting
- Abdominal distension

### Cardiovascular signs
- Tachycardia, bradycardia
- Hypotension
- Skin mottling, prolonged capillary refill time
- Pale or gray skin color

### Abnormal neurologic status
- Irritability
- Increased sleepiness
- Lethargy
- Hypotonia
- Seizures

### Abnormal skin findings
- Omphalitis
- Blisters on the skin
- Soft tissue swelling and redness
- Cellulitis
- Necrotic skin lesions

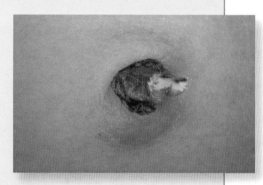

Mild omphalitis

## Laboratory Evaluation

### Prior to Transport

The following laboratory tests – the 4 B's – should be obtained prior to transport of the infant:

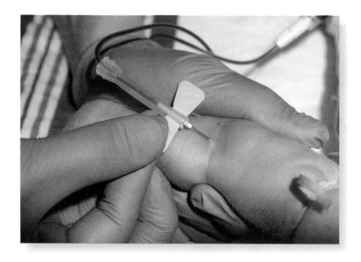

**B**lood Count (Complete Blood Count [CBC] with white blood cell [WBC] differential and platelet count)

### Blood Culture

- Use sterile technique when drawing the culture and transferring the blood into the culture bottle

- If possible, obtain at least one mL of blood per culture bottle[1,19,20]

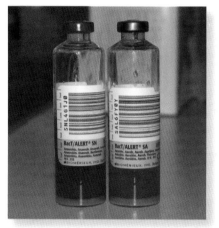

- Note: a volume of 2 to 3 mL of blood in the aerobic culture bottle will increase the likelihood of microorganism identification when there is a low colony-count bacterial sepsis present

- Obtain the culture before starting antibiotics

### Blood glucose

- Check early and follow closely as indicated based on risk factors

### Blood gas

- This is especially important if the infant is experiencing respiratory distress or if there is a history of shock, but in any neonate where infection is a consideration, measuring the pH and base deficit can be of value.

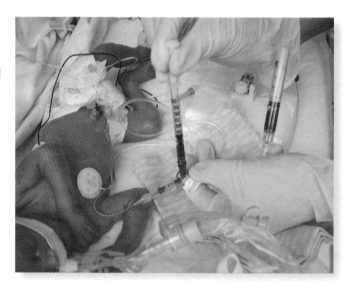

# Clinical Tip

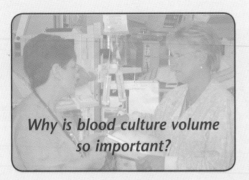

*Why is blood culture volume so important?*

The chance that bacteria will be detected in a blood culture goes up when an adequate amount of blood is placed in the culture bottle.[19,20] This is important because identifying the invading organism will guide selection of antibiotics and duration of therapy. As many as one quarter of all infants with sepsis have a very small amount of bacteria in their blood ($\leq$ 4 colony-forming units (CFU)/mL).[6] Modern microbial growth and detection technology equipment can detect these small amounts of bacteria providing the inoculum (blood culture volume) is sufficient. Therefore, a minimum of 1 mL of blood should be obtained, but 2 or 3 mL are preferred.[19] If you are only able to obtain 1 mL, do not split this volume between aerobic and anaerobic bottles; just place the entire 1 mL sample in the aerobic bottle. To avoid contamination of the culture sample, use sterile technique when obtaining the culture and transferring the blood to the culture bottle.

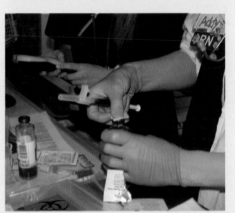

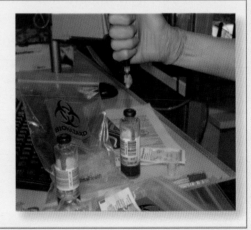

⚠ If you are having difficulty obtaining the blood culture, contact the infant's medical staff provider to report the situation and request assistance.

# Laboratory Tests to Obtain After Transport

Depending upon the infant's history, risk factors, and clinical presentation, additional laboratory tests may be indicated as part of the neonatal intensive care unit (tertiary center) evaluation. These tests are **usually not necessary prior to transport** unless directed by the transport control physician or tertiary center.

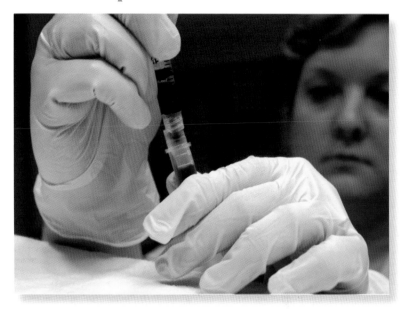

- **C-Reactive Protein (CRP)**[4,21-24]

  - A normal value (in most laboratories) is < 1.6 mg/dL for the first two days of life and then 1 mg/dL thereafter.[4] Be aware that various laboratories are available for CRP quantification. You must check with your hospital laboratory to determine the exact reference range for CRP measurement in newborn infants.

  - CRP does not cross the placenta, so results obtained reflect the infant's level.

  - CRP is a protein produced by liver cells during inflammation, infection, trauma, or tissue necrosis. CRP is considered an "acute-phase reactant" because of this property.

  - Blood concentrations of CRP generally increase during bacterial sepsis, meningitis, respiratory illnesses (meconium aspiration syndrome, respiratory distress syndrome, perinatal asphyxia); after surgery, following vacuum extraction or forceps delivery, following immunizations, and with bruising. In addition, CRP levels are higher following vaginal birth than cesarean birth. Thus, elevation of CRP can be non-specific and multifactorial.

  - The blood concentration of CRP is generally elevated within 4 to 8 hours following an inflammatory event or acute tissue injury, but it is important to know that it does not rise immediately.

  - The CRP remains elevated while inflammation or tissue destruction is ongoing and declines when inflammation or tissue destruction resolves.

  - CRP is not always elevated (even with proven sepsis), so the decision to not treat an infant for infection should **not** be based solely on CRP measurements.

## Laboratory Tests to Obtain After Transport (continued)

- Cerebrospinal fluid (CSF) to evaluate for meningitis:
  - Gram stain and culture
  - Cell count
  - Glucose and protein concentration
- Electrolytes:
  - To evaluate for hypo or hypernatremia, hypo or hyperkalemia
  - To calculate the anion gap when there is a metabolic acidosis

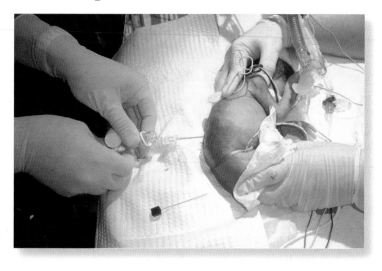

- Ionized calcium
- Renal function tests:
  - Blood urea nitrogen (BUN)
  - Creatinine
- Liver function tests:
  - Liver enzymes: aspartate aminotransferase (AST), alanine aminotransferase (ALT), and gamma-glutamyl transpeptidase (GGT)
  - Bilirubin (unconjugated and conjugated)
  - Coagulation studies:
    - Prothrombin time (PT)
    - Partial thromboplastin time (PTT)
    - Fibrinogen
    - D-dimer
- Magnesium:
  - If the mother was given magnesium during labor

# Complete Blood Count (CBC) Interpretation

WBCs are involved in protection against infective organisms and foreign substances and are produced in the bone marrow along with red blood cells and platelets. There are five main types of WBCs, as illustrated in Figure 5.1: neutrophils, eosinophils, basophils, lymphocytes, and monocytes. **Neutrophils** are the WBCs primarily responsible for killing and digesting bacteria. In neonates, and especially in preterm neonates, neutrophil chemotaxis (movement) is immature; in the face of serious bacterial infection, the neutrophils may not be capable of mounting an adequate response. The following discussion focuses on the neutrophil and how to calculate its concentration in the blood.

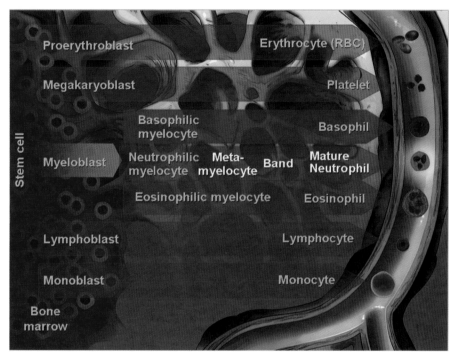

**Figure 5.1. Blood cell development – from the bone marrow to the bloodstream.** The stem cell differentiates into red blood cells, platelets, basophils, neutrophils, eosinophils, lymphocytes, and monocytes.

 A neonate with sepsis may have a completely normal CBC and a normal CRP in the early phase of illness.[12,25] The time between the onset of the infection and the first change in the CBC may be as long as 4 to 6 hours. The time between the onset of the infection and elevation in the CRP may be as long as 8 to 12 hours. During this "latent" period, the neonate is infected, and needs antibiotic treatment, but has a normal CBC and a normal CRP.

**Never withhold antibiotic treatment in an *ill* neonate on the sole basis that the CBC (or CRP) is normal.**

## Neutrophil Maturation

As shown in Figure 5.1, the neutrophil matures in the bone marrow, from the myeloblast, to the promyelocyte, to the myelocyte, to the metamyelocyte, to the band neutrophil, and finally to the mature **segmented neutrophil**. In the bone marrow, the metamyelocytes, band neutrophil, and segmented neutrophil comprise what is called the neutrophil storage pool (NSP). In neonates, the NSP is significantly smaller, per kilogram of body weight, than in adults; depletion of the NSP may occur with severe bacterial infection.[26,27] Under normal, non-infected, non-stressed, circumstances, mature segmented neutrophils are released from the NSP into the bloodstream where they circulate for a short period (6 to 8 hours) and then they migrate into the tissue where they live for approximately 24 hours.[28] In the presence of infection, immature forms of neutrophils – **bands and metamyelocytes** – are also released from the bone marrow into the blood stream as the body attempts to maximize the number of circulating neutrophils (illustrated in Figure 5.2). The term **left shift** refers to the appearance of immature neutrophils in the blood. The immature to total ratio (I/T ratio) calculation provides information about the proportion of immature to mature neutrophils in the blood. Interpretation of, and how to calculate the I/T ratio is discussed later in this module.

## Clinical Tip

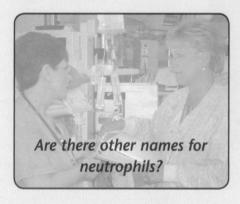

*Are there other names for neutrophils?*

Mature and immature neutrophil terminology are as follows:

- Segmented (mature) neutrophils may also be referred to as polymorphonuclear neutrophil, polys, PMNs, segs, and neuts.

- Band neutrophils are also called bands, juveniles, or stabs.

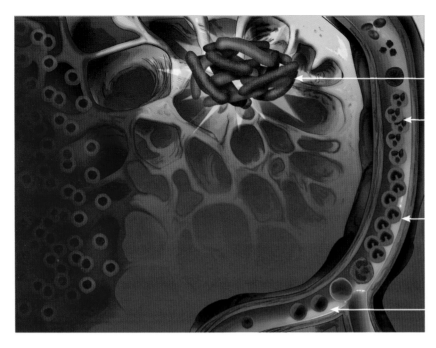

E. coli infection

Segmented neutrophils

Band neutrophils

Metamyelocytes

**Figure 5.2. Bone marrow response to bacterial infection.** In response to bacterial infection, the NSP released immature and mature neutrophils into the blood. Notice the increased numbers of band neutrophils and metamyelocytes with the appearance of a bacterial infection (Escherica coli bacteria is shown).

## The Absolute Neutrophil Count (ANC)

When evaluating the CBC for possible sepsis, it is useful to know the concentration of neutrophils in the blood. The ANC calculation will provide this information. Repeating the CBC at 12 to 24 hour intervals may be useful since the initial CBC may be normal and subsequent CBC results abnormal. However, the decision to treat with antibiotics should be made quickly and must be based upon clinical history, patient condition and signs, and not solely on CBC results!

 Remember, infection may still be present even if CBC results are normal. Conversely, abnormal CBC results do not always mean that an infant has an infection.[12,15,]

### Why is it helpful to calculate the ANC?

The ANC may be helpful when evaluating an infant for potential bacterial infection. Normally, the WBC count and neutrophil count rise for the first day after birth. In term infants, the neutrophil count peaks at about 8 hours after birth. Therefore, a declining neutrophil count, rather than the expected physiologic rise in count, should raise concern that the infant may be infected.[21]

Most concerning are infants who have a **low ANC** for their postnatal age, because this can indicate depletion of the NSP, or that the infant is not going to be able to mobilize enough neutrophils necessary to fight a bacterial infection.[13,21] Exhaustion of the NSP is very serious for the newborn.

Neonates who deplete their neutrophil reserves while fighting infection are at highest risk of dying from sepsis.[29] It should be noted that infants born to mothers with hypertension may have a low ANC compared with infants whose mothers are not hypertensive.[26] This maternal history is important to consider when evaluating ANC results. Other infants with abnormal WBC counts include infants with Trisomy 13, 18, and 21.[30,31]

Neutrophil counts vary with age; preterm infants have a lower ANC than term infants because their circulating neutrophil concentration is lower prior to term gestation.[26,30,32] Figures 5.3, 5.4 and 5.5 are graphs that demonstrate the ANC (i.e., the blood neutrophil concentration) for infants > 36-weeks gestation, 28- to 36-weeks gestation and < 28 weeks gestation.[30]

Notes:

1. The peak ANCs reported in the study by Schmutz[30] are higher than the peak ANCs reported by Manroe.[33] This is attributed to either different methodology used to count the neutrophils, versus the effect of the higher altitude of the Intermountain region study hospitals (average 4800 feet above sea level), compared to Manroe's study, which was conducted in Dallas, Texas (500 feet above sea level).

2. A recent study by Hornik[13] of infants admitted to 293 neonatal intensive care units in the U.S. evaluated the association between the WBC count, ANC and immature-to-total (I/T) ratio to blood culture results and the likelihood that early-onset infection was present. A low WBC count, low ANC and elevated I/T ratio were associated with increased odds that an infection was present, whereas an elevated WBC count was not associated with increased odds of an infection being present. **For this reason, the S.T.A.B.L.E. Program recommends use of the ANC charts published by Schmutz.**[30]

3. It should be noted that in the Hornik study,[13] the CBC was not useful for predicting that infection was *not* present, which underscores the recommendation that antibiotics be started based on clinical history, patient presentation, signs, and not solely on CBC results.

 When an infant's ANC falls into the neutropenic range for gestational age and postnatal age, the medical staff provider should be notified. Evaluation of risk factors, maternal pregnancy complications (i.e., pregnancy induced hypertension), clinical history, infant's presentation (current medical condition) and possibly follow up CBC (or additional) testing are recommended.

**Figure 5.3. Graph represents the normal range for the ANC in infants > 36-weeks gestation in the first 72 hours of life.**[30]

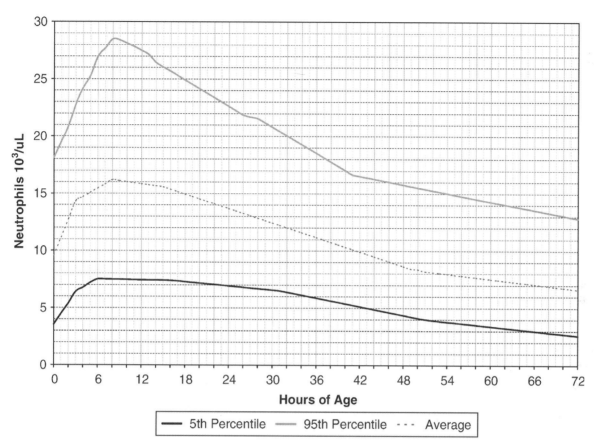

Notes (infants > 36 weeks):

1. Based on this data, at the time of birth, neutropenia would be defined as an ANC (or blood neutrophil concentration) less than 3500.

2. At 8 hours of life, in infants > 36 weeks' gestation, when the peak ANC occurs, neutropenia would be defined as an ANC less than 7500.

3. Data are based on 12,149 values that were analyzed using modern automated blood cell counting instrumentation.

4. Infants were excluded from the study if they had early-onset bacterial sepsis, congenital neutropenia, abnormally low or high neutrophil concentrations, trisomy 13, 18, or 21, or the mother had pregnancy induced hypertension.

*Reprinted by permission from Macmillan Publishers Ltd: Journal of Perinatology, Schmutz N, Henry E, Jopling J, Christensen RD. Expected ranges for blood neutrophil concentrations of neonates: the Manroe and Mouzinho charts revisited; Figure 1. 28:275-81, © 2008.*

**Figure 5.4. Graph represents the normal range for the ANC in infants 28- to 36-weeks gestation in the first 72 hours of life.**[30]

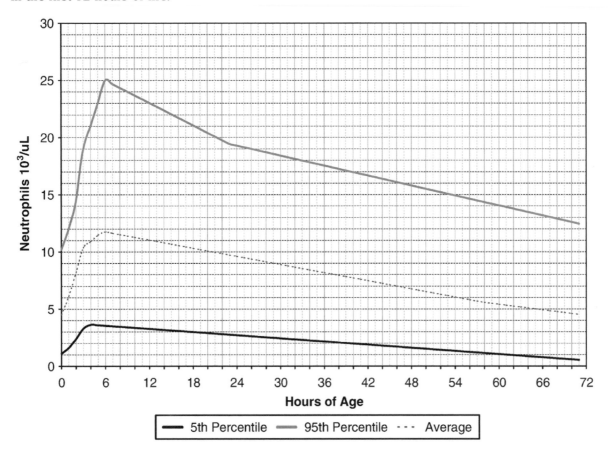

Notes (infants 28- to 36-weeks gestation):

1. Based on this data, at the time of birth, neutropenia would be defined as an ANC (or blood neutrophil concentration) less than 1000.

2. At 6 hours of life, when the peak ANC occurs, neutropenia would be defined as an ANC less than 3500.

3. Data are based on 8,896 values that were analyzed using modern automated blood cell counting instrumentation.

4. Infants were excluded from the study if they had early-onset bacterial sepsis, congenital neutropenia, abnormally low or high neutrophil concentrations, trisomy 13, 18, or 21, or the mother had pregnancy induced hypertension.

*Reprinted by permission from Macmillan Publishers Ltd: Journal of Perinatology, Schmutz N, Henry E, Jopling J, Christensen RD. Expected ranges for blood neutrophil concentrations of neonates: the Manroe and Mouzinho charts revisited; Figure 2. 28:275-81, © 2008.*

**Figure 5.5. Graph represents the normal range for the absolute neutrophil count (ANC) in infants <28-weeks gestation in the first 72 hours of life.**[30]

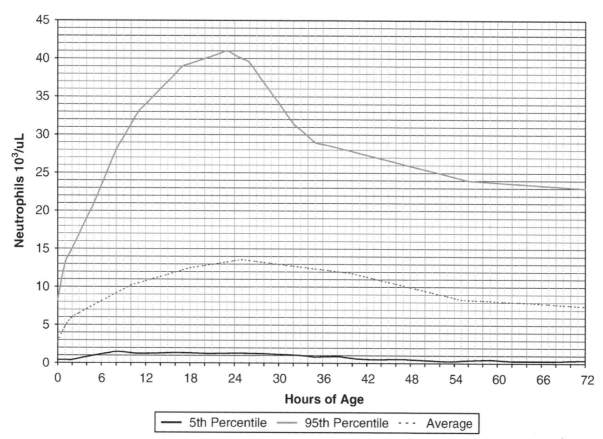

Notes (infants <28-weeks gestation):

1. Based on this data, at the time of birth, neutropenia would be defined as an ANC (or blood neutrophil concentration) less than 500.

2. At 24 hours of life, when the peak ANC occurs, neutropenia would be defined as an ANC less than 1500.

3. Data are based on 852 values that were analyzed using modern automated blood cell counting instrumentation.

4. Infants were excluded from the study if they had early-onset bacterial sepsis, congenital neutropenia, abnormally low or high neutrophil concentrations, trisomy 13, 18, or 21,[31] or the mother had pregnancy induced hypertension.

## Which cells are included in the ANC calculation?

As mentioned earlier, the total white blood cell (WBC) count is comprised of neutrophils, eosinophils, basophils, lymphocytes, and monocytes. When calculating the ANC, only the total white blood cell count and the mature and immature neutrophils are included in the calculation. The non-neutrophil cell types (eosinophils, basophils, lymphocytes, and monocytes) are not included.

## Understanding the calculation.

The neutrophils are a portion of the whole number of white blood cells. For example, a neutrophil count of "35" means 35 percent of the white blood cells are segmented neutrophils. A band count of "15" means 15 percent of the white blood cells are band neutrophils. Thus, 50% of the white blood cells in this scenario (35% segmented neutrophils plus 15% band neutrophils) are those primarily responsible for phagocytizing and killing bacteria. The remaining 50% of the white blood cells are a combination of eosinophils, basophils, lymphocytes, and monocytes, and are involved with other functions in the hematologic system.

## Example ANC calculation.

To obtain the ANC, multiply the white blood cell count by the neutrophil count as shown in the following example.

**History:** a **term** infant was delivered to a mother with poor prenatal care and foul smelling amniotic fluid. At four hours of life, the infant developed respiratory distress (cyanosis, tachypnea and retractions) and hypothermia. A CBC, blood culture and blood gas were ordered and obtained when the infant was five hours old.

| | |
|---|---|
| **White Blood Cell Count (WBC)** | **15,000 (15 x $10^3$/µL)** |
| Segmented neutrophils (segs) | 35 (%) |
| Band neutrophils (bands) | 15 (%) |
| Metamyelocytes (metas) | 3 (%) |
| Lymphocytes | 42 (%) |
| Basophils | 4 (%) |
| Eosinophils | 1 (%) |

## Directions to calculate the ANC.

Identify the immature and mature neutrophils on the CBC (highlighted in blue). Add the segmented neutrophils, band neutrophils, and metamyelocytes together. Multiply this number by the total white blood cell count.

1) 35 segs + 15 bands + 3 Metas = 53 (percent)

   (i.e, 53% of the white blood cell types are neutrophils)

2) 15,000 multiplied by 0.53 = 7950

3) The ANC is 7950

4) Plot this number (7950) for a 5-hour-old infant on the chart appropriate for this gestational age.

This means that the total neutrophil concentration is 7950 which, when plotted on the Schmutz ANC chart, is within normal range for an infant of this gestation and age.

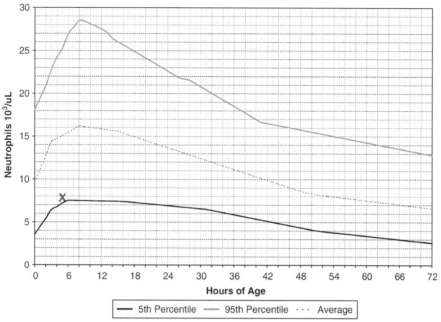

## The Immature to Total (I/T) Ratio

Another calculation used to evaluate neutrophils is the immature-to-total ratio (I/T ratio). This calculation will reveal what proportion of the circulating neutrophils, released from the NSP in the bone marrow, are the immature forms. The I/T ratio is the most sensitive for estimating the risk that infection may be present.[13]

## Why is it helpful to calculate the I/T ratio?

The majority of neutrophils that appear in the bloodstream should be mature cells, or segmented neutrophils. When more than 20 to 25% of the neutrophils in the blood are immature neutrophils, suspicion should increase that the infant is responding to a bacterial infection.[13,15]

## Directions to calculate the I/T ratio.

Identify the immature neutrophil forms (metamyelocytes and band neutrophils), and add them together. Place this number as the numerator. Next, add the mature (segmented neutrophils) and immature neutrophils (metamyelocytes and band neutrophils) together and place this number as the denominator. Divide the immature by the total neutrophil count.

$$\frac{\text{Immature (I)}}{\text{Total (T)}} = \text{I/ T ratio}$$

## Example I/T ratio calculation.

Using the previous CBC from the five-hour-old infant with respiratory distress and risk factors for sepsis, calculate the I/T ratio as follows:

| | |
|---|---|
| **White Blood Cell Count (WBC)** | **15,000 (15 x $10^3$/µL)** |
| Segmented neutrophils (segs) | 35 (%) |
| Band neutrophils (bands) | 15 (%) |
| Metamyelocytes (metas) | 3 (%) |
| Lymphocytes | 42 (%) |
| Basophils | 4 (%) |
| Eosinophils | 1 (%) |

1) 15 bands + 3 metas = 18 (%) of the neutrophils are immature

2) 15 bands + 3 metas + 35 segs = 53 (%) of the WBCs

3) 18 divided by 53 = 0.34

$$18 / 53 = .34$$

4) The I/T ratio is 0.34

This means that **34 percent** of the neutrophil types are the **immature forms**. This should raise concern that the NSP in the bone marrow is responding to a bacterial infection by sending immature forms into the bloodstream before they have had time to fully mature.

**I/T ratio > 0.20 raises index of suspicion for infection.**[13]

**I/T ratio > 0.8 correlated with a higher risk of death from sepsis.**[29]

## Platelet Count: *Interpreting the platelet count.*

A low platelet count is called thrombocytopenia. Thrombocytopenia may result from either decreased platelet production or increased platelet utilization (or destruction) as a result of various pathological conditions:[34-36]

- Infectious etiology: bacterial, fungal, or viral (e.g., CMV, HIV, rubella, herpes)

- Maternal medical conditions (e.g., pregnancy induced hypertension)

- Maternal auto- or isoimmunization: alloimmune or autoimmune thrombocytopenia (idiopathic thrombocytopenic purpura, systemic lupus erythematosus)

- Genetic etiology: chromosomal (trisomy 13, 18, 21, turner syndrome), familial thrombocytopenias, or specific mutations in the genes MPL, RUNX1, or PTPN11.

- Other etiologies: necrotizing enterocolitis, hyperviscosity, disseminated intravascular coagulation following perinatal asphyxia, metabolic (propionic methylmalonic, isovaleric acidemias)

Thrombocytopenia has traditionally been defined as a platelet count less than 150,000 per microliter ($\mu$L)[34,35] **Mild** thrombocytopenia is defined as a platelet count in the range 100,000/$\mu$L to 149,000/$\mu$L; **moderate** thrombocytopenia is between 50,000 and 100,000/$\mu$L and **severe** thrombocytopenia is when the platelet count is less than 50,000/$\mu$L.[36] New reference ranges for platelet counts for preterm and term infants at birth and the first 90 days of life may be found in Appendix 5.9.[37] These new reference ranges reveal that platelet counts advance with increasing gestational age. The 5th percentile for infants < 32 weeks gestation was 104,200/$\mu$L and for late preterm and term infants, 123,000/$\mu$L. Thus the traditional cutoff of 150,000/$\mu$L to define thrombocytopenia is a little higher value than the current data demonstrates.[37] Neonates previously judged to have "mild thrombocytopenia" because their count was in the range 100,000 to 149,000/$\mu$L actually fall within the reference range and therefore should not be considered thrombocytopenic.

## What number should I be concerned about?[38]

- **A platelet count less than 100,000/$\mu$L** is abnormal and needs to be re-evaluated, especially if there is a downward trend. In addition, the infant should be examined for signs of bleeding (oozing from puncture sites, bruising, petechiae, GI bleeding, etc.). Consult the tertiary center if any of these signs are present.

- **A platelet count less than 50,000/$\mu$L** in a neonate is termed "severe" thrombocytopenia and indicates that the risk of bleeding is increased.[34] If the platelet count is <50,000 in a neonate who has no petechiae and no signs of bleeding, consider repeating the count to make sure it is accurate (i.e., there is no platelet clumping). As mentioned above, evaluate for signs of bleeding and consult the tertiary center if any signs of bleeding are present.

- **Platelet counts less than 25,000/$\mu$L** are dangerously low. Consult the tertiary center for assistance with diagnosing the cause and treating this problem. As mentioned above, evaluate for signs of bleeding and be prepared to administer a platelet transfusion if instructed to do so.

# Initial Antibiotic Therapy for Sick Infants

## Begin Antibiotics Promptly

Once an adequate blood culture has been obtained, begin antibiotics promptly. The antibiotics of choice may vary from hospital to hospital, or region to region. However, ampicillin and gentamicin are commonly used for broad spectrum coverage against both Gram negative and Gram positive organisms.[39] Any delay in being able to carry out the order for antibiotics should be reported promptly to the infant's medical staff provider.

## Ampicillin

Varying doses of Ampicillin are recommended in current neonatal medication dosing references.[40-42] In the past, The S.T.A.B.L.E. Program recommended a dose of 100 mg/kg/dose every 12 hours. In this edition, the dose has been revised downward to be consistent with current dosing recommendations.

| Dose 50 mg/kilogram per dose[a] Gestational age-based dosing | | Interval | Route[b] |
|---|---|---|---|
| ≤ 29 weeks | 0 to 28 days old | Every 12 hours | IV slow push over 3 to 5 minutes. |
| 30 – 36 weeks | 0 to 14 days old | | |
| 37 – 44 weeks | 0 to 7 days old | | Not faster than 100 mg per minute. |

[a]  From reference NeoFax® 2011[41]p.14

[b]  May be given IM for a few doses, if having difficulty establishing IV access. For IM injection, mix to a final concentration of 250 mg/mL.

## Route

IV (preferred) over 3 to 5 minutes (not faster than 100 mg per minute).

- Use sterile water or normal saline to reconstitute medication.
- For IV infusion, maximum concentration is 100 mg/mL.
- Use reconstituted solutions within one hour of mixing to avoid loss of potency.

Notes about dosing:[40,41]

1. Some neonatal experts recommend infants with bacteremia receive a higher dose, such as 150 to 200 mg/kilogram per day in divided doses. The dosing interval should be decided with your neonatal pharmacist or neonatal specialist as it will vary depending upon the infants' clinical condition, gestational age, and post-natal age.

2. Infants with meningitis may require a dose of 300 to 400 mg/kilogram per day in divided doses at more frequent intervals. The dosing interval should be decided with your neonatal pharmacist or neonatal specialist as it will vary depending upon the infant's clinical condition, gestational age, and postnatal age.

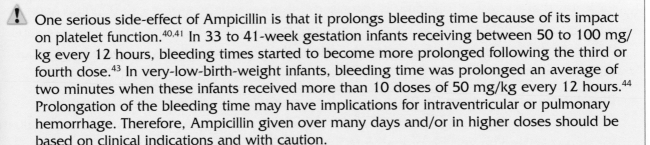

One serious side-effect of Ampicillin is that it prolongs bleeding time because of its impact on platelet function.[40,41] In 33 to 41-week gestation infants receiving between 50 to 100 mg/kg every 12 hours, bleeding times started to become more prolonged following the third or fourth dose.[43] In very-low-birth-weight infants, bleeding time was prolonged an average of two minutes when these infants received more than 10 doses of 50 mg/kg every 12 hours.[44] Prolongation of the bleeding time may have implications for intraventricular or pulmonary hemorrhage. Therefore, Ampicillin given over many days and/or in higher doses should be based on clinical indications and with caution.

## Gentamicin[40,42]

There are varying doses and intervals published for "higher dose, longer interval" gentamicin administration. In addition, tertiary care center experts (neonatologists and neonatal pharmacists) often modify the doses and/or intervals that are published in current neonatal drug handbooks. Therefore, both the NeoFax and Lexicomp dosing regimens are provided. Select the dose and interval that is recommended by your tertiary center. Traditional gentamicin dosing is also shown on page 252. It is strongly recommended that current drug handbooks are consulted on a regular basis, as dosing regimens may change in the future as new research becomes available.

**Extended Interval Dosing** *from NeoFax® 2011[41] p.50*

| Gestational age | Postnatal age (days) | Dose | Interval | Route (via infusion pump) |
|---|---|---|---|---|
| ≤ 29 weeks | 0 to 7 | 5 mg/kg | Every 48 hours | IV over 30 minutes |
| | 8 to 28 | 4 mg/kg | Every 36 hours | |
| | ≥ 29 | 4 mg/kg | Every 24 hours | |
| 30 – 34 weeks | 0 to 7 | 4.5 mg/kg | Every 36 hours | IV over 30 minutes |
| | ≥ 8 | 4 mg/kg | Every 24 hours | |
| ≥ 35 weeks | All | 4 mg/kg | Every 24 hours | IV over 30 minutes |

**Extended Interval Dosing** *from Lexicomp 2011[40] p.703*

| Gestational age-based dosing | Dose | Interval | Route [a] (via infusion pump) |
|---|---|---|---|
| < 32 weeks | 4 – 5 mg/kg | Every 48 hours | IV over 30 minutes |
| 32 – 36 weeks | 4 – 5 mg/kg | Every 36 hours | IV over 30 minutes |
| ≥ 37 weeks | 4 – 5 mg/kg | Every 24 hours | IV over 30 minutes |

| Weight-based dosing | Dose | Interval | Route [a] (via infusion pump) |
|---|---|---|---|
| **Postnatal age ≤ 7 days** | | | |
| < 1200 grams | 4 – 5 mg/kg | Every 48 hours | IV over 30 minutes |
| ≥ 1200 grams | 5 mg/kg | Every 36 hours | IV over 30 minutes |
| | *or* 4 mg/kg | Every 24 hours | IV over 30 minutes |

[a] Can be administered IM.

Notes:

1. Give gentamicin over 30 minutes on an infusion pump.

2. Use with caution if renal function is abnormal (urine output is less than 1 mL/kg/hour and/or serum creatinine is elevated).

## Gentamicin Levels (on extended interval schedule)

**Peak:**  Therapeutic range 6 – 12 mcg/mL (indication dependent)

**Trough:**  Therapeutic range 0.5 – 1 mcg/mL

- If there are concerns about renal function, a trough gentamicin level may be obtained prior to the second dose or at any point if renal function declines.

- When gentamicin is given for 3 days or less, it is usually unnecessary to obtain gentamicin levels unless there is a medical indication, as previously mentioned.

- When gentamicin is given for longer than 5 to 7 days, it is usually necessary to re-evaluate gentamicin levels.

## Traditional Gentamicin Dosing

**Dose:**  2.5 mg/kg/dose

**Interval:**  Every 12, 18 or 24 hours

The dosing interval depends upon gestational age and renal function.

**Route:**  IV over 30 minutes using an infusion pump.

## Gentamicin Levels (on a traditional dosing schedule)

**Trough:**  Therapeutic range 0.5 – 2 mcg/mL

**Peak:**  Therapeutic range 5 – 10 mcg/mL

- Evaluate the trough concentration 30 to 60 minutes before the 3rd dose.
  - If there are concerns about renal function, a trough gentamicin level may be obtained prior to the second dose or at any point if renal function declines.

- Evaluate the peak gentamicin concentration 30 minutes after the third dose has been administered over a 30-minute infusion period or one hour after an IM dose.

- When gentamicin is given for 3 days or less, it is usually unnecessary to obtain gentamicin levels.

- When gentamicin is given for longer than 5 to 7 days, it is usually necessary to re-evaluate gentamicin levels.

## Alternate Gentamicin Route

**Route:**  Intramuscular (IM)

If having difficulty establishing IV access, gentamicin may be given IM for a few doses. Absorption may be variable; IV administration is the preferred route.

# LAB WORK MODULE — Key Points

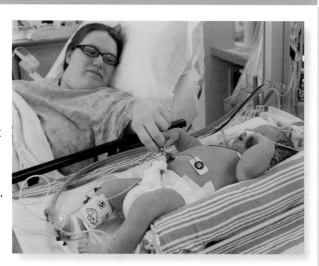

✧ Review the maternal and neonatal history for risk factors for infection.

✧ Be suspicious of subtle signs of infection.

✧ A neonate with sepsis can have a completely normal CBC and a normal CRP very early in the illness. Therefore, never withhold antibiotic treatment in an ill neonate on the basis that the CBC (and/or CRP) are normal.

✧ Draw an adequate volume of blood for culture.

✧ Initiate antibiotics promptly.

APPENDIX 5.1   **Evaluation of Asymptomatic Infants < 37 Weeks' Gestation with Risk Factors for Sepsis.**[6]

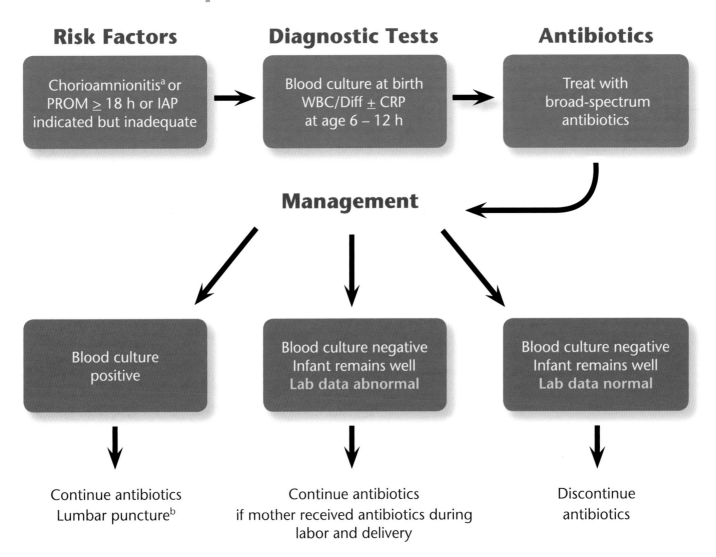

**Risk Factors**

Chorioamnionitis[a] or PROM ≥ 18 h or IAP indicated but inadequate

**Diagnostic Tests**

Blood culture at birth WBC/Diff ± CRP at age 6 – 12 h

**Antibiotics**

Treat with broad-spectrum antibiotics

**Management**

Blood culture positive

Blood culture negative Infant remains well Lab data abnormal

Blood culture negative Infant remains well Lab data normal

Continue antibiotics Lumbar puncture[b]

Continue antibiotics if mother received antibiotics during labor and delivery

Discontinue antibiotics

[a]   The diagnosis of chorioamnionitis is problematic and has important implications for the management of the newborn infant. Therefore, pediatric providers are encouraged to speak with their obstetrical colleagues whenever the diagnosis is made.

[b]   Lumbar puncture is indicated in any infant with a positive blood culture or in whom sepsis is highly suspected on the basis of clinical signs, response to treatment, and laboratory results.

IAP, intrapartum antimicrobial prophylaxis; WBC, white blood cell; Diff, differential white blood cell count.

*Reproduced with permission from Pediatrics, 129, 1006-1015, Copyright © 2012 by the AAP.*

APPENDIX 5.2  **Evaluation of Asymptomatic Infants ≥ 37 weeks' Gestation with Risk Factors for Sepsis.**[6]

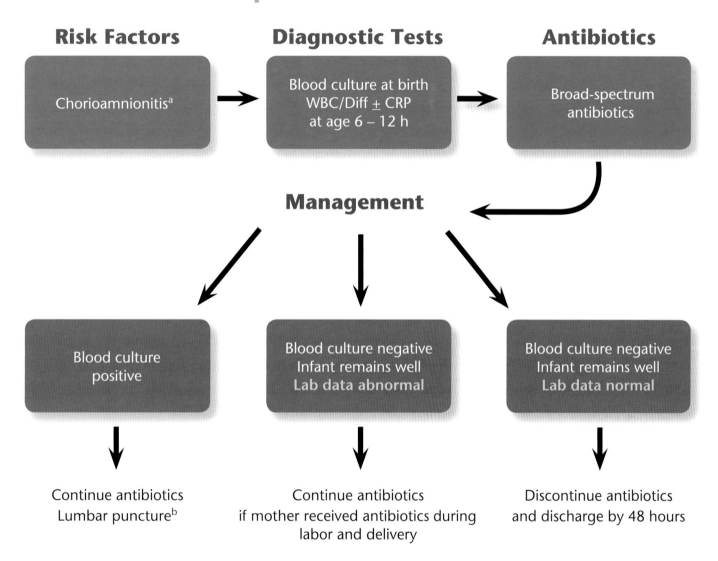

APPENDIX 5.3. **Evaluation of Asymptomatic Infants ≥ 37 Weeks' Gestation with Risk Factors for Sepsis (no chorioamnionitis).**[6]

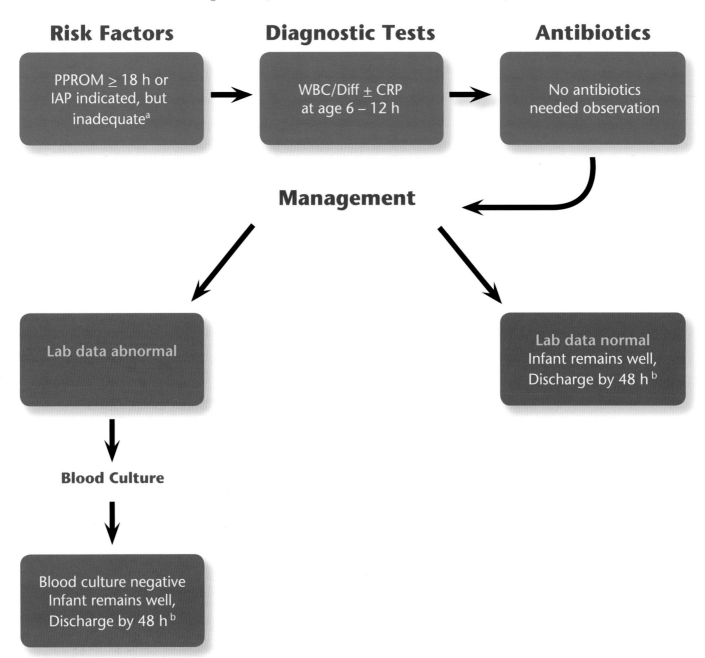

a   Inadequate treatment: Defined as the use of an antibiotic other than penicillin, ampicillin, or cefazolin or if the duration of antibiotics before delivery was <4 hours.

b   Discharge at 24 hours is acceptable if other discharge criteria have been met, access to medical care is readily accessible, and a person who is able to comply fully with instructions for home observation will be present. If any of these conditions is not met, the infant should be observed in the hospital for at least 48 hours and until discharge criteria are achieved.

IAP, intrapartum antimicrobial prophylaxis; WBC, white blood cell; Diff, differential white blood cell count

## Appendix 5.4 Algorithm for Secondary Prevention of Early-Onset Group B Streptococcal Disease Among Newborns[7]

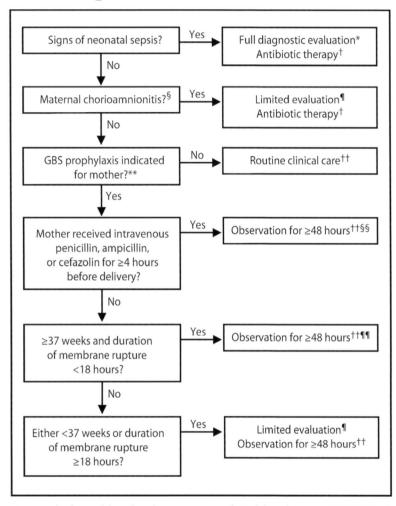

\* Full diagnostic evaluation includes a blood culture, a complete blood count (CBC) including white blood cell differential and platelet counts, chest radiograph (if respiratory abnormalities are present), and lumbar puncture (if patient is stable enough to tolerate procedure and sepsis is suspected).

† Antibiotic therapy should be directed toward the most common causes of neonatal sepsis, including intravenous ampicillin for GBS and coverage for other organisms (including *Escherichia coli* and other gram-negative pathogens) and should take into account local antibiotic resistance patterns.

§ Consultation with obstetric providers is important to determine the level of clinical suspicion for chorioamnionitis. Chorioamnionitis is diagnosed clinically and some of the signs are nonspecific.

¶ Limited evaluation includes blood culture (at birth) and CBC with differential and platelets (at birth and/or at 6–12 hours of life).

\*\* See **Appendix 5.5** for indications for intrapartum GBS prophylaxis.

†† If signs of sepsis develop, a full diagnostic evaluation should be conducted and antibiotic therapy initiated.

§§ If ≥37 weeks' gestation, observation may occur at home after 24 hours if other discharge criteria have been met, access to medical care is readily available, and a person who is able to comply fully with instructions for home observation will be present. If any of these conditions is not met, the infant should be observed in the hospital for at least 48 hours and until discharge criteria are achieved.

¶¶ Some experts recommend a CBC with differential and platelets at age 6–12 hours.

*Excerpt from: Centers for Disease Control and Prevention. Prevention of Perinatal Group B Streptococcal Disease. Revised Guidelines from CDC, 2010. MMWR, 2010,59 (No RR-10); 1-32.*
*Available at: http://www.cdc.gov/groupbstrep/guidelines/index.html*

## Appendix 5.5 Indications and Nonindications for Intrapartum Antibiotic Prophylaxis to Prevent Early-Onset Group B Streptococcal (GBS) Disease[7]

| Intrapartum GBS prophylaxis indicated | Intrapartum GBS prophylaxis not indicated |
|---|---|
| • Previous infant with invasive GBS disease<br><br>• GBS bacteriuria during any trimester of the current pregnancy*<br><br>• Positive GBS vaginal-rectal screening culture in late gestation[†] during current pregnancy*<br><br>• Unknown GBS status at the onset of labor (culture not done, incomplete, or results unknown) and any of the following:<br>  – Delivery at <37 weeks' gestation§<br>  – Amniotic membrane rupture ≥18 hours<br>  – Intrapartum temperature ≥100.4°F (≥38.0°C)[A]<br>  – Intrapartum NAAT** positive for GBS | • Colonization with GBS during a previous pregnancy (unless an indication for GBS prophylaxis is present for current pregnancy)<br><br>• GBS bacteriuria during previous pregnancy (unless an indication for GBS prophylaxis is present for current pregnancy)<br><br>• Negative vaginal and rectal GBS screening culture in late gestation[†] during the current pregnancy, regardless of intrapartum risk factors<br><br>• Cesarean delivery performed before onset of labor on a woman with intact amniotic membranes, regardless of GBS colonization status or gestational age |

**Abbreviation:** NAAT = Nucleic acid amplification tests

\* Intrapartum antibiotic prophylaxis is not indicated in this circumstance if a cesarean delivery is performed before onset of labor on a woman with intact amniotic membranes.

† Optimal timing for prenatal GBS screening is at 35–37 weeks' gestation.

§ Recommendations for the use of intrapartum antibiotics for prevention of early-onset GBS disease in the setting of threatened preterm delivery are presented in Appendices 5.6 and 5.7.

A If amnionitis is suspected, broad-spectrum antibiotic therapy that includes an agent known to be active against GBS should replace GBS prophylaxis.

\*\* NAAT testing for GBS is optional and might not be available in all settings. If intrapartum NAAT is negative for GBS but any other intrapartum risk factor (delivery at <37 weeks' gestation, amniotic membrane rupture at ≥18 hours, or temperature ≥100.4°F [≥38.0°C]) is present, then intrapartum antibiotic prophylaxis is indicated.

*Excerpt from: Centers for Disease Control and Prevention. Prevention of Perinatal Group B Streptococcal Disease. Revised Guidelines from CDC, 2010. MMWR, 2010,59 (No RR-10); 1-32. Available at: http://www.cdc.gov/groupbstrep/guidelines/index.html*

Appendix 5.6 **Algorithm for Screening for Group B Streptococcal (GBS) Colonization and Use of Intrapartum Prophylaxis for Women with Preterm\* Labor (PTL)[7]**

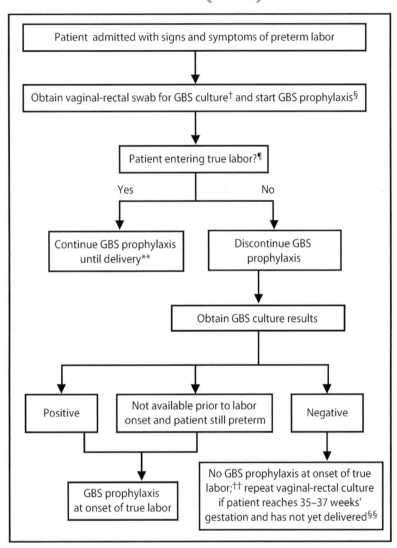

\*   At <37 weeks and 0 days' gestation.

†   If patient has undergone vaginal-rectal GBS culture within the preceding 5 weeks, the results of that culture should guide management. GBS-colonized women should receive intrapartum antibiotic prophylaxis. No antibiotics are indicated for GBS prophylaxis if a vaginal-rectal screen within 5 weeks was negative.

§   See Appendix 5.8 for recommended antibiotic regimens.

¶   Patient should be regularly assessed for progression to true labor; if the patient is considered not to be in true labor, discontinue GBS prophylaxis.

\*\*   If GBS culture results become available prior to delivery and are negative, then discontinue GBS prophylaxis.

††   Unless subsequent GBS culture prior to delivery is positive.

§§   A negative GBS screen is considered valid for 5 weeks. If a patient with a history of PTL is re-admitted with signs and symptoms of PTL and had a negative GBS screen >5 weeks prior, she should be rescreened and managed according to this algorithm at that time.

*Excerpt from: Centers for Disease Control and Prevention. Prevention of Perinatal Group B Streptococcal Disease. Revised Guidelines from CDC, 2010. MMWR, 2010,59 (No RR-10); 1-32.*
*Available at: http://www.cdc.gov/groupbstrep/guidelines/index.html*

Appendix 5.7 **Algorithm for Screening for Group B Streptococcal (GBS) Colonization and Use of Intrapartum Prophylaxis for Women with Preterm\* Premature Rupture of Membranes (pPROM)**[7]

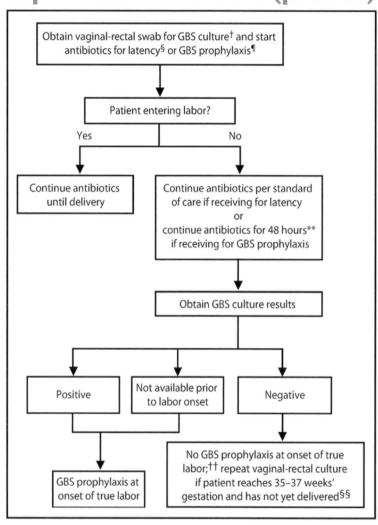

\*  At <37 weeks and 0 days' gestation.

†  If patient has undergone vaginal-rectal GBS culture within the preceding 5 weeks, the results of that culture should guide management. GBS-colonized women should receive intrapartum antibiotic prophylaxis. No antibiotics are indicated for GBS prophylaxis if a vaginal-rectal screen within 5 weeks was negative.

§  Antibiotics given for latency in the setting of pPROM that include ampicillin 2 g intravenously (IV) once, followed by 1 g IV every 6 hours for at least 48 hours are adequate for GBS prophylaxis. If other regimens are used, GBS prophylaxis should be initiated in addition.

¶  See Appendix 5.8 for recommended antibiotic regimens.

\*\*  GBS prophylaxis should be discontinued at 48 hours for women with pPROM who are not in labor. If results from a GBS screen performed on admission become available during the 48-hour period and are negative, GBS prophylaxis should be discontinued at that time.

††  Unless subsequent GBS culture prior to delivery is positive.

§§  A negative GBS screen is considered valid for 5 weeks. If a patient with pPROM is entering labor and had a negative GBS screen >5 weeks prior, she should be rescreened and managed according to this algorithm at that time.

*Excerpt from: Centers for Disease Control and Prevention. Prevention of Perinatal Group B Streptococcal Disease. Revised Guidelines from CDC, 2010. MMWR, 2010,59 (No RR-10); 1-32.*
*Available at: http://www.cdc.gov/groupbstrep/guidelines/index.html*

## Appendix 5.8 Recommended Regimens for Intrapartum Antibiotic Prophylaxis for Prevention of Early-Onset Group B Streptococcal (GBS) Disease*[7]

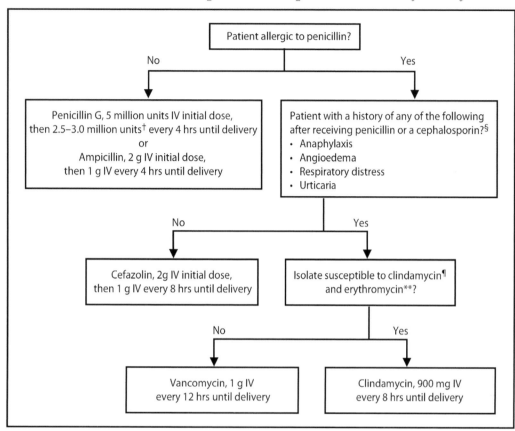

**Abbreviation:** IV = intravenously.

\* Broader spectrum agents, including an agent active against GBS, might be necessary for treatment of chorioamnionitis.

† Doses ranging from 2.5 to 3.0 million units are acceptable for the doses administered every 4 hours following the initial dose. The choice of dose within that range should be guided by which formulations of penicillin G are readily available to reduce the need for pharmacies to specially prepare doses.

§ Penicillin-allergic patients with a history of anaphylaxis, angioedema, respiratory distress, or urticaria following administration of penicillin or a cephalosporin are considered to be at high risk for anaphylaxis and should not receive penicillin, ampicillin, or cefazolin for GBS intrapartum prophylaxis. For penicillin-allergic patients who do not have a history of those reactions, cefazolin is the preferred agent because pharmacologic data suggest it achieves effective intraamniotic concentrations. Vancomycin and clindamycin should be reserved for penicillin-allergic women at high risk for anaphylaxis.

¶ If laboratory facilities are adequate, clindamycin and erythromycin susceptibility testing (Box 3) should be performed on prenatal GBS isolates from penicillin-allergic women at high risk for anaphylaxis. If no susceptibility testing is performed, or the results are not available at the time of labor, vancomycin is the preferred agent for GBS intrapartum prophylaxis for penicillin-allergic women at high risk for anaphylaxis.

\*\* Resistance to erythromycin is often but not always associated with clindamycin resistance. If an isolate is resistant to erythromycin, it might have inducible resistance to clindamycin, even if it appears susceptible to clindamycin. If a GBS isolate is susceptible to clindamycin, resistant to erythromycin, and testing for inducible clindamycin resistance has been performed and is negative (no inducible resistance), then clindamycin can be used for GBS intrapartum prophylaxis instead of vancomycin.

*Excerpt from: Centers for Disease Control and Prevention. Prevention of Perinatal Group B Streptococcal Disease. Revised Guidelines from CDC, 2010. MMWR, 2010,59 (No RR-10); 1-32.*
*Available at: http://www.cdc.gov/groupbstrep/guidelines/index.html*

# Appendix 5.9 **Hematologic Reference Ranges**

## Introduction and reference ranges contributed by:

*Robert D. Christensen, MD*
*Director, Neonatology Research*
*Intermountain Healthcare*
*Salt Lake City, Utah*
*Medical Director, Newborn Intensive Care Unit*
*McKay Dee Medical Center*
*Ogden, Utah*

Interpreting the complete blood count (CBC) in adult patients involves comparing their measured values with "normal ranges". Such ranges were established by drawing blood on large numbers of healthy volunteers. In contrast, because of ethical concerns for newborn infants, blood is not drawn on healthy normal neonates for the purpose of establishing normal ranges and therefore another approach must be used to permit proper interpretation of their CBC results. That approach involves the concept of "reference ranges". These ranges consist of 5th to 95th percentile values compiled from laboratory tests that were performed on neonates for clinical purposes. Data is compiled retrospectively from neonates thought to have minimal pathology relevant to the laboratory test, or with pathology unlikely to significantly affect the test results. The premise on which the reference range concept is based is that these values approximate normal ranges, although they were admittedly obtained for a clinical reason and not from healthy volunteers. "Normal ranges" for most laboratory in adult medicine, are those encompassing 95% of values drawn from healthy volunteers, thus the normal range falls between the 2.5th percentile value as the lower limit of normal, and the 97.5th percentile value as the upper limit of normal. Because "reference ranges" are not obtained from healthy volunteers, it is the usual convention to narrow the range to that incorporating 90% of values, and thus the reference ranges are those that fall between the 5th and the 95th percentile values.

### Normal range for ANC in infants > 36-weeks gestation in the first 72 hours of life[30]

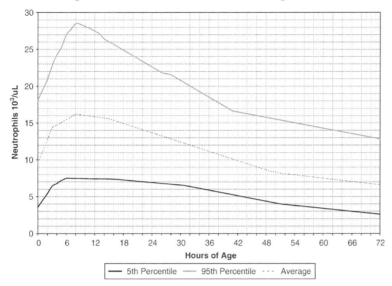

### Normal range for ANC in infants 28- to 36-weeks gestation in the first 72 hours of life[30]

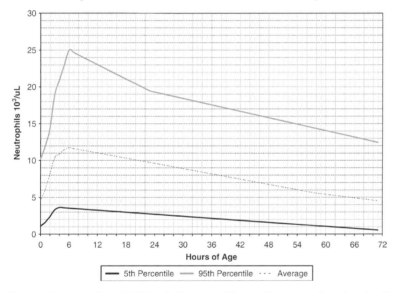

### Normal range for ANC in infants < 28-weeks gestation in the first 72 hours of life[30]

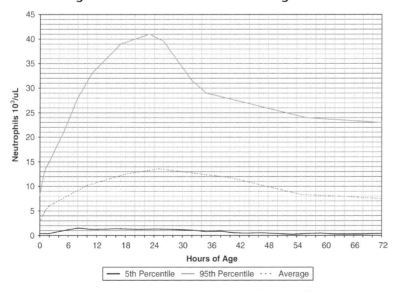

Reprinted by permission from Macmillan Publishers Ltd: Journal of Perinatology, Schmutz N, Henry E, Jopling J, Christensen RD. Expected ranges for blood neutrophil concentrations of neonates: the Manroe and Mouzinho charts revisited; Figure 3. 28:275-81, © 2008.

# Appendix 5.9 **Hematologic Reference Ranges** (continued)

**Lymphocyte counts at birth as a function of gestational age**

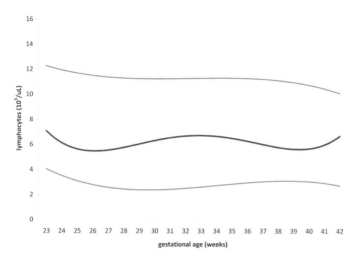

## Lymphocyte counts in the first 12 hours of life

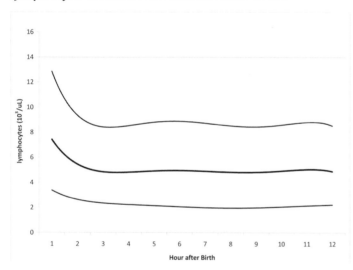

## Lymphocyte counts in the first 28 days, term and preterm

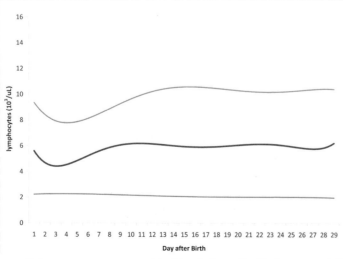

Reference ranges provided by Robert D. Christensen, MD and reproduced with permission.

Eosinophil counts at birth as a function of gestational age

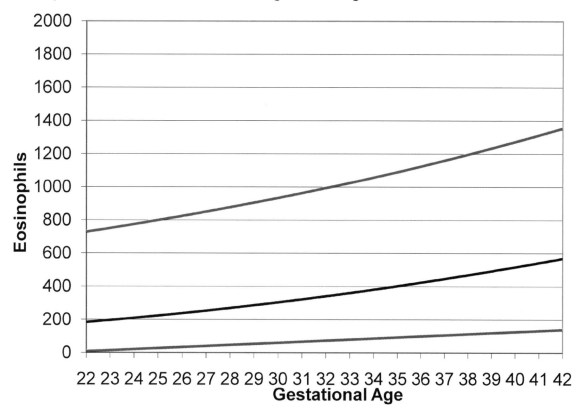

Eosinophil counts in the first 28 days of life, term and preterm

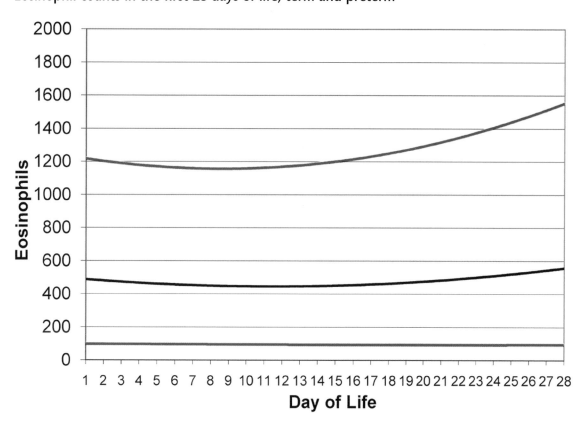

Reference ranges provided by Robert D. Christensen, MD and reproduced with permission.

# Appendix 5.9  **Hematologic Reference Ranges** (continued)

**Monocyte count at birth as a function of gestational age**

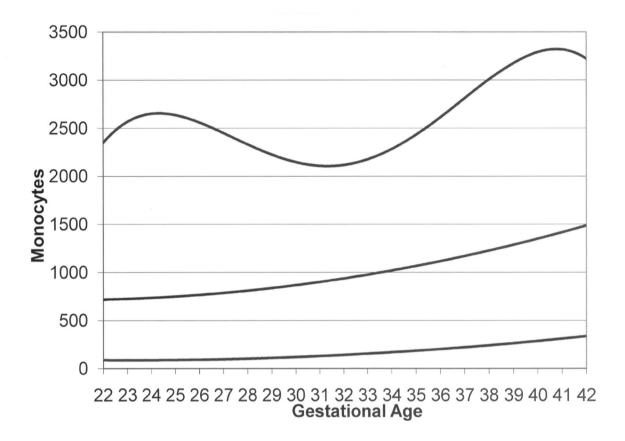

Reference ranges provided by Robert D. Christensen, MD and reproduced with permission.

## Platelet count at birth as a function of gestational age

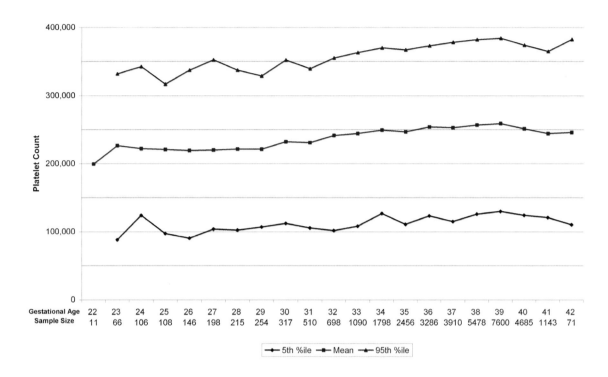

## Platelet counts in the 90 days after birth, term and preterm

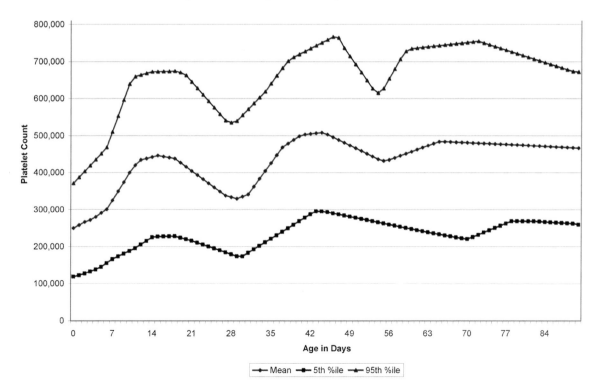

Reference ranges provided by Robert D. Christensen, MD and reproduced with permission.

# Appendix 5.10 **Case Study: Baby Smith**

*This case study was based upon an actual patient account. Some of the infant and maternal characteristics have been changed to maintain anonymity.*

A 36-week gestation AGA infant was delivered vaginally following spontaneous rupture of membranes five hours prior to delivery. The mother was a gravida 3, para 2 (full-term deliveries in prior pregnancies) woman with good prenatal care. Aside from a urinary tract infection treated with oral antibiotics two weeks prior to delivery, the mother's pregnancy was uncomplicated. APGAR scores were 6 at one minute and 8 at five minutes. Resuscitation included drying, suctioning of the oropharynx, tactile stimulation and blow-by oxygen for a brief period. The infant appeared stable, so was bundled in warm blankets and held by his mother.

Ninety minutes later the nurse was preparing to bathe the infant, when she noted the infant appeared cyanotic. She immediately took the infant to the observation nursery and placed him under a radiant warmer and attached an oximeter to his right hand.

His vital signs were:

◇ Axillary temperature 36.1°C (97°F)

◇ Heart rate 160 beats per minute

◇ Respiratory rate 80 per minute

$O_2$ saturation on room air was 82%. 30% oxygen was provided by hood, with improvement in the saturation to 92%.

The infant's physician was notified and a CBC was ordered. The results were:

◇ WBC 11,000 (11 x 10³/µL)

◇ Segmented neutrophils 31%

◇ Band neutrophils 6%

◇ Lymphocytes 57%

◇ Monocytes 6%

◇ Platelet count 30,000

**Activity**: Evaluate the CBC results and calculate the I/T ratio and the ANC.

The nurse evaluated the CBC and decided it was "normal because there were very few bands" and so she did not call the physician to report the results. One hour later the infant was maintaining $O_2$ saturation above 90% on room air and the mother was requesting the infant be brought back to her room. Vital signs at this point are: 37°C (98.6°F) axillary, respiratory rate 60. The infant was then taken to his mother who reported a short while later, that he breast fed with "fair interest" and that he seemed very sleepy.

### Case Study · Baby Smith

- › G3, P2, 36 weeks, good prenatal care
- › History of UTI treated 2 weeks prior to delivery
- › SVD following SROM of AGA male infant
- › APGAR 6 at 1 minute and 8 at 5 minutes
  - ▪ Tactile stimulation and blow-by $O_2$ briefly
- › Wrapped in blankets – held by mother
- › Infant assessed as stable and remained with mother

269

### Case Study · Baby Smith

- › Cyanosis noted 90 minutes later → placed under radiant warmer
- › VS → T 36.1°C (97°F), HR 160, RR 80
- › $O_2$ saturation 82% on room air
- › 30% $O_2$ by hood → $SaO_2$ ↑ 92%
- › Physician notified → CBC ordered
- › CBC: WBC 11,000, 31% segs, 6% bands, 57% lymphs, 6% monos, platelets 30,000
  - ▪ Because I/T ratio 'normal', physician not notified

*Calculate I/T ratio and Absolute Neutrophil Count*

269

### Case Study · Baby Smith

- › 1 hour later weaned to room air
  - ▪ T 37°C (98.6°F), RR 60, $SaO_2$ > 90%
  - ▪ To mother's room for breast-feeding (fair interest)

- › 6 hours of age T 36°C (96.8°F) → placed in incubator
- › Bottle fed with encouragement 15 – 20 ml per feeding
  - ▪ Regurgitation after a few feedings
- › Intermittently required $O_2$ for desaturation to low 80s

269

At six hours of age the infant was again hypothermic (36°C or 96.8°F) and was placed in an incubator. This action occurred shortly before a change of nursing shift; the physician was also not notified that the infant required an incubator. Throughout the evening, the infant remained in the incubator and the mother came to the nursery to breast feed. The infant would not latch and so he was offered formula. He took between 15 and 25 mL per feeding. The blood glucose was not evaluated at any point.

Towards the morning, the infant became less responsive and when offered formula, he vomited. He again looked cyanotic ($O_2$ saturation was evaluated and found to be 80%) and he was given supplemental oxygen. At 16 hours of life, his respiratory status deteriorated further and he began grunting and retracting. The oxygen was increased to 50% to maintain an $O_2$ saturation > 90%. The on-call pediatrician was notified at this point and ordered a CBC, CRP, CBG, and chest x-ray.

When the x-ray was being taken, the infant deteriorated and became apneic and bradycardic. Bag and mask positive pressure ventilation was given and the heart rate improved to > 100. The pediatrician arrived shortly thereafter to the bedside.

> ### Case Study · Baby Smith
>
> › 16 hours of life → increased respiratory distress
>   - Grunting and retractions
>   - 50% $O_2$ to keep SaO2 > 90%
> › On-call physician notified
>   - Chest x-ray → pneumonia
>   - CBC: WBC 1,800, 9% segs, 31% bands, platelets 22K
> › During chest x-ray → apnea, bradycardia, mottled
>   - Bag-mask PPV
> › Intubated, mechanical ventilation, normal saline bolus x 2 for poor perfusion and hypotension
> › Dopamine 10 mcg/kg/min, blood glucose 20 mg/dL
>
> 269
> S.T.A.B.L.E.
> © K. Karlsen 2013

The chest x-ray was consistent with pneumonia and the second CBC revealed significant neutropenia and left shift with the following results:

✧ WBC 1,800 (1.8 x 10³/µL)

✧ Segmented neutrophils 9%

✧ Band neutrophils 31%

✧ Platelet count 22,000

   **Activity**: Evaluate the CBC results and calculate the I/T ratio and the ANC.

The infant required endotracheal intubation, assisted ventilation, and aggressive cardiopulmonary support including two normal saline boluses for poor perfusion and hypotension. Dopamine was initiated at 10 mcg/kg/minute. The blood glucose (first one obtained since birth), was 20 mg/dL (1.1 mmol/L). Blood cultures were drawn and ampicillin and gentamicin antibiotics were started. The low blood glucose was treated with an IV glucose bolus of 2 mL/kg of $D_{10}W$ and a continuous infusion of $D_{10}W$. The blood sugar remained stable above 50 mg/dL (2.8 mmol/L) thereafter.

Shortly after arrival of the neonatal transport team, the infant again became bradycardic (heart rate 50) and was given five minutes of chest compressions and two doses of epinephrine. He was then transported to the tertiary neonatal intensive care unit without incident.

The blood culture grew Group B Streptococcus within 12 hours. Over the next two weeks the infant was critically ill, and required treatment for pulmonary hypertension, disseminated intravascular coagulation, and poor cardiac output. At five weeks of age, the infant improved sufficiently to allow discharge to home. The parents remained very concerned about their ability to care for the infant at home because he still required supplemental oxygen and gavage feedings. Follow-up over the next three years revealed marked motor and developmental delay.

> ### Case Study · Baby Smith
>
> › Blood cultures drawn, antibiotics started
>   - Cultures positive at 12 hours for Group B Strep
> › Transport team arrived – infant became bradycardic – chest compressions and 2 rounds of resuscitation drugs required
> › Transported to tertiary center
> › Critically ill for 2 weeks – seizures, PPHN, DIC, hypotension
> › Discharged at 5 weeks of age – still requiring supplemental $O_2$ and gavage feedings
> › Poor neurodevelopmental status on follow-up
>
>
>
> 269
> S.T.A.B.L.E.
> © K. Karlsen 2013

# Practice Session: Lab Work

1.  For the following CBC results, calculate the ANC and the I/T ratio.

2.  Plot the ANC on the Schmutz charts provided with each CBC example.

3.  For each CBC, is the platelet count low, normal or high?

---

## ANC Calculation
WBC (may be reported as WBC x $10^3/\mu L$) multiplied by [(%) (segs + bands + metas)]

## Immature to Total (I/T) ratio calculation
(%) metamyelocytes + bands **(Immature)** divided by (%) metamyelocytes + bands + segs **(Total)**

---

## CBC 1

**Age 8 hours**
**39 weeks gestation**

| | |
|---|---|
| WBC (mm³) | 10.4 |
| Metamyelocytes (%) | 0 |
| Band Neutrophils (%) | 14 |
| Segmented Neutrophils (%) | 5 |
| Monocytes (%) | 6 |
| Basophils (%) | 2 |
| Eosinophils (%) | 3 |
| Lymphocytes (%) | 70 |
| Platelets | 141,000 |

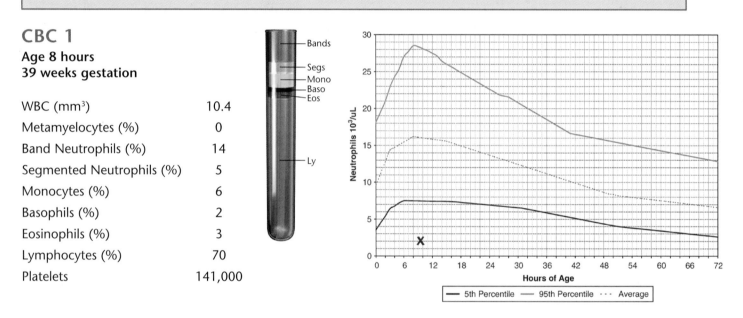

## ANC calculation

The ANC is 1976 (plot on the appropriate chart for gestational age for the patient's age)

| 10,400 | x | 19% or .19 | = | 1976 |
|---|---|---|---|---|

## I/T ratio calculation

$$\frac{\boxed{0}\ \text{metas} + \boxed{14}\ \text{bands} = \text{Immature}}{\boxed{0}\ \text{metas} + \boxed{14}\ \text{bands} + \boxed{5}\ \text{segs} = \text{Total}}$$

$\dfrac{\boxed{14}}{\boxed{19}} = 0.74$ The I/T ratio is 0.74

For the I/T and ANC calculations, disregard the lymphocyte, monocyte, eosinophil, and basophil percentages, but do include any metamyelocytes or myelocytes as immature cells if present on the CBC report.

## CBC 2

**Age 24 hours**
**34 weeks gestation**

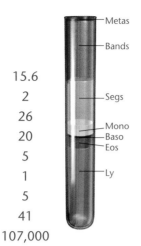

| | |
|---|---|
| WBC (mm³) | 15.6 |
| Metamyelocytes (%) | 2 |
| Band Neutrophils (%) | 26 |
| Segmented Neutrophils (%) | 20 |
| Monocytes (%) | 5 |
| Basophils (%) | 1 |
| Eosinophils (%) | 5 |
| Lymphocytes (%) | 41 |
| Platelets | 107,000 |

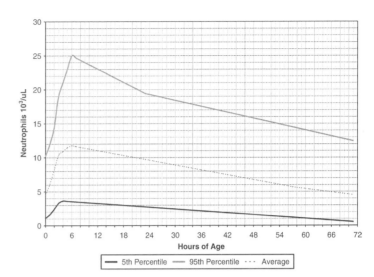

### ANC calculation

15,600 x _____ (%) neutrophils = _____ (ANC)

### I/T ratio calculation

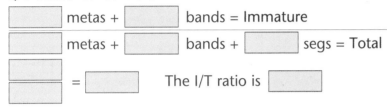

_____ metas + _____ bands = Immature

_____ metas + _____ bands + _____ segs = Total

_____ / _____ = _____     The I/T ratio is _____

---

## CBC 3

**Age 18 hours**
**30 weeks gestation**

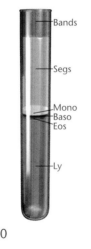

| | |
|---|---|
| WBC (mm³) | 15.4 |
| Metamyelocytes (%) | 0 |
| Band Neutrophils (%) | 12 |
| Segmented Neutrophils (%) | 33 |
| Monocytes (%) | 2 |
| Basophils (%) | 1 |
| Eosinophils (%) | 1 |
| Lymphocytes (%) | 51 |
| Platelets | 171,000 |

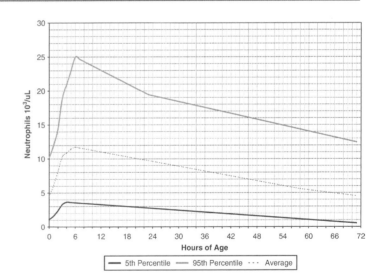

### ANC calculation

_____ x _____ (%) neutrophils = _____ (ANC)

### I/T ratio calculation

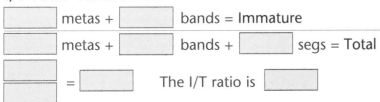

_____ metas + _____ bands = Immature

_____ metas + _____ bands + _____ segs = Total

_____ / _____ = _____     The I/T ratio is _____

## CBC 4

**Age 4 hours**
**26 weeks gestation**

| | |
|---|---|
| WBC (mm³) | 1.3 |
| Metamyelocytes (%) | 2 |
| Band Neutrophils (%) | 17 |
| Segmented Neutrophils (%) | 42 |
| Monocytes (%) | 4 |
| Basophils (%) | 1 |
| Eosinophils (%) | 1 |
| Lymphocytes (%) | 33 |
| Platelets | 226,000 |

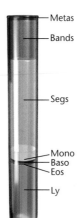

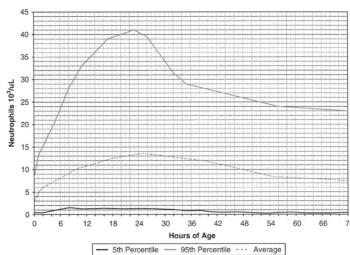

### ANC calculation

[   ] x [   ] (%) neutrophils = [   ] (ANC)

### I/T ratio calculation

[   ] metas + [   ] bands = Immature

[   ] metas + [   ] bands + [   ] segs = Total

[   ] / [   ] = [   ]    The I/T ratio is [   ]

---

## CBC 5

**Age 10 hours**
**36 weeks gestation**

| | |
|---|---|
| WBC (mm³) | 3.1 |
| Metamyelocytes (%) | 0 |
| Band Neutrophils (%) | 37 |
| Segmented Neutrophils (%) | 27 |
| Monocytes (%) | 2 |
| Basophils (%) | 1 |
| Eosinophils (%) | 4 |
| Lymphocytes (%) | 29 |
| Platelets | 72,000 |

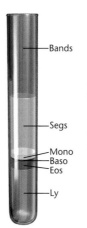

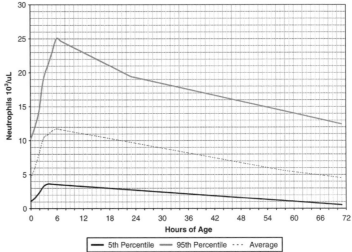

### ANC calculation

[   ] x [   ] (%) neutrophils = [   ] (ANC)

### I/T ratio calculation

[   ] metas + [   ] bands = Immature

[   ] metas + [   ] bands + [   ] segs = Total

[   ] / [   ] = [   ]    The I/T ratio is [   ]

## CBC 6

**Age 36 hours**
**38 weeks gestation**

| | |
|---|---|
| WBC (mm³) | 26.5 |
| Metamyelocytes (%) | 0 |
| Band Neutrophils (%) | 10 |
| Segmented Neutrophils (%) | 60 |
| Monocytes (%) | 4 |
| Basophils (%) | 1 |
| Eosinophils (%) | 1 |
| Lymphocytes (%) | 24 |
| Platelets | 280,000 |

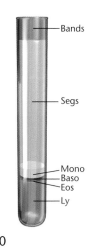
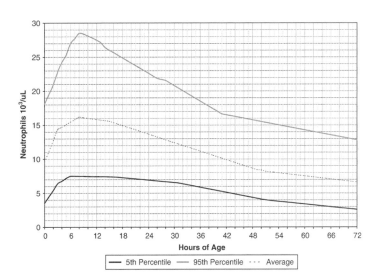

### ANC calculation

☐ x ☐ (%) neutrophils = ☐ (ANC)

### I/T ratio calculation

☐ metas + ☐ bands = Immature

☐ metas + ☐ bands + ☐ segs = Total

$\dfrac{☐}{☐}$ = ☐   The I/T ratio is ☐

---

## CBC 7

**Age 60 hours** – same patient as
CBC 6 – **24 hours later**

| | |
|---|---|
| WBC (mm³) | 10.4 |
| Metamyelocytes (%) | 0 |
| Band Neutrophils (%) | 4 |
| Segmented Neutrophils (%) | 73 |
| Monocytes (%) | 7 |
| Basophils (%) | 1 |
| Eosinophils (%) | 1 |
| Lymphocytes (%) | 14 |
| Platelets | 240,000 |

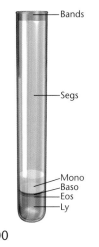
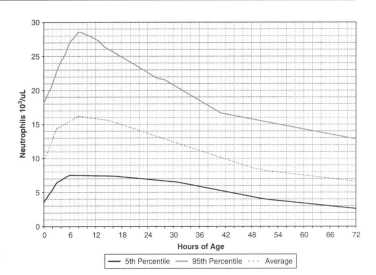

### ANC calculation

☐ x ☐ (%) neutrophils = ☐ (ANC)

### I/T ratio calculation

☐ metas + ☐ bands = Immature

☐ metas + ☐ bands + ☐ segs = Total

$\dfrac{☐}{☐}$ = ☐   The I/T ratio is ☐

## CBC 8

**Age 48 hours**
**30 weeks gestation**

| | |
|---|---|
| WBC (mm³) | 6.3 |
| Metamyelocytes (%) | 6 |
| Band Neutrophils (%) | 44 |
| Segmented Neutrophils (%) | 23 |
| Monocytes (%) | 6 |
| Basophils (%) | 1 |
| Eosinophils (%) | 2 |
| Lymphocytes (%) | 18 |
| Platelets | 95,000 |

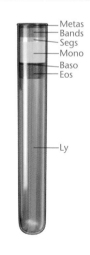

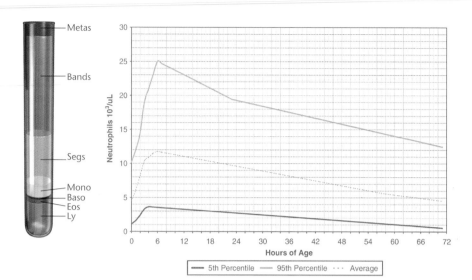

### ANC calculation

[ ] x [ ] (%) neutrophils = [ ] (ANC)

### I/T ratio calculation

[ ] metas + [ ] bands = Immature

[ ] metas + [ ] bands + [ ] segs = Total

[ ] / [ ] = [ ] The I/T ratio is [ ]

---

## CBC 9

**Age 60 hours** – same patient as CBC 8, **12 hours later**

| | |
|---|---|
| WBC (mm³) | 0.8 |
| Metamyelocytes (%) | 2 |
| Band Neutrophils (%) | 4 |
| Segmented Neutrophils (%) | 2 |
| Monocytes (%) | 9 |
| Basophils (%) | 1 |
| Eosinophils (%) | 6 |
| Lymphocytes (%) | 76 |
| Platelets | 24,000 |

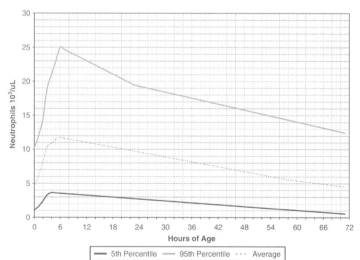

### ANC calculation

[ ] x [ ] (%) neutrophils = [ ] (ANC)

### I/T ratio calculation

[ ] metas + [ ] bands = Immature

[ ] metas + [ ] bands + [ ] segs = Total

[ ] / [ ] = [ ] The I/T ratio is [ ]

## CBC 10

**Age 12 hours**
**35 weeks gestation**

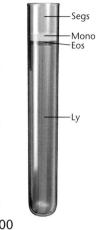

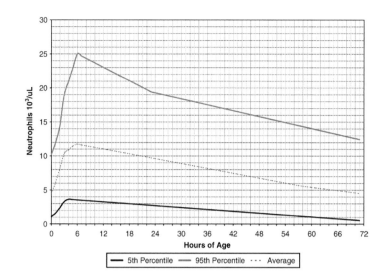

| | |
|---|---|
| WBC (mm³) | 1.1 |
| Metamyelocytes (%) | 0 |
| Band Neutrophils (%) | 0 |
| Segmented Neutrophils (%) | 13 |
| Monocytes (%) | 3 |
| Basophils (%) | 0 |
| Eosinophils (%) | 2 |
| Lymphocytes (%) | 82 |
| Platelets | 46,000 |

## ANC calculation

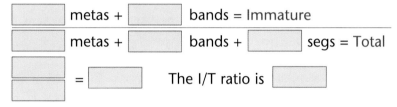

[    ] x [    ] (%) neutrophils = [    ] (ANC)

## I/T ratio calculation

[    ] metas + [    ] bands = Immature

[    ] metas + [    ] bands + [    ] segs = Total

[    ] / [    ] = [    ]     The I/T ratio is [    ]

# References

1. Ferrieri P, Wallen LD. Neonatal Bacterial Sepsis. In: Gleason CA, Devaskar SU, eds. Avery's Diseases of the Newborn. 9th ed. Philadelphia: Elsevier Saunders; 2012:538-50.

2. Gerdes JS. Diagnosis and management of bacterial infections in the neonate. Pediatr Clin North Am 2004;51:939-59, viii-ix.

3. Koenig JM, Yoder MC. Neonatal neutrophils: the good, the bad, and the ugly. Clin Perinatol 2004;31:39-51.

4. Edwards MS. Postnatal Bacterial Infections. In: Martin RJ, Fanaroff AA, Walsh MC, eds. Fanaroff and Martin's Neonatal-Perinatal Medicine: Diseases of the Fetus and Infant. 9th ed. St. Louis: Elsevier Mosby; 2011:793-829.

5. Stoll BJ, Hansen N, Fanaroff AA, et al. Changes in pathogens causing early-onset sepsis in very-low-birth-weight infants. N Engl J Med 2002;347:240-7.

6. Polin RA. Management of neonates with suspected or proven early-onset bacterial sepsis. Pediatrics 2012;129:1006-15.

7. Verani JR, McGee L, Schrag SJ. Prevention of perinatal group B streptococcal disease--revised guidelines from CDC, 2010. MMWR Recomm Rep 2010;59:1-36.

8. Tita AT, Andrews WW. Diagnosis and management of clinical chorioamnionitis. Clin Perinatol 2010;37:339-54.

9. Venkatesh MP, Adams KM, Weisman LE. Infection in the Neonate. In: Gardner SL, Carter BS, Enzman-Hines M, Hernandez JA, eds. Merenstein & Gardner's Handbook of Neonatal Intensive Care. 7th ed. St. Louis: Mosby Elsevier; 2011:553-80.

10. Burchett SK. Viral Infections. In: Cloherty JP, Eichenwald EC, Hansen AR, Stark AR, eds. Manual of Neonatal Care. 7th ed. Philadelphia: Lippincott, Williams & Wilkins; 2012:588-623.

11. Puopolo K. Bacterial and Fungal Infections. In: Cloherty JP, Eichenwald EC, Hansen AR, Stark AR, eds. Manual of neonatal care. 7th ed. Philadelphia: Wolters Kluwer / Lippincott Williams & Wilkins; 2012:624-55.

12. Ottolini MC, Lundgren K, Mirkinson LJ, Cason S, Ottolini MG. Utility of complete blood count and blood culture screening to diagnose neonatal sepsis in the asymptomatic at risk newborn. Pediatr Infect Dis J 2003;22:430-4.

13. Hornik CP, Benjamin DK, Becker KC, et al. Use of the Complete Blood Cell Count in Early-onset Neonatal Sepsis. Pediatr Infect Dis J 2012;31:799-802.

14. Eichenwald EC. Care of the Extremely Low-Birthweight Infant. In: Gleason CA, Devaskar SU, eds. Avery's Diseases of the Newborn. 9th ed. Philadelphia: Elsevier Saunders; 2012:390-404.

15. Hornik CP, Benjamin DK, Becker KC, et al. Use of the Complete Blood Cell Count in Late-onset Neonatal Sepsis. Pediatr Infect Dis J 2012;31:803-7.

16. Engelkirk PG, Duben-Engelkirk J. Burton's Microbiology for the Health Sciences. 9th ed. Baltimore: Lippincott Williams & Wilkins, Wolters Kluwer; 2011.

17. Schleiss MR, Patterson JC. Viral Infections of the Fetus and Newborn and Human Immunodeficiency Virus Infection During Pregnancy. In: Gleason CA, Devaskar SU, eds. Avery's Diseases of the Newborn 9th ed. Philadelphia: Elsevier Saunders; 2012:468-512.

18. Anderson BL, Gonik B. Perinatal Infections. In: Martin RJ, Fanaroff AA, Walsh MC, eds. Fanaroff and Martin's Neonatal-Perinatal Medicine: Diseases of the Fetus and Infant. 9th ed. St. Louis: Elsevier Mosby; 2011:399-422.

19. Schelonka RL, Chai MK, Yoder BA, Hensley D, Brockett RM, Ascher DP. Volume of blood required to detect common neonatal pathogens. J Pediatr 1996;129:275-8.

20. Connell TG, Rele M, Cowley D, Buttery JP, Curtis N. How reliable is a negative blood culture result? Volume of blood submitted for culture in routine practice in a children's hospital. Pediatrics 2007;119:891-6.

21. Papoff P. Use of Hematologic Data to Evaluate Infections in Neonates. In: Christensen RD, ed. Hematologic Problems of the Neonate. Philadelphia: W.B. Saunders Company; 2000:389-404.

22. Kaapa P, Koistinen E. Maternal and neonatal C-reactive protein after interventions during delivery. Acta Obstet Gynecol Scand 1993;72:543-6.

23. Black S, Kushner I, Samols D. C-reactive Protein. J Biol Chem 2004;279:48487-90.

24. Weitkamp JH, Aschner JL. Diagnostic use of C-Reactive Protein (CRP) in assessment of neonatal sepsis. NeoReviews 2005;6:e508-e15.

25. Christensen RD, Rothstein G, Hill HR, Hall RT. Fatal early onset group B streptococcal sepsis with normal leukocyte counts. Pediatr Infect Dis 1985;4:242-5.

26. Schibler K. Leukocyte Development and Disorders During the Neonatal Period. In: Christensen RD, ed. Hematology of the Neonate. Philadelphia: W.B. Saunders Company; 2000:311-42.

27. Strauss RG. Blood Banking and Transfusion Issues in Perinatal Medicine. In: Christensen RD, ed. Hematology of the Neonate. Philadelphia: W.B. Saunders Company; 2000:405-25.

28. Kapur R, Yoder MC, Polin RA. Developmental Immunology. In: Martin RJ, Fanaroff AA, Walsh MC, eds. Fanaroff and Martin's Neonatal-Perinatal Medicine: Diseases of the Fetus and Infant. 9th ed. St. Louis: Elsevier Mosby; 2011:761-93.

29. Christensen RD, Bradley PP, Rothstein G. The leukocyte left shift in clinical and experimental neonatal sepsis. J Pediatr 1981;98:101-5.

30. Schmutz N, Henry E, Jopling J, Christensen RD. Expected ranges for blood neutrophil concentrations of neonates: the Manroe and Mouzinho charts revisited. J Perinatol 2008;28:275-81.

31. Wiedmeier SE, Henry E, Christensen RD. Hematological abnormalities during the first week of life among neonates with trisomy 18 and trisomy 13: data from a multi-hospital healthcare system. Am J Med Genet A 2008;146:312-20.

32. Mouzinho A, Rosenfeld CR, Sanchez PJ, Risser R. Revised reference ranges for circulating neutrophils in very-low-birth-weight neonates. Pediatrics 1994;94:76-82.

33. Manroe BL, Weinberg AG, Rosenfeld CR, Browne R. The neonatal blood count in health and disease. I. Reference values for neutrophilic cells. J Pediatr 1979;95:89-98.

34. Sola MC. Evaluation and treatment of severe and prolonged thrombocytopenia in neonates. Clin Perinatol 2004;31:1-14.

35. McPherson RJ, Juul S. Patterns of thrombocytosis and thrombocytopenia in hospitalized neonates. J Perinatol 2005;25:166-72.

36. Saxonhouse MA, Sola-Visner MC. Thrombocytopenia in the Neonatal Intensive Care Unit. NeoReviews 2009;10:e435-e45.

37. Wiedmeier SE, Henry E, Sola-Visner MC, Christensen RD. Platelet reference ranges for neonates, defined using data from over 47,000 patients in a multihospital healthcare system. J Perinatol 2009;29:130-6.

38. Sola MC, Christensen RD. Developmental Aspects of Platelets and Disorders of Platelets in the Neonatal Period. In: Christensen RD, ed. Hematologic Problems of the Neonate. Philadelphia: W.B. Saunders Co.; 2000:273-309.

39. Puopolo KM. Bacterial and Fungal Infections. In: Cloherty JP, Eichenwald EC, Hansen AR, Stark AR, eds. Manual of Neonatal Care. 7th ed. Philadelphia: Lippincott, Williams & Wilkins; 2012:624-55.

40. Taketomo CK, Hodding JH, Kraus DM. Pediatric & Neonatal Dosage Handook. 18th ed. Hudson: Lexicomp; 2011.

41. Thomson Reuters Editorial Staff. NeoFax. 24th ed. Montvale: Thomson Reuters; 2011.

42. Douma CE, Schonen Gardner J. Common Neonatal Intensive Care Unit (NICU) Medication Guidelines. In: Cloherty JP, Eichenwald EC, Hansen AR, Stark AR, eds. Manual of Neonatal Care. 7th ed. Philadelphia: Lippincott, Williams & Wilkins; 2012:886-931.

43. Sheffield MJ, Lambert DK, Henry E, Christensen RD. Effect of ampicillin on the bleeding time of neonatal intensive care unit patients. J Perinatol 2010;30:527-30.

44. Sheffield MJ, Lambert DK, Baer VL, et al. Effect of ampicillin on bleeding time in very low birth-weight neonates during the first week after birth. J Perinatol 2011;31:477-80.

**S**ugar and **S**afe Care

**T**emperature

**A**irway

**B**lood Pressure

**L**ab Work

**E**motional Support

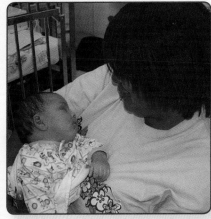

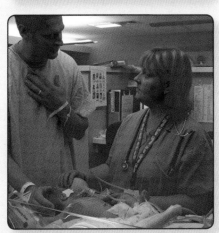

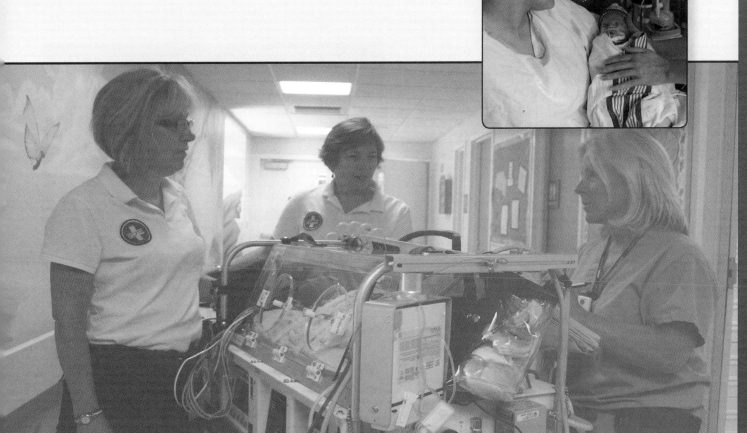

# Emotional Support – Module Objectives

Upon completion of this module, participants will gain an increased understanding of:

1. The crisis families experience when an infant requires transport to, or care in, a neonatal intensive care unit.

2. Ways healthcare providers can support parents of sick infants.

3. Methods neonatal healthcare providers can use to facilitate parenting in the NICU.

## Introduction

### When a newborn or young infant is born preterm or sick, parents experience a complicated crisis.[1]

It is helpful when caregivers recognize that each family brings a unique and potentially complicated history, as well as a diverse cultural background to each childbirth experience.[2,3] Parental reactions are sometimes hard to interpret and styles of coping vary, as do responses seen from the parents of the same baby. It is important to approach the family in a nonjudgmental manner and to activate support systems as necessary.

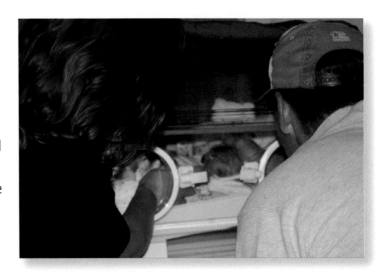

Emotions parents may experience when their infant is sick and/or preterm include guilt, anger, disbelief, sadness, a sense of failure, powerlessness, fear, blame, uncertainty, and depression.[1,4,5] Commonly, however, in the early period following onset of the baby's illness, the parents may not express any specific emotion, but may appear "numb".[1] They may not know what questions to ask, or what to do in a situation they did not expect or for which they were unprepared. Guilt and a sense of responsibility for the situation are likely the first and strongest emotions experienced by mothers.[6] Whenever possible, provide support and assistance to help the family cope with this crisis and their grief. Help the family to understand their infant's medical situation and involve them in decision making as this is critically important.[4]

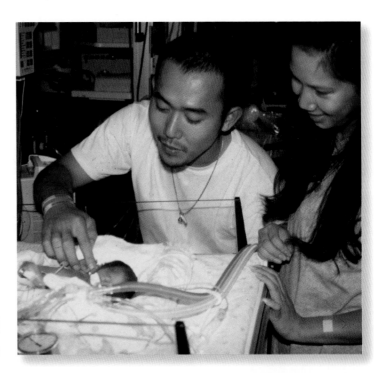

# Helpful Ideas for When the Infant Requires Transport

## Initial Stabilization Period

In the community hospital, nurses are in an ideal position to offer support to the family. The following are suggestions to guide this initial care.

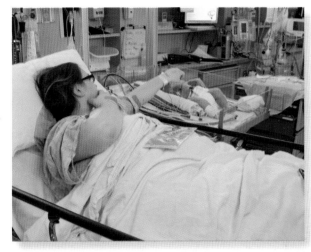

- If the mother is alone, inquire about her support system and encourage her to call or allow you to help call those whom she identifies – clergy, friends, and family members.

- If the mother's medical condition permits, take the mother to the nursery so she can be with the infant before the transport team arrives. Encourage the mother to talk to and touch her baby. If the mother's condition does not allow for her to be at the bedside, the transport team customarily will take the baby to the mother's room for a brief visit before their departure. It is helpful for at least one of the infant's nursery caregivers to accompany the transport team to the mother's room. When the team has departed, the caregiver can then answer any additional questions as well as help the mother understand the situation and what may happen next. The father or mother's significant other should also be encouraged to be with the infant as much as possible prior to transport. Allow and encourage photos and videotaping as both may be very comforting to the mother during her separation from the baby.

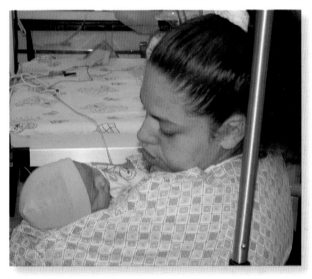

- Although analgesics are important for maternal care post-delivery, they may also interfere with the mother's ability to remember her time with the infant. Therefore, if you explain this fact to the mother, she may agree that it is best to receive an analgesic after the visit is over. The mother will appreciate that you helped her understand how an analgesic may affect her later recall of this important time with the infant.

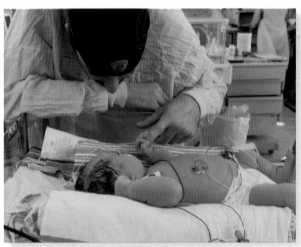

- Ask the parent(s) if the infant has been given a name and if yes, call the infant by name.

- In some cultures, names are not given in the immediate post-birth period; name selection and timing of naming the baby varies with different cultures; remain sensitive to these cultural differences.[3]

- Use the correct gender when referring to the infant.

- Referring to the infant with terms such as "your son" or "your daughter" will help the parents to identify as the parent of this infant.

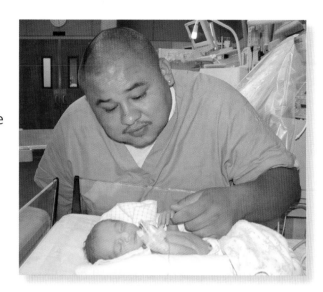

## Clinical Tip

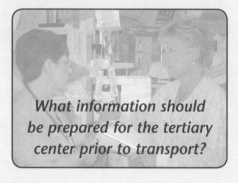

*What information should be prepared for the tertiary center prior to transport?*

- Complete maternal records
  - ✧ Prenatal (including consultations, laboratory and ultrasound results)
  - ✧ Labor and delivery (including medications administered to the mother)
- Complete neonatal records
  - ✧ Physician orders and notes, nurses and respiratory therapists notes, medication record, laboratory results
  - ✧ Copy of radiographs or other diagnostics tests

## When the Transport Team Arrives

- Accompany the transport team to the mother's room and listen to explanations of the infant's condition and likely medical treatments.

- Observe parental reactions, both before transport of the infant and once the infant has been transported, to enable specific interventions and consultations.

- Very frequently, this situation is overwhelming for parents. Because of the large amount of information they hear, parents may have difficulty remembering what was explained to them. Help parents to understand information; ask if they have questions, be prepared to repeat explanations, and be aware that explanations are easily misinterpreted or misunderstood.

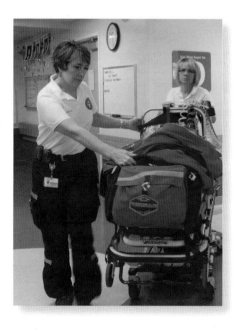

- Recommend to parents that they write down questions as they arise. Often it is difficult for them to remember questions and information when talking with the infant's healthcare providers.

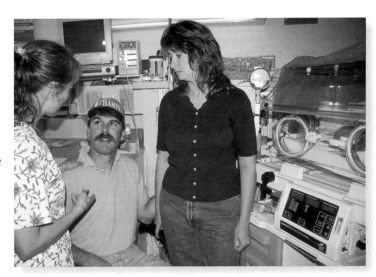

- Most parents have limited background in healthcare and many have no prior experience with sick newborns. Keep explanations simple, but accurate. Provide illustrations and written material when possible.

- Be aware of reading limitations. If this problem is identified, provide appropriate alternative resources.

- If there is a language barrier, avoid using family members or friends to interpret. Rather, use interpreters with medical expertise, or over-the-phone interpretation/translation services such as Language Line (account information may be found at www.LanguageLine.com). This is also applicable for care provided in the neonatal intensive care unit.

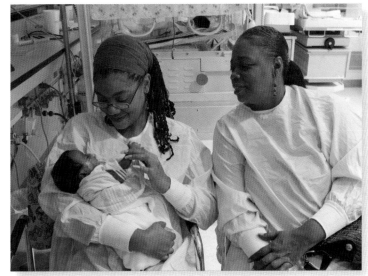

- Even though this is a very difficult experience for the family, congratulate the parents on the birth of their infant. Grandparents are often present, but overlooked; they should also receive congratulations on the birth of their grandchild. Often grandparents are grieving not only for their new grandchild, but for their own child. Discuss feelings and concerns with both the parents and grandparents whenever possible, recognizing that the parents must always receive medical information about their baby first. Privacy laws must be observed at all times, therefore, unless the parents give permission, do not discuss the infant's medical condition with anyone other than the parents.

- Part of the congratulations you provide to parents can involve comments about the physical attributes of the infant. For example, if the infant looks well-nourished, tell the parents how nice and big the infant is, and compliment the mother on this achievement. Other examples might be to notice a full head of hair, or a beautiful petite face, or the long toes. Attachment to the infant will be enhanced as you direct attention to specifics about the baby.

- If you are the postpartum nurse, try to go to the nursery to see the infant before transfer. If the infant has already departed, ask the parents if they have a photo that you can see. This shows your interest in their situation and may open the door for dialogue about their infant and understanding of the situation.

- Often, the transport team will provide specific information regarding how to locate the hospital and NICU where the infant will be transported, as well as the name of the physician who will be responsible for the infant's care. This is very helpful for parents because they often fear separation from their infant.

## Care of the Family after Transport of the Infant

In the community hospital.

- If the infant is in very critical condition, and if at all possible, call the newborn intensive care nurse who will be caring for the infant and request that you or the infant's birth physician or practitioner be notified if "bad news" is given to the family, so that you can offer increased levels of support. This is especially helpful if the mother is going to be alone when sad or distressing news is delivered.

- Investigate the parents' feelings and sources of coping. If the parents express overwhelming fear or anxiety, reassure them that you can help them to obtain and interpret information. If the parents seem to be in denial or unusually calm, don't be surprised. Sometimes reality sinks in slowly and every individual within a family has their own approach to coping and dealing with a crisis. It may be that the family had no warning that their infant would be anything but healthy and normal. Remember that we, as caregivers, may only gain a small amount of insight into the parent's feelings and style of coping. However, it is important to notify the NICU hospital staff with new information you learn that may be relevant to the ongoing care of the infant and the family.

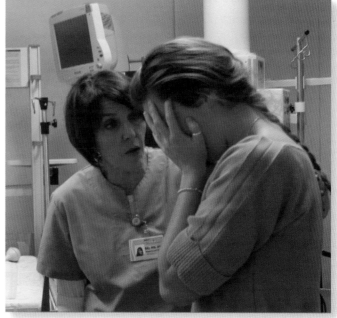

- Find out if the mother had planned to breast feed and whether she's now ambivalent given the crisis she's experiencing. In most cases, it is best to encourage the mother to proceed with pumping rather than to wait. Early initiation of pumping will help to establish her milk supply, which in the long run may be less frustrating or discouraging for the mother. Realize also that many mothers feel that providing breast milk for the infant is a significant way to contribute to the infant's care, and that this is reassuring to them. If in doubt about the best approach and whether or not breast feeding instruction is indicated, consult with the infant's caregivers at the neonatal intensive care unit.

- Once the infant is transported, the parents may need assistance with calling the neonatal intensive care unit to check on the baby's status. Facilitate communication with the neonatal intensive care unit nursing and/or medical staff when needed.

## In the neonatal intensive care unit.

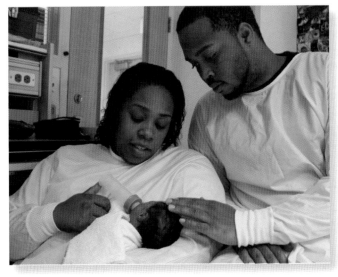

- Remember that adults are accustomed to having control over events in their lives. This situation takes their control away. They are not able to "parent" their baby the way that they had dreamed of. Depending upon the infant's state of health, the parents may not be able to do much or any of the normal "parenting" activities without asking permission; for example, hold or feed their baby, or change their baby's diaper. By being aware of these feelings, healthcare providers will be better able to empathize with what the family is experiencing, especially if they seem angry toward healthcare providers, or the situation.

- Facilitate parenting in the neonatal intensive care unit by involving parents in the infant's care and medical decision-making. Help the family become aware of the many support groups that are available within the NICU, such as parent and sibling support groups, breastfeeding support, social worker support, clergy, and if necessary, grief support groups.

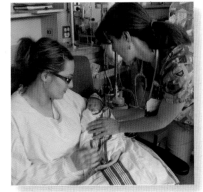

- Recognize that men and women may cope and respond very differently with stress and the illness experience. Fathers may find it difficult to balance the stress of caring for the mother, spending time with the baby, caring for other children at home, and work obligations. They may not verbalize their thoughts and feelings as openly as the mother. Oftentimes, family and friends flock to the mother's side, while the father is left somewhat alone and unsupported.

- Encourage the parents to communicate often with each other about their stress, the infant, and their feelings.

- This is *their* infant, not ours. When we, as healthcare providers, refer to an infant as "my baby", we mean, "my patient"; however, parents may not understand that is our intent. Rather, refer to the infant by name: "baby Smith" or "Nicole", for example.

- Explain the infant's condition in simple, accurate, and honest terms. Be consistent with explanations and the plan of care. Oftentimes, parents complain that "everyone is telling me something different" and "no-one seems to agree with the plan of care". Encourage parents to participate in patient rounds so they may hear the discussions that take place and also so they may be more involved in decision making. It is important to collaborate with other members of the healthcare team on the plan of care and to encourage the family to speak up if they are hearing conflicting information.

- If there is a language barrier, avoid using family members or friends to interpret. Rather, use interpreters with medical expertise, or over-the-phone interpretation/translation services such as Language Line (account information may be found at **www.LanguageLine.com**).

- Be supportive, non-judgmental, and culturally sensitive at all times.

# Appendix 6.1  **Providing Relationship-Based Care to Babies and Their Parents**[7-18]

## Contributed by Deborah L. Davis, Ph.D and Mara Tesler Stein, Psy.D.

Relationship-based care for critically ill newborns and their parents is a philosophy of care that is holistic, gentle, and developmentally supportive. Intensive care can pose physical and emotional hardships, but when health care professionals focus on providing sensitive, responsive, supportive care, infants are protected rather than overstimulated, and parents feel respected, rather than ignored. Technical expertise is essential, but using that expertise in the context of relationships forms the cornerstone of quality healthcare.

## For Babies

As a nurse, your technical expertise can save lives, but your relationship expertise contributes to the quality of those lives in the NICU. Relationship expertise is your ability to be attuned and responsive to an individual patient's unique needs, not just for medical intervention, but also for soothing and comfort. As you provide intensive medical care, reflect on how you carry out intensive medical procedures. Do you find that you tune out the baby's distress, or do you strive to prevent, reduce, or eliminate it? When you only focus on carrying out the technical aspects of medical procedures as quickly and effectively as possible, you may compound the baby's stress level. "Stressful but quick" may seem efficient and necessary to you, but for the baby, it may set off a chain reaction of hormonal and metabolic sequelae that are not conducive to medical stabilization, nor to recovery and healing. Even simple or routine caregiving tasks, such as diaper changes, heel sticks, or tubing adjustments can cause unnecessary stress to a sick or premature baby when they are done in ways that are invasive, painful, or intrusive. Any time a baby is physiologically overwhelmed, this may create a significant stress response that can be difficult to recover from.

In contrast, by attending and responding to the infant's subtle signs of stress, even during a medical crisis, you can approach the baby with a nurturing mindset. You can be efficient and effective without being hurried or insensitive to the baby's suffering. Depending on the infant's unique sensitivities and thresholds, you can soothe or circumvent distress with:

- Gentle touch
- Soft, soothing voice
- Measured pacing
- Appropriate timing
- Shielding the eyes from bright lights
- Covering the ears to block out sharp or loud sounds
- Warmth and containment or swaddling
- Supportive positioning, and
- Adequate pain medication

Your relationship, however fleeting, with each baby is what enables you to tune in to signs of discomfort as well as calm, and to respond to his or her unique cues, preferences, tolerance levels, and needs. In the past decade or so, some research has provided clinical evidence that this type of relationship-based care (also called individualized developmental care, as advocated and practiced by the Newborn Individualized Developmental Care and Assessment Program, NIDCAP) may improve growth, healing, and long-term outcome for NICU infants.

There is one more piece to allaying an infant's distress, and it is perhaps the most important piece: enlisting the parents' soothing presence. In fact, involving the parents in their baby's care is a key component of providing relationship-based care to babies. The parents' touch and soothing presence can promote their baby's weight gain, temperature maintenance, and oxygen saturation level. Bringing baby and parent together benefits the parent, as it promotes bonding, parental identity, involvement, confidence, competence, and emotional coping. Kangaroo care (laying the diapered baby on the parent's bare chest) and breast-feeding let parents feel how intimately necessary they are to their baby's recovery. Actively and implicitly encouraging supportive, close contact is central to providing relationship-based care to the baby and the parents.

## For Parents

Just as intensive care can be stressful for babies, it is stressful for parents. When a preterm or sick infant is first admitted to intensive care, parents may feel helpless and incompetent, knowing that their baby's care must be handed over to medical professionals. Hospitalization and critical medical conditions are barriers that can feel insurmountable. It is normal for parents to feel distressed, overwhelmed, disoriented, fearful, and uncertain about how to approach their baby.

## How can you effectively involve these parents?

Just as your relationship with each baby enables you to attend and respond in ways that support

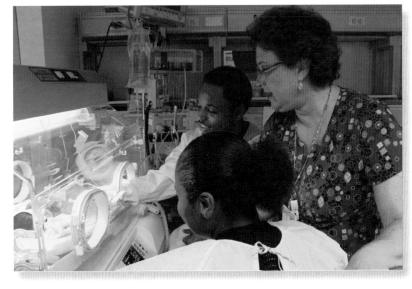

healing, growth, and development, your relationship with each baby's parents is what enables you to support them as they grow into their role as mother or father to this child. In fact, your attitude toward parents and toward their involvement with their baby is key to their success as parents in the NICU and beyond. As you strive to build relationships with parents, here are some tips to remember:

Assume that even though parents may be emotionally numb or overwhelmed at times, they are competent and devoted to their baby, and with your support, they can adjust to the situation, cope with their grief, and learn the caregiving skills that match their baby's special needs.

◇ As you build a warm rapport with parents, you can support them in their struggles, which builds their trust in you and enhances your ability to teach and model caregiving skills.

◇ Your responsive, soothing care of their baby is reassuring to parents, because your sensitivity reinforces their own nurturing instincts, and helps them feel good about leaving their baby in your care.

◇ Reach out in a spirit of collaboration, as this welcomes and includes parents as central members of their baby's caregiving team.

◇ Stop thinking of parents as "visitors," and integrate them as partners in their baby's care.

◇ As you become attuned to their baby, share what you've observed, and ask them for their observations and ideas.

◇ Make room for their parenting abilities, and facilitate their growth into effective soothers, competent decision-makers, and confident caregivers for their baby.

◇ When you facilitate the parents' relationship with their baby, you are fortifying their competence, attunement, and confidence, which provide the foundation for a successful transition to home after discharge.

Just as it is for babies, relationship-based care for parents is a framework and philosophy for how you approach working with families. And again, it is the relationships you form— with babies and parents alike— that enable you to provide responsive, individualized care that supports growth, health and development. Your goal is not simply to discharge a healthy baby, but to discharge a healthy baby to parents who feel connected and are competent to assume total care of their infant.

Deborah L. Davis, Ph.D. is a developmental psychologist, researcher, and writer; whose books include *Empty Cradle, Broken Heart* (Fulcrum, 1996) and Loving and Letting Go (Centering, 2002). Mara Tesler Stein, Psy.D. is a clinical psychologist in private practice, speaker, and consultant. Both Davis and Stein specialize in the emotional aspects of coping with crisis and adjustment around pregnancy and parenting, and are co-authors of *Parenting Your Premature Baby and Child: The Emotional Journey*[4]

# References

1. Siegel R, Gardner SL, Dickey LA. Families in Crisis: Theoretical and Practical Considerations. In: Gardner SL, Carter BS, Enzman-Hines M, Hernandez JA, eds. Merenstein & Gardner's Handbook of Neonatal Intensive Care. 7th ed. St. Louis: Mosby Elsevier; 2011:849-97.

2. National Perinatal Association. Transcultural Aspects of Perinatal Health Care. Elk Grove Village: American Academy of Pediatrics; 2004.

3. Lynch EW, Hanson MJ. Developing Cross-Cultural Competence: A Guide for Working with Children and Their Families. 3rd ed. Baltimore: Paul H. Brookes Publishing Co.; 2004.

4. Davis DL, Stein MT. Parenting Your Premature Baby and Child: The Emotional Journey. Golden: Fulcrum 2004.

5. Klaus MH, Kennell JH, Edwards WH. Care of the Mother, Father, and Infant. In: Martin RJ, Fanaroff AA, Walsh MC, eds. Fanaroff and Martin's Neonatal-Perinatal Medicine: Diseases of the Fetus and Infant. 9th ed. St. Louis: Elsevier Mosby; 2011:615-27.

6. Garcia-Prats JA, Hornfischer SS. What To Do When Your Baby is Premature. New York: Three Rivers Press; 2000.

7. Aita M, Snider L. The art of developmental care in the NICU: a concept analysis. J Adv Nurs 2003;41:223-32.

8. Als H, Duffy FH, McAnulty GB. Effectiveness of individualized neurodevelopmental care in the newborn intensive care unit (NICU). Acta Paediatr Suppl 1996;416:21-30.

9. Als H, Gilkerson L. The role of relationship-based developmentally supportive newborn intensive care in strengthening outcome of preterm infants. Semin Perinatol 1997;21:178-89.

10. Als H, Lawhon G, Duffy FH, McAnulty GB, Gibes-Grossman R, Blickman JG. Individualized developmental care for the very low-birth-weight preterm infant. Medical and neurofunctional effects. Jama 1994;272:853-8.

11. Byers JF. Components of developmental care and the evidence for their use in the NICU. MCN Am J Matern Child Nurs 2003;28:174-80; quiz 81-2.

12. Griffin T, Wishba C, Kavanaugh K. Nursing interventions to reduce stress in parents of hospitalized preterm infants. J Pediatr Nurs 1998;13:290-5.

13. Kledzik T. Holding the very low birth weight infant: skin-to-skin techniques. Neonatal Netw 2005;24:7-14.

14. Lawhon G. Facilitation of parenting the premature infant within the newborn intensive care unit. J Perinat Neonatal Nurs 2002;16:71-82.

15. Maroney DI. Recognizing the potential effect of stress and trauma on premature infants in the NICU: how are outcomes affected? J Perinatol 2003;23:679-83.

16. Robison LD. An organizational guide for an effective developmental program in the NICU. J Obstet Gynecol Neonatal Nurs 2003;32:379-86.

17. Spatz DL. Ten steps for promoting and protecting breastfeeding for vulnerable infants. J Perinat Neonatal Nurs 2004;18:385-96.

18. White RD. Mothers' arms--the past and future locus of neonatal care? Clin Perinatol 2004;31:383-7, ix.

**S**ugar and **S**afe Care

**T**emperature

**A**irway

**B**lood Pressure

**L**ab Work

**E**motional Support

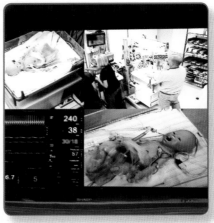

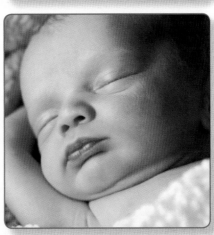

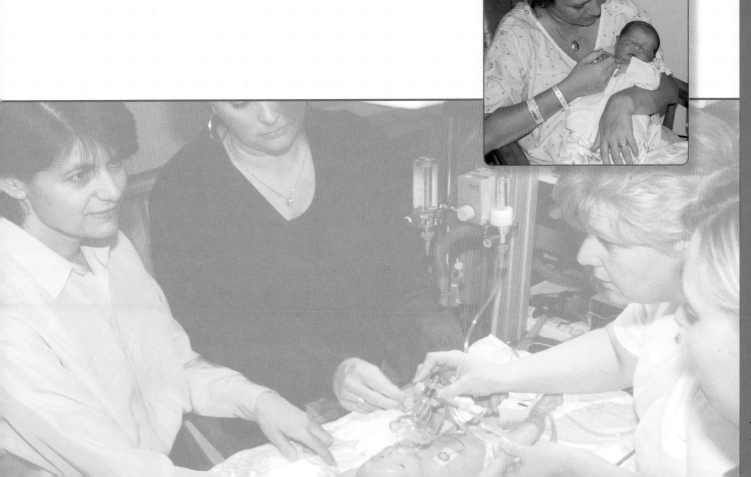

## Quality Improvement – Module Objectives

Upon completion of this module, participants will gain an increased understanding of:

1. Concerns regarding patient safety and methods to reduce medical errors and preventable adverse events in this vulnerable population.

2. The importance of effective communication and teamwork to prevent harm and to improve patient safety.

3. Simulation-based education as a strategy to improve patient safety.

4. The importance of self-assessment and debriefing to evaluate care provided in the post-resuscitation/pre-transport stabilization period.

## Introduction

A uniform, standardized process of care and comprehensive team approach can improve patient safety and ultimately, infant outcomes. The six S.T.A.B.L.E. modules you just completed focused on the importance of assessing patient history, signs, laboratory and test data, and developing a team plan of care. It is important to remember that care of sick infants requires continual re-assessment because infant status may change very rapidly. The goal of this program is to provide important, evidenced-based information that can be used to improve delivery of quality care to sick, vulnerable infants in the safest manner.

Mechanisms known to reduce errors include standardizing processes of care, avoiding reliance on memory, and communicating in clear, direct ways. The Situation, Background, Assessment, Recommendation (SBAR) form of structured communication is a strategy used to reduce potential errors associated with miscommunication or lack of information. The SBAR technique also achieves an important goal of standardizing communication regarding an infant's condition. SBAR had its roots in the military and was designed to allow for quick communication of critical information to the leader. Table 7.1 contains a summary of the components of SBAR communication. The S.T.A.B.L.E. Program added an additional "R" to represent repeat back orders received or the plan of care agreed upon with the medical staff provider.

| | **Start interaction by INTRODUCING yourself and the patient you are calling about.** | |
|---|---|---|
| | Example:<br>*Hi Dr. Smith, this is **your name** and I'm the nurse taking care of baby girl Jones in Bed 16. She's the 39 week gestation baby that was admitted for TEF last night. I'm calling because I'm concerned about her increased respiratory distress. At the beginning of my shift, she was on 40% oxygen and saturating in the mid-90's, but ever since we started her IV an hour ago, her oxygen requirement has gone up to 60% and she has started to retract"...* | |

| | **INFORMATION TO PROVIDE** | |
|---|---|---|
| **S**ITUATION<br><br>Concise statement of the problem – what is happening with the patient? | Admitting diagnosis or reason for admission | |
| | Age | |
| | Weight | |
| | Gender | |
| | Brief summary of significant medical history | |
| | Signs/symptoms of concern (**the reason you are calling**) | |
| **B**ACKGROUND<br><br>Information pertinent to your concern – what is the clinical background? | Vital signs and status | |
| | Labs- normal & critical findings | |
| | Medications or treatments given | |
| | Previous orders received | |
| | Tests – ordered and results known or pending | |
| | IV status and fluids | |
| | Maternal history (if applicable) | |
| | Other information pertinent to present illness | |
| **A**SSESSMENT<br><br>Synthesis of relevant information you have analyzed – what you think the problem is or what you have found | Respiratory | Neurological |
| | Cardiovascular | GI / GU |
| | Endocrine / Labs | Infection |
| | Family psychosocial / social | Lines/tubes |
| | Other systems pertinent to present illness | |
| **R**ECOMMENDATION<br><br>Action requested or recommended to address the problem | Overall impressions and / or concerns – be specific | |
| | Make recommendations for change in plan of care or new orders needed | |
| | Identify the plan of care | |
| | Wrap Up: When does the physician or HCP want follow up? | |
| | For what changes does HCP want to be notified? | |
| | **If you want the medical staff provider to come to the bedside, state that request and ask when you can expect them to arrive** | |
| **R**EAD BACK of all verbal orders or repeating back understanding of expectations | | |

**Table 7.1. Components of SBARR communication.** Adapted from TeamSTEPPS
www.ahrq.gov/teamsteppstools

The S.T.A.B.L.E. Program, when applied by all members of the healthcare team, can help everyone to work together and in the same direction. Appropriate, timely, and correctly executed actions can impact short and long term neonatal outcomes.

# The Importance of Teamwork and Team Training

Improving patient outcomes and reducing errors and adverse events is the goal of everyone involved with delivery of health care. Some suggestions to realize this goal include knowing how to invoke the "chain of command"; using clear, unambiguous communication at all times; using simple, standardized processes of care; being prepared with knowledge, equipment, and skills for scenarios that will arise; and post-assessment evaluation of care that was delivered.

## Communication

Written and verbal communication must be clear, unambiguous, and timely. When a verbal order is given, it should be repeated back to the person giving the order to be sure that it was heard correctly. A written order should be legible and should not include medical abbreviations that may be easily mistaken for other words. In the United States, the hospital accreditation agency, The Joint Commission published a Sentinel Event report[1] of 93 cases of infant death and 16 cases of permanent disability. Communication issues topped the list of identified root causes (72 percent), with 55% of the facilities citing organizational culture as a barrier to effective communication and teamwork (i.e., intimidation and hierarchy, failure to function as a team, and failure to follow the chain-of-communication). Numerous risk reduction strategies were identified by the Joint Commission which included conducting team training in perinatal areas to teach staff to work together and communicate more effectively.

## Chain of Command

Every healthcare facility has a "chain-of-command" or a "chain-of-communication" in place to help employees resolve disputes and advocate for patients. This chain is designed to identify personnel with progressively higher authority within a department or facility, who can be approached to help resolve disputes. For example, a nurse who is concerned about a physician order would first discuss her concern with the physician. If she was not satisfied with the response and felt carrying out the order would not be in the best interest of the patient, she could then discuss her concern with the charge nurse. The charge nurse can help the nurse discuss the problem with the physician, and if both are not satisfied that the problem is being addressed, the charge nurse can then notify the nursing supervisor, who can then go to the medical director of the nursery, and so on up the chain, until the dispute is satisfactorily resolved. Knowing how to access the chain-of-command includes knowing when to invoke it, the line of authority, and steps to move up. Most hospitals have safety initiatives in place that you should become familiar with, such as safety rounds, safety committees, anonymous reporting phone lines or anonymous electronic reporting (of concerns), and quality department personnel who are available for private consultation should you have concerns that you would like to discuss.

## Simulation-Based Training: Being prepared for situations that will arise

Neonatology and newborn care is a dynamic and ever-changing field. One of the newest and most exciting changes in recent years is the integration of simulation-based education into neonatal training.[2,3] Although more complex and expensive to accomplish than lecture-based education, simulation allows for comprehensive practice of cognitive, technical, and behavioral skills by interprofessional participants – nurses, physicians, respiratory therapists, licensed practical nurses, nurse aides and other allied health professionals.[2,4]

Simulation-based education offers a valuable opportunity to improve patient safety.[5,6] By practicing realistic clinical scenarios, participants will be challenged with dynamic decision-making under stress, experience firsthand the impact of communication and interactions between team members on patient care and outcomes, and understand the challenges of selecting and correctly using resources and information during time-pressured emergencies.[6,7]

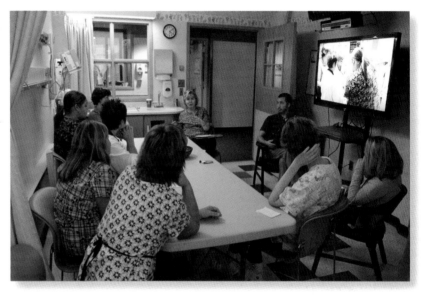

One of the most valuable aspects of simulation-based training is the opportunity for participants to **debrief** at the conclusion of each clinical scenario. During debriefing, the participants analyze, discuss and make sense of what just happened.[8,9] It is important for the debriefer, (the person facilitating the debriefing), to seek training in simulation methodology and debriefing, since the effect of a poorly run simulation experience, or poorly conducted debriefing, will dilute the intended effect of the simulation experience, and may even be harmful to the participants.[10,11]

Universally, confidentiality is maintained for events that occur in the simulation lab. This allows participants to feel safe to make mistakes, and to learn from them, without any consequence of patient harm. It is true we learn more from our mistakes than our successes. Simulation training is a powerful way to learn and practice teamwork which, when applied in the clinical arena, will improve patient care and safety.

## Human Factors

Human factors are known to play a part in the occurrence of adverse critical clinical events and include areas such as:

- Lack of effective leadership;

- Lack of effective teamwork as evidenced by individuals working independently of each other, without coordination;

- Use of hierarchical methods of communication that inhibit contributions from less experienced or less confident staff.

These human factors must be taken into account if educational strategies such as simulation are to be successful.[12,13] Effective stabilization of the infant requires all those involved to work respectfully and collaboratively. There is increasing evidence that an understanding of human behavior under stressful conditions may also give further insight into how further improvements can be made.[14]

In 2012, The S.T.A.B.L.E. Program introduced challenging and realistic resuscitation and stabilization scenarios as an optional, adjunct component to the existing didactic/interactive program. One or more of the S.T.A.B.L.E. modules are the basis for each scenario. The goals for the S.T.A.B.L.E. simulation-based-training are:

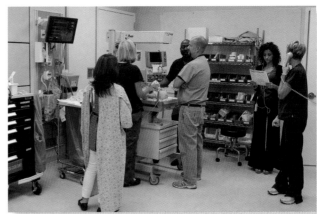

- For interprofessional caregivers to demonstrate understanding of postresuscitation care principles.

- To practice clinical decision making while at the same time managing challenging behavioral and technical components of time-pressured emergencies.

- To have an opportunity to practice realistic team interactions that will ultimately increase understanding of how other disciplines view and process information while responding to a clinical event.

The ultimate goal of the S.T.A.B.L.E. Program simulation-based education is to improve patient care and safety. Simulation is a golden opportunity to take what is learned theoretically and practice in the safe environment of a simulated scenario. In addition, the development of scenarios based on real life situations facilitates the further development of teamwork and communication skills.[15] This dynamic way of learning through simulation will translate to more effective handling of challenging clinical situations and emergencies when they are encountered. For more information, visit the S.T.A.B.L.E. website at www.stableprogram.org.

## Simple, Standardized, Processes of Care: The S.T.A.B.L.E. Program

Training maternal-child and neonatal healthcare providers in The S.T.A.B.L.E. Program will help achieve several goals. First, it will help promote teamwork by bringing everyone together on the same page so that the team can work effectively and in concert with each other. Second, it will allow for evaluation of care, as well as enable identification of deviations from program guidelines. At times, it is necessary to change or modify care provided to sick infants, however, inappropriate deviations are easier to identify when everyone is using the same general approach.

### Post-assessment evaluation of care / debriefing

Evaluation of care is an important aspect of improving care and patient safety. Developing strategies to improve care within the context of a specific situation includes looking at causes of poor or inadequate care and types of errors that were committed. The process includes medical record review, involving all members of the healthcare delivery team in debriefing discussions, and consultation with neonatal experts when necessary.[16] The S.T.A.B.L.E. Program recommends case review for the following situations:

- An infant is expected to be well, but is unexpectedly sick, and requires transport.

- An error occurs during delivery of care.

- An error is defined as use of a wrong plan to achieve an aim (an error of planning); or failure of a planned action to be completed as intended (an error of execution).[17]

- A preventable adverse event is identified.

  - This is defined as injury that was caused by the medical and/or nursing management rather than the underlying disease or condition.[17]

- Patient care should be reviewed when an infant becomes sicker than was expected, or when other unanticipated issues arise, including complications that lengthen hospitalization.

In addition, other situations may arise that merit review of patient care.

When an infant requires transport, it is helpful to comprehensively assess the stabilization care provided prior to transport. Again, it is most effective and beneficial if the infant's caregivers are involved with the assessment. The Pre-Transport Stabilization Self-Assessment Tool (PSSAT), found on page 299, is a form that may be of use during debriefing of neonatal caregivers involved with a transport. The PSSAT data collection tool may also be utilized to assess timeliness and completeness of stabilization care. The time "A" and "B" recordings should be completed by the birth hospital providers (referring) and the time "C" recordings should be completed by the transport team and the referring facility together. Directions for using the PSSAT are found on page 298. The PSSAT form may also be downloaded from the S.T.A.B.L.E. website at **http://www.stableprogram.org/ stabilizationtool.php**

## Questions to ask when evaluating stabilization care

- Was the patient well-stabilized?

- Did we encounter problems that affected our ability to stabilize the infant?

  - Lack of equipment or knowledge about how to use equipment?

  - Lack of necessary personnel?

  - Education deficits?

  - Lack of experience or skills?

  - Lack of protocols or procedures to guide care?

- How did we perform as a team?

- What could we do to improve our performance?

- Did we provide safe patient care?

- Can we identify any preventable errors or adverse events?

- What was the patient outcome?

Asking yourself and your team whether anything could have been done differently or better will promote discussion about how to improve care the next time an infant is sick and needs to be stabilized and/or transported to a neonatal intensive care unit. In addition, this important review process is very helpful for identifying simulation education activities that may help prepare for similar future events.

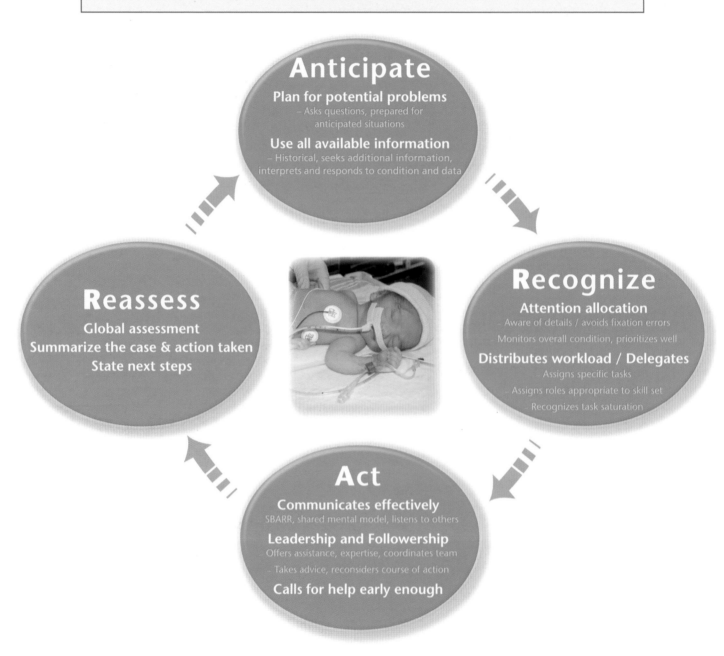

While providing care to sick infants, the goal is to . . .

Anticipate problems that may arise,

Recognize the problems when they occur, and then

Act on them promptly and effectively.

Reassess and summarize the case and actions taken.

**Anticipate**

**Plan for potential problems**
– Asks questions, prepared for anticipated situations

**Use all available information**
– Historical, seeks additional information, interprets and responds to condition and data

**Recognize**

**Attention allocation**
– Aware of details / avoids fixation errors
– Monitors overall condition, prioritizes well

**Distributes workload / Delegates**
– Assigns specific tasks
– Assigns roles appropriate to skill set
– Recognizes task saturation

**Reassess**

**Global assessment**
**Summarize the case & action taken**
**State next steps**

**Act**

**Communicates effectively**
SBARR, shared mental model, listens to others

**Leadership and Followership**
Offers assistance, expertise, coordinates team
– Takes advice, reconsiders course of action

**Calls for help early enough**

# S.T.A.B.L.E. Model of Care

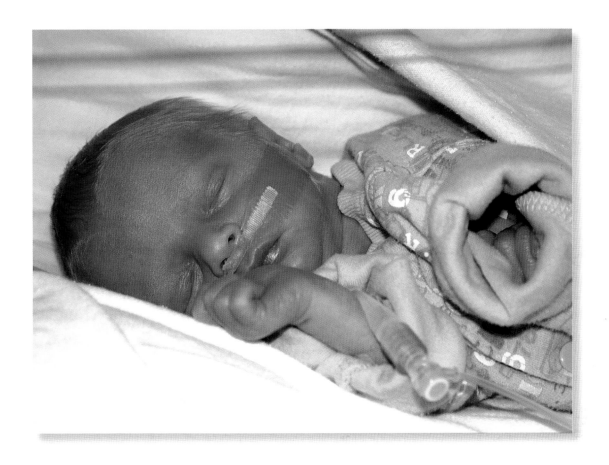

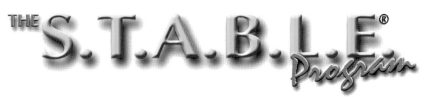

## Improving Outcomes – With Education

## Directions for using the Pre-transport Stabilization Self-Assessment Form

1. Either during pre-transport stabilization care, or immediately after the infant is transported, complete the demographic information in the Patient Information section of the form.

2. Under Indications for Referral, select all of the suspected or confirmed diagnoses that apply at the time of referral.

3. Times A, B, and C are used repetitively on the first and second pages of the form.

   Record the vital signs, physical exam, and stabilization procedures that were performed:

   • At the time the transport team was called (transport was requested) = **Time A**

   • Upon arrival of the transport team in your nursery = **Time B**

   • Upon departure of the transport team = **Time C**

     ◦ The transport team should help complete the Time C items, unless the infant is unstable and time does not allow. In that case, if at all possible, ask the team to leave a copy of their stabilization record so you can complete the Time C items.

4. Completion of this form will allow evaluation of stabilization care by looking at three specific time intervals:

   • What stabilization actions were taken at the time it was determined the infant was sick?

   • What stabilization actions were taken while awaiting the team's arrival?

   • What stabilization actions were completed by the team?

   The following scenarios are possible:

     ◦ The team arrives and stabilization is complete so they do not need to do more than assess the baby, attach the transport equipment and move the baby into the incubator.

     ◦ The team arrives quickly and completes the stabilization procedures that you did not have time to complete.

     ◦ The team arrives and determines that additional care is needed, and therefore, additional actions are taken (such as intubating the patient, inserting lines, changing an ET tube, administering certain medications, etc.).

   • By recording these actions, it is hoped that the nursing and medical leadership team will be able to assess adequacy of pre-transport (or transfer) stabilization care.

   • In addition, this important review process may be very helpful for identifying simulation education activities that may help prepare for similar future events.

If you have trouble filling out the form, or you need additional expertise to answer the questions on the third page of the form, then your transport team should be consulted for assistance. An optimally performed stabilization is the goal of community caregivers and transport teams alike!

## Pre-transport Stabilization Self-Assessment Tool (PSSAT)

**PARENT INFORMATION**

**Birth weight:** ☐☐☐☐ grams   **Birth order:** ____ of ____

**Growth:** AGA  SGA  LGA       **Gender:** Male  Female  Ambiguous

**Estimated Gest. Age:** ☐☐ - ☐ / ☐ weeks/days (ex: 34-3/7)

**Baby admitted from:** ☐ Labor & Delivery   ☐ Mother-baby unit
☐ Nursery   ☐ Emergency room

**Indications for referral** (circle all that apply)

Prematurity   Respiratory distress   Sepsis   Cardiac   Metabolic   Genetic   Neurologic   Hematologic   Surgical   Birth depression

Other (explain): _____

**Resuscitation at birth:**   Suction   Blow-by oxygen   CPAP
CPAP & PPV   Intubation & PPV   Chest compressions

Resuscitation meds (list): _____
_____

Other meds (list): _____

**Apgar** at 1 minute: ☐☐   5 min: ☐☐   10 min: ☐☐
15 min: ☐☐   20 min: ☐☐

**TIME**

**Age of baby** in Days and Hours after birth – **at time transport team called** _____ Days _____ Hours

**A** **Transport team called** _____ AM PM

**B** **Transport team arrived at nursery** _____ AM PM

**C** **Transport team departed nursery** _____ AM PM

*Note: these times will be used throughout this form. When answering questions, evaluate the parameter closest to time A, B, and C.*

Time patient died; transport aborted _____ AM PM (complete remainder of form even if patient died)

**VITAL SIGNS**

| | Temperature °C °F | Axillary or Rectal | Heart Rate | Respiratory Rate | Blood Pressure Systolic/Diastolic | Mean | Method (RA, LA, RL, LL) or Arterial |
|---|---|---|---|---|---|---|---|
| Time A | _____ | _____ | ☐ | ☐ | ☐ / ☐ | ☐ | _____ |
| Time B | _____ | _____ | ☐ | ☐ | ☐ / ☐ | ☐ | _____ |
| Time C | _____ | _____ | ☐ | ☐ | ☐ / ☐ | ☐ | _____ |

**PHYSICAL EXAM**

**Perfusion/Pulses**

| | Capillary Refill Time (sec.) over chest | over knee | | Pulses | Pulses equal upper & lower | (If no, explain) |
|---|---|---|---|---|---|---|
| Time A | _____ | _____ sec. | | Normal  Decreased  Increased | YES  NO | _____ |
| Time B | _____ | _____ sec. | | Normal  Decreased  Increased | YES  NO | _____ |
| Time C | _____ | _____ sec. | | Normal  Decreased  Increased | YES  NO | _____ |

**Retractions**

| | Severity (circle all that apply) | Location (circle all that apply) | O₂ Saturation | FiO₂ |
|---|---|---|---|---|
| Time A | Mild  Moderate  Severe  Gasping | Substernal  Intercostal  Subcostal | ☐ % | ☐ % |
| Time B | Mild  Moderate  Severe  Gasping | Substernal  Intercostal  Subcostal | ☐ % | ☐ % |
| Time C | Mild  Moderate  Severe  Gasping | Substernal  Intercostal  Subcostal | ☐ % | ☐ % |

**Level of consciousness**      Response to noxious stimuli (circle all that apply)                Other (explain)

| | | |
|---|---|---|
| Time A | Withdraws/good tone, cries   Lethargic, no cry   Seizure(s)   No response, comatose | _____ |
| Time B | Withdraws/good tone, cries   Lethargic, no cry   Seizure(s)   No response, comatose | _____ |
| Time C | Withdraws/good tone, cries   Lethargic, no cry   Seizure(s)   No response, comatose | _____ |

Paralytic used (i.e. pavulon)?   Yes   No   Reason given: _____

Time/dose of all Opioids given past 24 hrs (list type) _____

Time/dose of all Sedatives given past 24 hrs (list type) _____

## Pre-transport Stabilization Self-Assessment Tool (PSSAT)

| STABILIZATION PROCEDURES | Use Time **A B C** from page 1 | **Time A** _____ | **Time B** _____ | **Time C** _____ |
|---|---|---|---|---|
| | IV in place? | Y  N  Location _____ | Y  N  Location _____ | Y  N  Location _____ |
| | IV fluid infusing? | Y  N  Type _____ <br> Rate ml/kg/day _____ | Y  N  Type _____ <br> Rate ml/kg/day _____ | Y  N  Type _____ <br> Rate ml/kg/day _____ |
| | UVC in place? | Y  N  Tip location _____ | Y  N  Tip location _____ | Y  N  Tip location _____ |
| | UAC in place? | Y  N  Tip location _____ | Y  N  Tip location _____ | Y  N  Tip location _____ |
| | Glucose – closest to 15 – 30 minutes of this time | Y  N  Value mg/dL _____ | Y  N  Value mg/dL _____ | Y  N  Value mg/dL _____ |
| | Glucose bolus given? | Y  N  Fluid _____ <br> Amount _____ | Y  N  Fluid _____ <br> Amount _____ | Y  N  Fluid _____ <br> Amount _____ |
| | Oxygen in use? | Y  N  % _____ | Y  N  % _____ | Y  N  % _____ |
| | Pulse oximetry on? | Y  N  $O_2$ sat _____ | Y  N  $O_2$ sat _____ | Y  N  $O_2$ sat _____ |
| | CPAP in use? | Y  N  Type _____ <br> Pressure _____ | Y  N  Type _____ <br> Pressure _____ | Y  N  Type _____ <br> Pressure _____ |
| | PPV provided? | Y  N  Pressures _____ <br> Rate _____ | Y  N  Pressures _____ <br> Rate _____ | Y  N  Pressures _____ <br> Rate _____ |
| | Tracheal intubation? | Y  N  Cm at lip _____ | Y  N  Cm at lip _____ | Y  N  Cm at lip _____ |
| | ET tube properly secured? | Y  N | Y  N | Y  N |
| | Chest tube in place? | Y  N | Y  N | Y  N |
| | Chest needle or cath placed? | Y  N | Y  N | Y  N |
| | Volume bolus? | Y  N  Type _____ <br> Amount _____ | Y  N  Type _____ <br> Amount _____ | Y  N  Type _____ <br> Amount _____ |
| | On dopamine? | Y  N  Dose mcg/kg/min _____ | Y  N  Dose mcg/kg/min _____ | Y  N  Dose mcg/kg/min _____ |
| | CBC with differential done? | Y  N | Y  N | Y  N |
| | Blood culture drawn? | Y  N | Y  N | Y  N |
| | Antibiotics given? | Y  N | Y  N | Y  N  Additional antibiotic or dose given? |
| | On radiant warmer on ISC? | Y  N | Y  N | Y  N |
| | In incubator on ISC? | Y  N | Y  N | Y  N |
| | In incubator on air temp? | Y  N | Y  N | Y  N |

### BLOOD GASSES

| Time | Indicate <u>C</u>BG, <u>A</u>BG, Venous | | | | | | Ventilation settings <br> PIP/PEEP | Rate | $FiO_2$ | Method <br> B/M? Prongs? <br> Hood Intubated |
|---|---|---|---|---|---|---|---|---|---|---|
| ____ AM/PM | ☐ | pH ____ | $pCO_2$ ____ | $pO_2$ ____ | $HCO_3$ ____ | BE ____ | ____ / ____ | ____ | ____ % | ____ |
| ____ AM/PM | ☐ | pH ____ | $pCO_2$ ____ | $pO_2$ ____ | $HCO_3$ ____ | BE ____ | ____ / ____ | ____ | ____ % | ____ |
| ____ AM/PM | ☐ | pH ____ | $pCO_2$ ____ | $pO_2$ ____ | $HCO_3$ ____ | BE ____ | ____ / ____ | ____ | ____ % | ____ |

Confidential report for improvement of hospital facility and patient care – Not part of medical record and not to be used in litigation pursuant to (state)_____ code _____

## Pre-transport Stabilization Self-Assessment Tool (PSSAT)

**SPECIFIC INTERVENTIONS**

### Airway

ET tube location (cm marking **at the lip**) when Team arrived: _____cm

Was ET tube location readjusted **prior** to the transport team arrival?   Y   N   Explain:_____

Was ET tube location readjusted **after** transport team arrival?   Y   N   Explain:_____

Was patient **re-intubated** by the transport team?   Y   N   Explain:_____

Other: _____

### Antibiotics

Time _____ AM/PM   Order for antibiotics given   Order was (Circle one)   Written   Verbally given

Time _____ AM/PM   Blood culture obtained

Time _____ AM/PM   Antibiotic 1 begun (name/dose) _____

Time _____ AM/PM   Antibiotic 2 begun (name/dose) _____

**Other stabilization efforts not yet described:** _____
_____

**Healthcare providers involved with this stabilization** (to be completed by initial healthcare facility providers). Healthcare provider who requested the transport: ☐ Family practice ☐ Pediatrician ☐ Neonatologist ☐ Midwife ☐ Nurse Practitioner ☐ Physician Assistant

Was physician or primary healthcare provider PRESENT at patient's bedside or in nursery at the time of transport team arrival?

☐ Yes ☐ No (If no, explain):_____

**TIME consultations made:** _____ AM/PM Family practice called   _____ AM/PM Pediatrician called   _____ AM/PM Neonatologist called

**Provide name or initials of other healthcare providers involved with this stabilization:**

**SELF-EVALUATION QUESTIONS**

Nurse (RN) _____

RT_____ LPN _____ Nurse Assistant_____ Other:_____

1. We feel our strengths with this stabilization effort were: _____
_____

   The following people should be commended: _____
_____

2. We feel our weaknesses with this stabilization effort were: _____
_____

3. We encountered the following barriers that altered our ability to work as a team:_____
_____

4. We wish we had the opportunity to learn more about (list all educational needs):_____
_____

5. We encountered the following problems that affected our ability to perform the stabilization we would like to perform (include equipment malfunction or equipment not available, slow response times from other healthcare departments, uncertainty about the diagnosis, communication issues, etc). _____
_____
_____

6. The next time we have to stabilize a sick neonate, we would change the following:_____
_____

   NAME OF PERSON completing this form & date: _____

# References

1. Sentinel event alert issue 30--July 21, 2004. Preventing infant death and injury during delivery. Adv Neonatal Care 2004;4:180-1.

2. Anderson JM, Warren JB. Using simulation to enhance the acquisition and retention of clinical skills in neonatology. Semin Perinatol 2011;35:59-67.

3. Draycott TJ, Crofts JF, Ash JP, et al. Improving neonatal outcome through practical shoulder dystocia training. Obstet Gynecol 2008;112:14-20.

4. Merien AE, van de Ven J, Mol BW, Houterman S, Oei SG. Multidisciplinary team training in a simulation setting for acute obstetric emergencies: a systematic review. Obstet Gynecol 2010;115:1021-31.

5. Miller KK, Riley W, Davis S, Hansen HE. In situ simulation: a method of experiential learning to promote safety and team behavior. J Perinat Neonatal Nurs 2008;22:105-13.

6. Fioratou E, Flin R, Glavin R. No simple fix for fixation errors: cognitive processes and their clinical applications. Anaesthesia 2010;65:61-9.

7. Salas E, Wilson KA, Burke CS, Priest HA. Using simulation-based training to improve patient safety: what does it take? Jt Comm J Qual Patient Saf 2005;31:363-71.

8. Gaba DM, Howard SK, Fish KJ, Smith BE, Sowb YA. Simulation-Based Training in Anesthesia Crisis Resource Management (ACRM): A Decade of Experience. Simulation & Gaming 2001;32:175-93.

9. Rudolph JW, Simon R, Raemer DB, Eppich WJ. Debriefing as formative assessment: closing performance gaps in medical education. Acad Emerg Med 2008;15:1010-6.

10. Owen H, Follows V. GREAT simulation debriefing. Med Educ 2006;40:488-9.

11. Rudolph JW, Simon R, Dufresne RL, Raemer DB. There's no such thing as "nonjudgmental" debriefing: a theory and method for debriefing with good judgment. Simul Healthc 2006;1:49-55.

12. Reason J. Human error: models and management. West J Med 2000;172:393-6.

13. Berwick DM, Leape LL. Reducing errors in medicine. Qual Health Care 1999;8:145-6.

14. Shepherd M. Improving health care systems following an incident investigation. Conf Proc IEEE Eng Med Biol Soc 2004;5:3500-2.

15. Bush MC, Jankouskas TS, Sinz EH, Rudy S, Henry J, Murray WB. A method for designing symmetrical simulation scenarios for evaluation of behavioral skills. Simul Healthc 2007;2:102-9.

16. Fanning RM, Gaba DM. The role of debriefing in simulation-based learning. Simul Healthc 2007;2:115-25.

17. Kohn LT, Corrigan JM, Donaldson MS, Committee on Quality of Health Care in America. To Err is Human: Building a Safer Health Care System. Washington, DC: National Academy Press 2000.

## Peripheral IV Insertion and Taping the IV

### PIV Insertion

▸ Getting started
- Wash and dry hands
- Apply gloves
- Clean skin with antiseptic solution

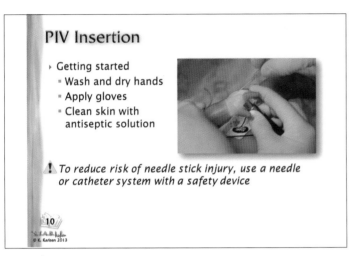

⚠ *To reduce risk of needle stick injury, use a needle or catheter system with a safety device*

slide 1

### PIV Insertion

*Catheter Selection*
▸ 24 gauge IV catheter

▸ 23 or 25 gauge butterfly needle

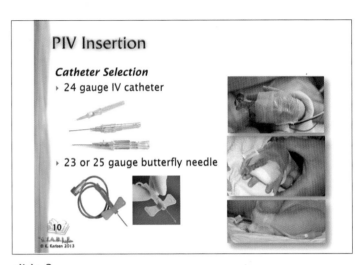

slide 2

### PIV Insertion

▸ A transilluminating light may help locate veins
▸ *Optional:* place non-latex tourniquet on extremity above area where needle or catheter will be inserted
▸ Insert needle or catheter in vein
▸ Ensure good blood return → if tourniquet used, loosen or remove

⚠ *Activate sheathing system to protect needle and promptly dispose stylet or needle in regulation sharps container*

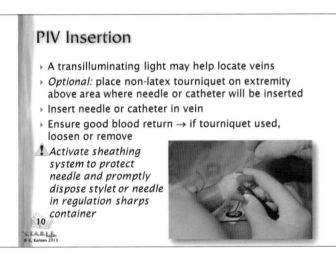

slide 3

### PIV Insertion

*Taping an IV*
▸ Place small piece of transparent dressing over catheter from hub to below insertion site
- If clear dressing not available, secure hub with 1/2 inch tape
- If using butterfly needle, secure butterfly wings with tape

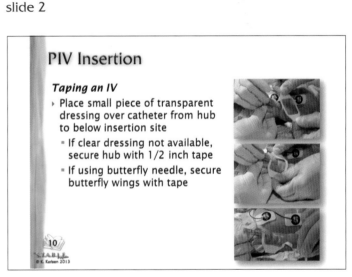

slide 4

### PIV Insertion

*Taping an IV*
▸ Periodically flush IV with small amount of sterile normal saline while taping
▸ Wrap 1/2 inch piece of tape over hub of catheter
▸ To enable observation for redness or infiltration, do not cover needle insertion site with tape

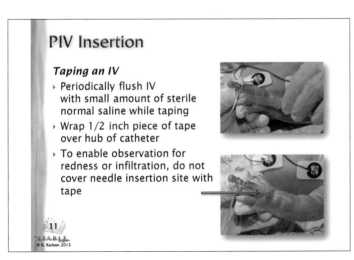

slide 5

### IV Infiltration

▸ Monitor site closely for swelling or redness → infiltration, phlebitis
▸ Document hourly
- Appearance of IV
- Amount of fluid infused

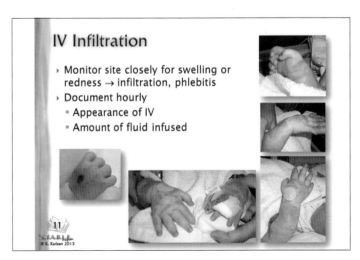

slide 6

# Positive Pressure Ventilation with Bag and Mask or T-Piece Resuscitator

## Positive Pressure Ventilation (PPV)

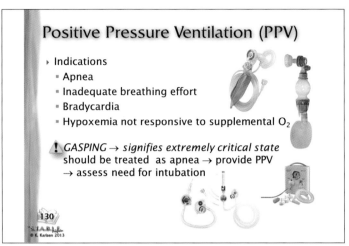

- ‣ Indications
  - ▪ Apnea
  - ▪ Inadequate breathing effort
  - ▪ Bradycardia
  - ▪ Hypoxemia not responsive to supplemental $O_2$

  **!** *GASPING → signifies extremely critical state should be treated as apnea → provide PPV → assess need for intubation*

130

S.T.A.B.L.E.
© K. Karlsen 2013

slide 1

## T-Piece Resuscitator

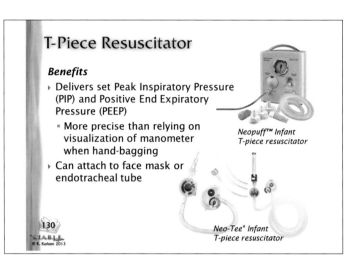

***Benefits***
- ‣ Delivers set Peak Inspiratory Pressure (PIP) and Positive End Expiratory Pressure (PEEP)
  - ▪ More precise than relying on visualization of manometer when hand-bagging
- ‣ Can attach to face mask or endotracheal tube

*Neopuff™ Infant T-piece resuscitator*

*Neo-Tee® Infant T-piece resuscitator*

130

S.T.A.B.L.E.
© K. Karlsen 2013

slide 2

## Positive Pressure Ventilation (PPV)

***Mask Selection***
- ‣ Use cushioned, anatomically shaped mask
- ‣ Mask must cover nose and mouth completely
- ‣ Bottom rim should cover edge of chin

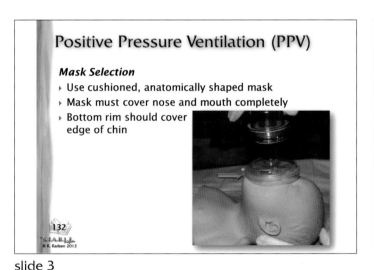

132

S.T.A.B.L.E.
© K. Karlsen 2013

slide 3

## Positive Pressure Ventilation (PPV)

***Mask Position***
- ‣ Avoid pressure over eyes
- ‣ A well-fitting mask will help ensure a good seal

132

S.T.A.B.L.E.
© K. Karlsen 2013

slide 4

## Positive Pressure Ventilation (PPV)

***Technique***
- ‣ Place thumb and index finger over top of mask to form a "C"
- ‣ Use 3rd, 4th and 5th fingers to form an "E" → allows good control of chin
  - ▪ Lift chin up toward mask
- ‣ Use light downward pressure

**!** Do not press head into bed
Avoid pressure on trachea

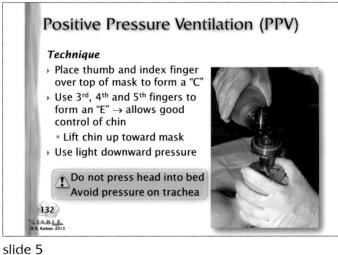

132

S.T.A.B.L.E.
© K. Karlsen 2013

slide 5

## Positive Pressure Ventilation (PPV)

- ‣ Watch for chest rise while squeezing bag or occluding T-piece
  - ▪ If bradycardic, watch for ↑ in heart rate

**!** Avoid excessive chest rise

132

S.T.A.B.L.E.
© K. Karlsen 2013

slide 6

# Positive Pressure Ventilation with Bag and Mask or T-Piece Resuscitator (continued)

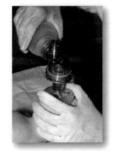

slide 7

# Endotracheal Intubation: Assisting, Verifying Placement and Securing ET Tube

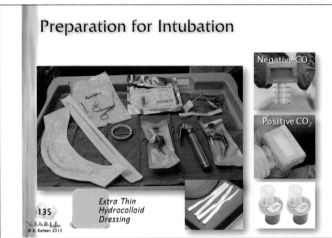

slide 1

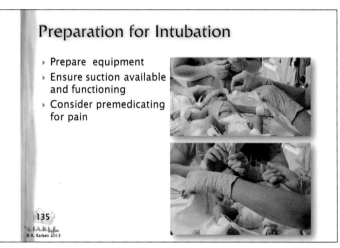

slide 2

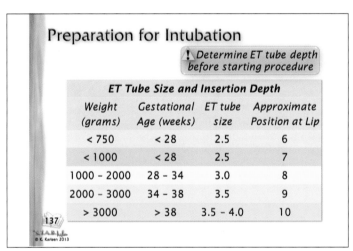

slide 3

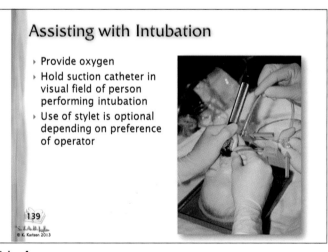

slide 4

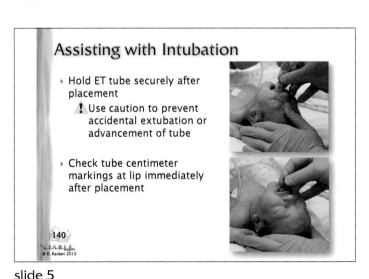

slide 5

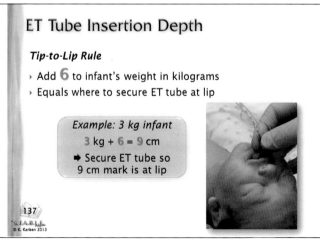

slide 6

The following text appears within the slides:

**Slide 1 — Preparation for Intubation**
Negative CO₂ / Positive CO₂
Extra Thin Hydrocolloid Dressing
135
S.T.A.B.L.E. © K. Karlsen 2013

**Slide 2 — Preparation for Intubation**
- Prepare equipment
- Ensure suction available and functioning
- Consider premedicating for pain
135
S.T.A.B.L.E. © K. Karlsen 2013

**Slide 3 — Preparation for Intubation**
! Determine ET tube depth before starting procedure

### ET Tube Size and Insertion Depth

| Weight (grams) | Gestational Age (weeks) | ET tube size | Approximate Position at Lip |
|---|---|---|---|
| < 750 | < 28 | 2.5 | 6 |
| < 1000 | < 28 | 2.5 | 7 |
| 1000 – 2000 | 28 – 34 | 3.0 | 8 |
| 2000 – 3000 | 34 – 38 | 3.5 | 9 |
| > 3000 | > 38 | 3.5 – 4.0 | 10 |

137
S.T.A.B.L.E. © K. Karlsen 2013

**Slide 4 — Assisting with Intubation**
- Provide oxygen
- Hold suction catheter in visual field of person performing intubation
- Use of stylet is optional depending on preference of operator
139
S.T.A.B.L.E. © K. Karlsen 2013

**Slide 5 — Assisting with Intubation**
- Hold ET tube securely after placement
  ! Use caution to prevent accidental extubation or advancement of tube
- Check tube centimeter markings at lip immediately after placement
140
S.T.A.B.L.E. © K. Karlsen 2013

**Slide 6 — ET Tube Insertion Depth**
*Tip-to-Lip Rule*
- Add 6 to infant's weight in kilograms
- Equals where to secure ET tube at lip

Example: 3 kg infant
3 kg + 6 = 9 cm
➡ Secure ET tube so 9 cm mark is at lip
137
S.T.A.B.L.E. © K. Karlsen 2013

# Endotracheal Intubation: Assisting, Verifying Placement and Securing ET Tube (continued)

### Securing Endotracheal Tubes

- Cut two pieces of adhesive tape
  - One "V"
  - One "X"

- If possible, prepare cheeks and upper lip with base layer of hydrocolloid material

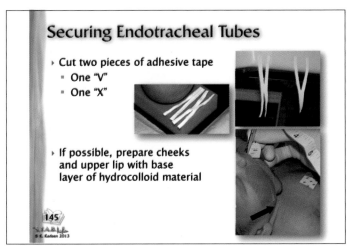

145

slide 7

### Securing Endotracheal Tubes

- Hold ET tube entire time
- Apply "X" piece first to upper lip

145

slide 8

### Securing Endotracheal Tubes

- Wrap lower tape around tube – moving up slightly onto tube
- Wrap other side of tape
- Make tab

146

slide 9

### Securing Endotracheal Tubes

- Apply upper part of "V" over upper lip tape
- Wrap lower piece around tube – working up slightly

146

slide 10

### Securing Endotracheal Tubes

- Wrap until ½ inch of tape remains
- Make a tab → allows easier unfastening if tube needs to be repositioned

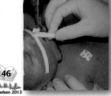
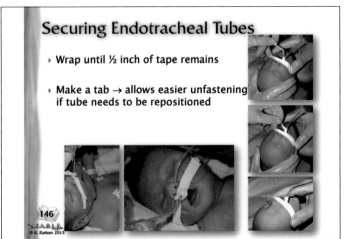

146

slide 11

### Securing Endotracheal Tubes

- Place a gastric tube to decompress stomach
- Trim ET tube as needed

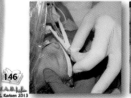
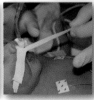
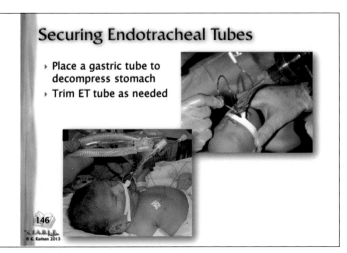

146

slide 12

**308**

# Endotracheal Intubation: Assisting, Verifying Placement and Securing ET Tube (continued)

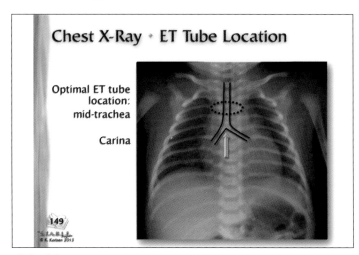

slide 13

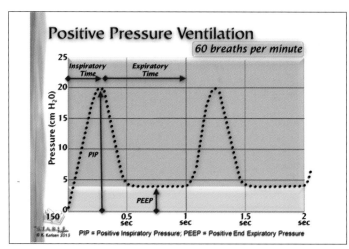

slide 14

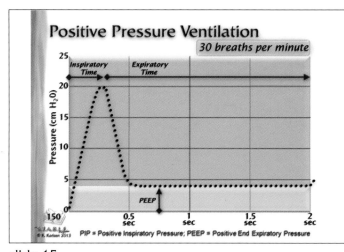

slide 15

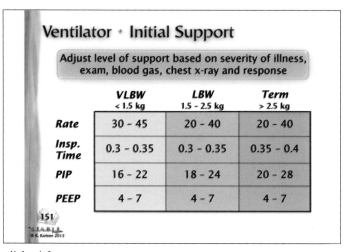

slide 16

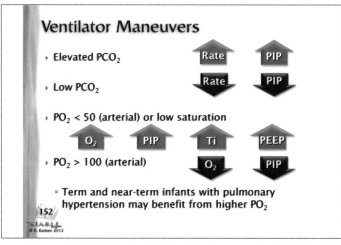

slide 17

# Umbilical Venous Catheter Insertion

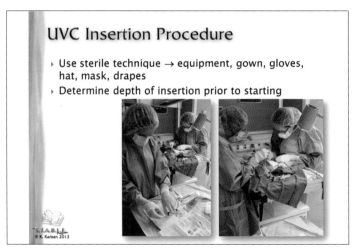

slide 1

slide 2

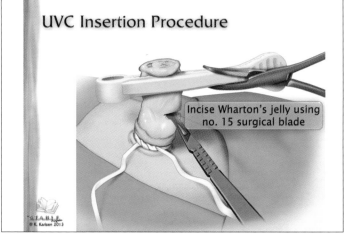

slide 3

slide 4

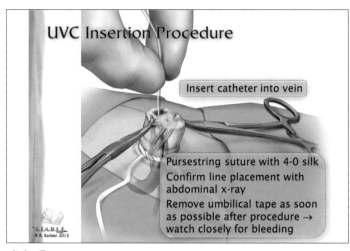

slide 5

slide 6

# Umbilical Venous Catheter Insertion (continued)

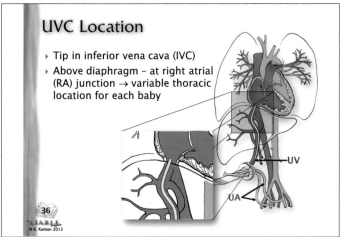

slide 7

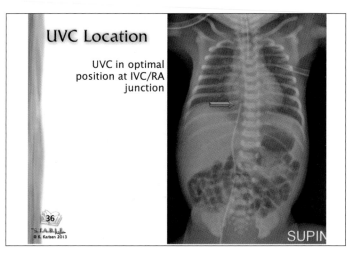

slide 8

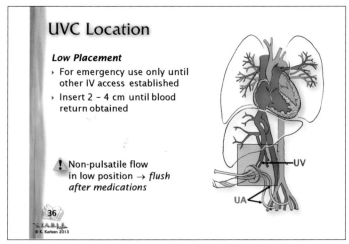

slide 9

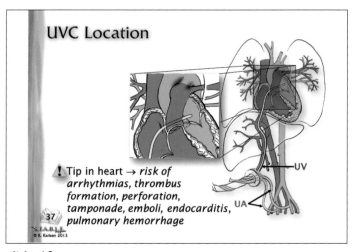

slide 10

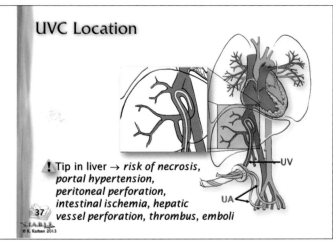

slide 11

# Umbilical Venous Catheter Insertion (continued)

## Line Malposition Series

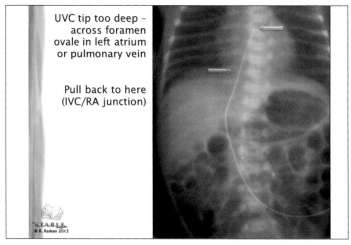

UVC tip too deep – across foramen ovale in left atrium or pulmonary vein

Pull back to here (IVC/RA junction)

slide 12

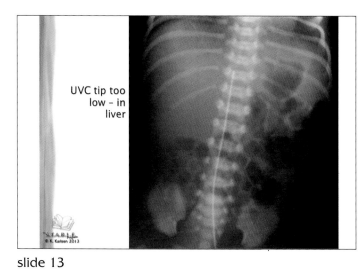

UVC tip too low – in liver

slide 13

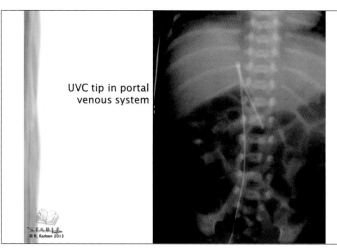

UVC tip in portal venous system

slide 14

# Umbilical Artery Catheter Insertion

### Umbilical Artery Catheterization

*Use sterile technique* → equipment, gown, gloves, hat, mask, drapes

*Catheter size*
› Under 1.5 kg → 3.5 French
› Over 1.5 kg → 5 French

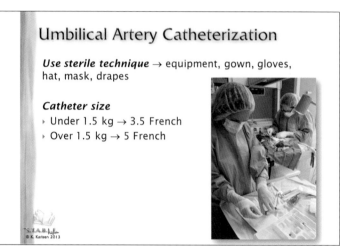

slide 1

### Umbilical Artery Catheterization

*Location*
› High line → tip located between T6 and T9
› Low line → tip located between L3 and L4
› Confirm placement with x-ray

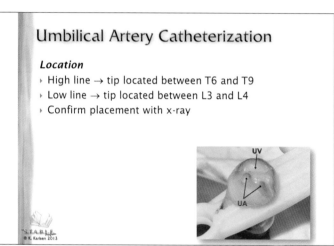

slide 2

### Umbilical Artery Catheterization

*Calculating insertion depth**
› Determine distance before starting procedure
› Refer to graph in Learner Manual p. 57 or calculate
*High UAC*
› UA catheter length (in cm) =
  [3 X birth weight (in kg)] + 9
*UVC*
› UV catheter length (in cm) =
  [0.5 X high line UA catheter length (in cm)] + 1

⚠ *May overestimate insertion depth → confirm placement with x-ray

From Sigman (2012)
The Harriet Lane Handbook

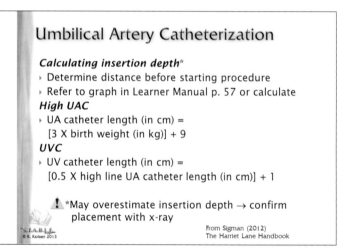

slide 3

### Umbilical Artery Catheterization

› Catheter size
  ▪ Under 1.5 kg → 3.5 French
  ▪ Over 1.5 kg → 5 French

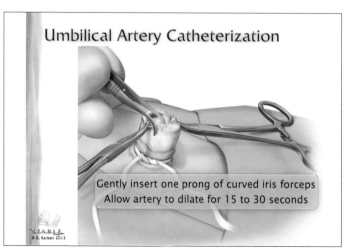

slide 4

### Umbilical Artery Catheterization

Securely hold umbilical cord through Wharton's jelly with curved hemostats

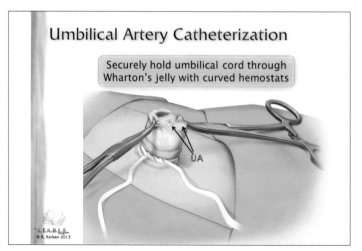

slide 5

### Umbilical Artery Catheterization

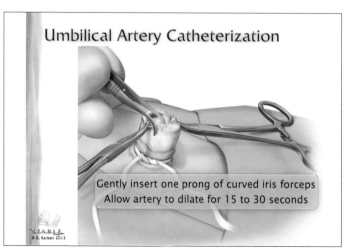

Gently insert one prong of curved iris forceps
Allow artery to dilate for 15 to 30 seconds

slide 6

# Umbilical Artery Catheter Insertion   (continued)

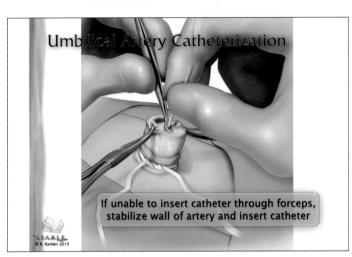

slide 7

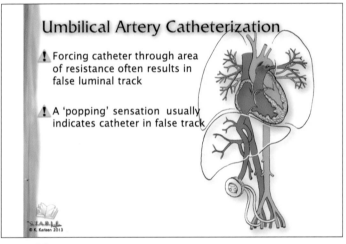

slide 8

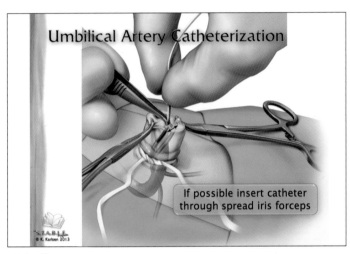

slide 9

## Umbilical Artery Catheterization

- Resistance may be met at intersection of umbilical artery / iliac artery → approximately 6 to 8 centimeters from umbilical stump
  - Apply steady gentle pressure for 30 to 60 seconds
  - ! Do not force catheter through areas of obstruction

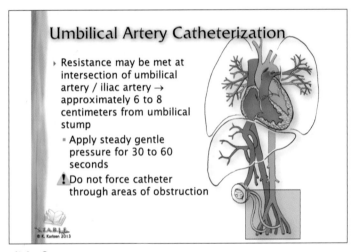

slide 10

## Umbilical Artery Catheterization

- ! Forcing catheter through area of resistance often results in false luminal track

- ! A 'popping' sensation usually indicates catheter in false track

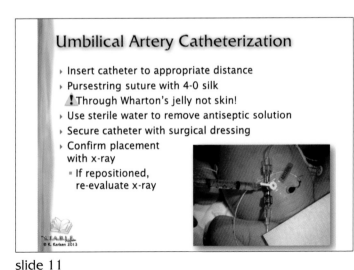

slide 11

## Umbilical Artery Catheterization

- Insert catheter to appropriate distance
- Pursestring suture with 4-0 silk
  - ! Through Wharton's jelly not skin!
- Use sterile water to remove antiseptic solution
- Secure catheter with surgical dressing
- Confirm placement with x-ray
  - If repositioned, re-evaluate x-ray

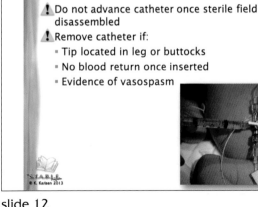

slide 12

## Umbilical Artery Catheterization

- ! Do not advance catheter once sterile field disassembled
- ! Remove catheter if:
  - Tip located in leg or buttocks
  - No blood return once inserted
  - Evidence of vasospasm

# Umbilical Artery Catheter Insertion (continued)

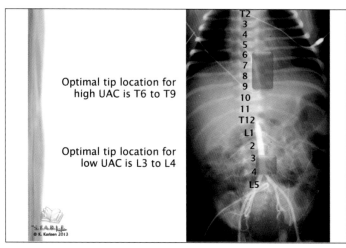

Optimal tip location for high UAC is T6 to T9

Optimal tip location for low UAC is L3 to L4

(T2, 3, 4, 5, 6, 7, 8, 9, 10, 11, T12, L1, 2, 3, 4, L5)

slide 13

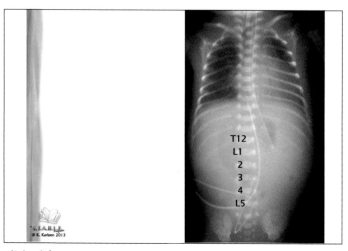

**Note origin of:**
- Spinal arteries off thoracic aorta
- Celiac trunk arteries T11 – L1
- Superior mesenteric artery T12 – L1
- Renal arteries L1 – L2
- Inferior mesenteric artery L2 – L3/4
- Bifurcation of aorta L3/4 – L5

(T2, 3, 4, 5, 6, 7, 8, 9, 10, 11, T12, L1, 2, 3, 4, L5)

slide 14

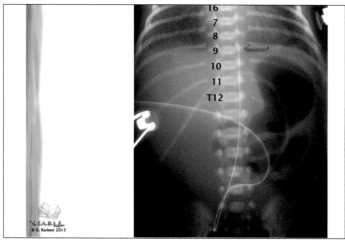

(T6, 7, 8, 9, 10, 11, T12)

slide 15

slide 16

(T12, L1, 2, 3, 4, L5)

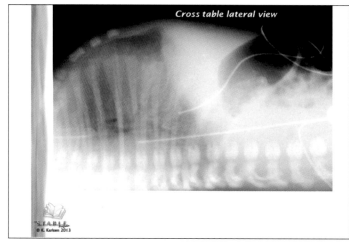

*Cross table lateral view*

slide 17

# Umbilical Artery Catheter Insertion (continued)

## Line Malposition Series

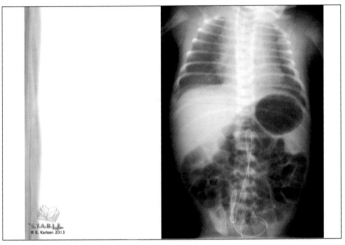

slide 18

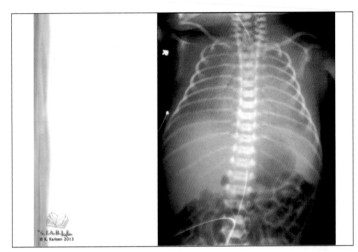

slide 19

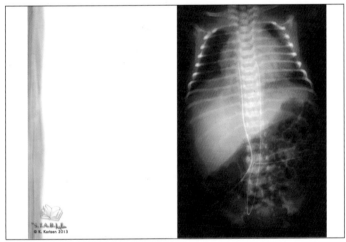

slide 20

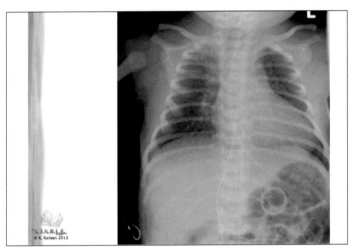

slide 21

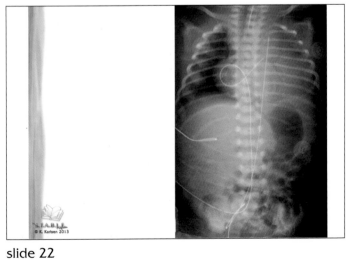

slide 22

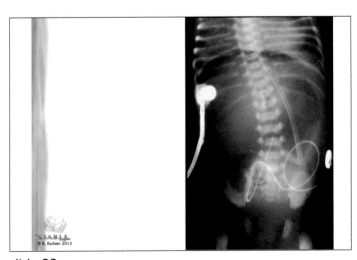

slide 23

# Pneumothorax Evacuation: Needle Aspiration of the Chest[1-4]

There are two options for needle insertion. The first is a **lateral** approach and the second is an **anterior** approach. The lateral approach is recommended because of the reduced risk for hitting major blood vessels in the anterior medial region of the chest. Prior to starting the procedure, decide which landmarks will be used.

## Lateral approach and landmarks

Turn the infant 45 degrees with the affected (pneumothorax) side up and support the back with a small blanket. Move the arm up and away from the catheter insertion site. The needle or catheter will be inserted into the 4th intercostal space (the space between the 4th and 5th rib) in the mid-axillary or anterior axillary line. This location is usually adjacent to the nipple line and down approximately one centimeter. Care must be taken to avoid the breast tissue.

## Anterior approach and landmarks

If using the anterior approach, position the infant supine with the head of the bed slightly elevated (so that air will rise). The needle or catheter will be inserted into the 2nd intercostal space (the space between the 2nd and 3rd rib) in the midclavicular line. The 3rd intercostal space (between the 3rd and 4th rib) may also be used.[4] Take care to avoid inserting the needle into breast tissue.

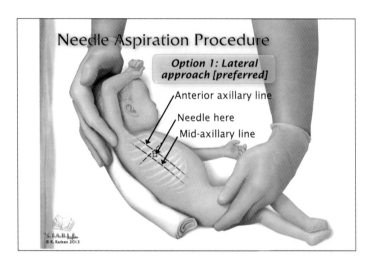

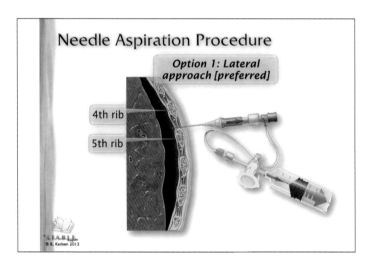

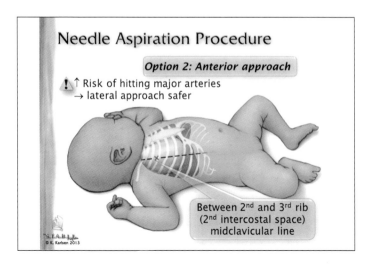

# Pneumothorax Evacuation: Needle Aspiration of the Chest[1-4]
(continued)

## Step by Step Procedure for Either the Lateral or Anterior Approach

1. Gather all of the equipment that will be needed:

   a) 18, 20, or 22-gauge angiocatheter (preferred), or 19, 21, or 23-gauge butterfly needle. Use the smaller angiocatheter or butterfly needle for the preterm infant.

   b) 20 or 30 mL syringe.

   c) 3-way stopcock.

   d) T-connector or short IV extension tubing (if using an angiocatheter).

   e) Antiseptic solution to clean the skin.

   f) Sterile gloves.

2. If possible, time allows, and appropriate cardiorespiratory and oxygen saturation monitoring can be performed, pre-medicate the infant with an analgesic medication. Assemble the needle aspiration kit. Open the stopcock and aspirate on the syringe to make sure air can pass easily into the syringe.

3. Apply sterile gloves and cleanse the skin with antiseptic solution. Use sterile technique throughout the procedure.

4. The catheter or needle will be inserted into the pleural space, above the rib to avoid the intercostal artery and nerve which are located on the inferior surface of the rib. Avoid excessive insertion depth of the stylet or butterfly needle.

> ⚠ Be careful to insert the needle as close to the **top** of the rib as possible to avoid hitting the blood vessels and nerve that are located on the underside surface of the rib.

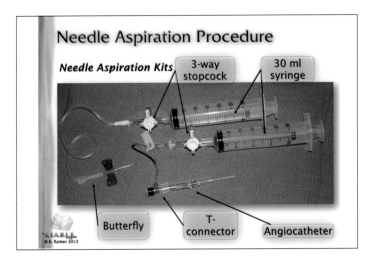

**Needle Aspiration Procedure**

‣ Needle aspiration
  ▪ 18, 20 or 22-gauge angiocatheter (preferred) or 19, 21 or 23-gauge butterfly needle
  ▪ 30 mL syringe
  ▪ 3-way stopcock
  ▪ T-connector or short IV extension tubing → if using angiocatheter
  ▪ Antiseptic solution to cleanse skin
‣ Chest tube → 10 or 12 French
  ▪ Heimlich one-way flutter valve or chest tube drainage system

**Needle Aspiration Procedure**

Needle Aspiration Kits — 3-way stopcock — 30 ml syringe — Butterfly — T-connector — Angiocatheter

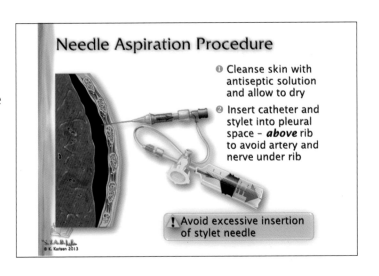

**Needle Aspiration Procedure**

❶ Cleanse skin with antiseptic solution and allow to dry

❷ Insert catheter and stylet into pleural space – *above* rib to avoid artery and nerve under rib

⚠ Avoid excessive insertion of stylet needle

# Pneumothorax Evacuation: Needle Aspiration of the Chest[1-4]
(continued)

### If using an IV catheter (angiocatheter)

Remove the stylet once the catheter enters the pleural space (avoid excessive insertion depth of the stylet). Advance the catheter further into the pleural space. With the stylet removed, attach the catheter hub to the pre-assembled T-connector, stopcock, and syringe set-up. Ask the assistant to gently aspirate on the syringe. If no air is obtained, the catheter may need to be inserted further.

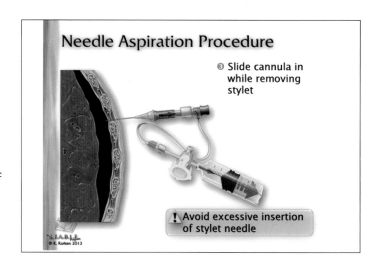

Note: some centers recommend leaving the IV catheter in place to allow for periodic aspiration to check whether air is re-accumulating.

However, this is a short-term measure. If the air leak is ongoing, the infant will most likely need a chest tube placed. Remember that the IV catheter is soft and flexible; if it is secured in place after insertion, there is the risk of kinking and obstruction, which may result in an inability to successfully aspirate air from the pleural space.

### If using a butterfly needle

Before inserting the butterfly needle into the chest, attach the IV tubing to the pre-assembled three-way stopcock and syringe. Aspirate on the syringe to make sure air is obtained. This will ensure the stopcock is open from the IV needle tip to the syringe. As the needle is inserted into the pleural space, ask the assistant to gently aspirate on the syringe. When a gush of air is obtained, stop advancing the needle (to avoid piercing lung tissue). If no air is obtained at the point you think you are already in the pleural space, stop inserting the sharp needle tip further. Try repositioning the patient to allow air to rise to the area beneath the needle and consider changing needle insertion sites. The butterfly needle is sharp and will therefore need to be removed when the procedure is finished.

# Pneumothorax Evacuation: Needle Aspiration of the Chest[1-4]
(continued)

5. If not done already, open the stopcock to the patient.

6. Gently aspirate on the plunger until resistance is met, or until the syringe is full of air.

7. Turn the stopcock off to the patient.

8. Rapidly push the air out of the syringe into the air. Be careful not to spray this air, which may contain body fluids. Repeat this process until all of the air is evacuated.

9. If air is rapidly re-accumulating, then it may be necessary to insert a chest tube.

10. When the procedure is completed, transilluminate the chest again to obtain another baseline assessment. A chest x-ray will also help identify whether the pneumothorax has been drained completely.

11. Frequently reassess the infant's condition to monitor for re-accumulation of the pneumothorax.

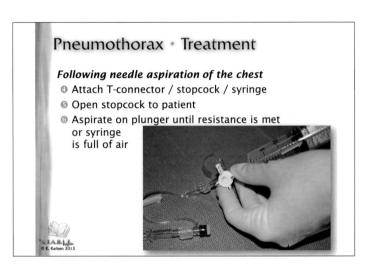

Pneumothorax · Treatment

*Following needle aspiration of the chest*
④ Attach T-connector / stopcock / syringe
⑤ Open stopcock to patient
⑥ Aspirate on plunger until resistance is met or syringe is full of air

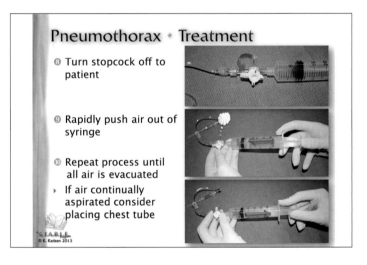

Pneumothorax · Treatment

⑧ Turn stopcock off to patient

⑨ Rapidly push air out of syringe

⑩ Repeat process until all air is evacuated
  ‣ If air continually aspirated consider placing chest tube

# Pneumothorax Evacuation: Chest Tube Insertion[1-6]

### Preparation

A size 8, 10, and 12 Fr. thoracostomy tube should be available. Use the size appropriate to the patient's size and gestational age. Alternatively, a pigtail catheter, inserted percutaneously may be utilized. The selection of a thoracostomy tube versus pigtail catheter should depend upon the experience and comfort level of the person performing the procedure.

The following description is for placement of a thoracostomy tube for drainage of a pneumothorax (tube placed in an anterior position to rest above the affected lung).

- Attach cardiorespiratory and pulse oximeter equipment in locations that will not interfere with the surgical field.

- Provide fentanyl analgesic medication since fentanyl has a more rapid onset of action than morphine. Be careful to not give the fentanyl too quickly or the infant may experience negative side effects including rigid chest. Provide comfort measures to the infant.

- Maintain sterile technique throughout the surgical procedure. Use sterile gloves, gown, and drapes, and wear a surgical cap or hat, and mask.

**If the patient condition allows,** prior to sterile skin cleansing and draping, identify the intended insertion landmark, clean the skin with alcohol and infiltrate the skin with 1% lidocaine to locally anesthetize the skin. This will allow time for the lidocaine to take effect. If the patient is experiencing severe cardiorespiratory compromise just proceed quickly with cleansing, sterile draping, infiltrating with lidocaine, and incising the skin.

# Pneumothorax Evacuation: Chest Tube Insertion[1-6] (continued)

## Step by Step Procedure for Inserting a Chest Tube Using a Lateral Approach

1. Turn the infant 45 degrees with the **affected (pneumothorax) side *up***. Place a roll behind infant's back to support the infant. Move the arm up over the head or lateral so that it is clear of the surgical field.

2. Cleanse the skin with antiseptic solution.

3. If not already done, infiltrate the skin at the incision site with 1% lidocaine to locally anesthetize the skin.

4. Use a surgical blade to make a small skin incision (parallel to the rib) at approximately the 6th rib in the anterior axillary or mid-axillary line. **Be sure to avoid incising into the areola and surrounding breast tissue.**

5. Enter the incision with a curved mosquito hemostat.

6. Perform blunt dissection of the subcutaneous tissue overlying the rib. Tunnel over the top of the 5th rib toward the 4th rib until the tips are located at the 4th intercostal space.

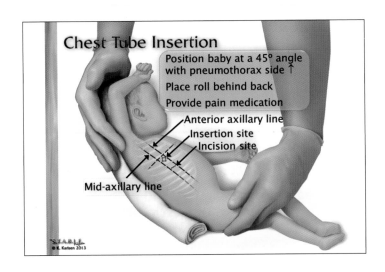

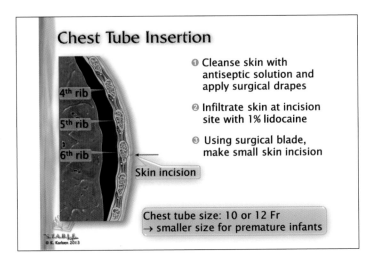

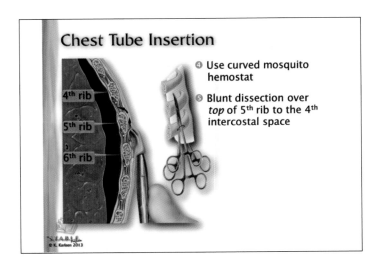

# Pneumothorax Evacuation: Chest Tube Insertion[1-6] (continued)

7. Apply steady pressure on the tips of the hemostat until the tips pass through the intercostal muscle and parietal pleura. Be careful to stay close to the top of the rib to avoid hitting the blood vessels and nerve that are located on the underside of the rib. A rush of air may be heard when the pleural space is entered.

8. To prevent injury to the lung, be careful to not insert the tips of the hemostat any more than necessary, which is usually less than 1 centimeter, to reach the pleural space.

9. Spread the hemostat enough to open the puncture space and to allow insertion of the chest tube.

10. If possible, insert the chest tube between the spread hemostat tips. Advance the chest tube while aiming anteriorly toward the midclavicular line.

> ⚠ Avoid using a trocar or other sharp instrument during insertion of the tube since these instruments may increase risk for lung injury (lung puncture, phrenic nerve damage that paralyzes the diaphragm, and bleeding).

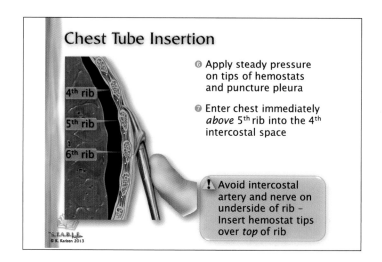

**Chest Tube Insertion**

- 4th rib
- 5th rib
- 6th rib

6 Apply steady pressure on tips of hemostats and puncture pleura

7 Enter chest immediately *above* 5th rib into the 4th intercostal space

⚠ Avoid intercostal artery and nerve on underside of rib – Insert hemostat tips over *top* of rib

© K. Karlsen 2013

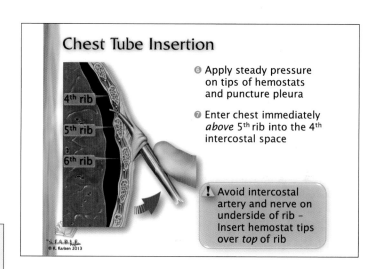

**Chest Tube Insertion**

- 4th rib
- 5th rib
- 6th rib

6 Apply steady pressure on tips of hemostats and puncture pleura

7 Enter chest immediately *above* 5th rib into the 4th intercostal space

⚠ Avoid intercostal artery and nerve on underside of rib – Insert hemostat tips over *top* of rib

© K. Karlsen 2013

# Pneumothorax Evacuation: Chest Tube Insertion[1-6] (continued)

11. Ensure that all side holes of the chest tube are within the thorax.

12. Close the skin with one suture and wrap the suture around the tube. A purse-string suture may create more scar tissue so should be avoided if possible.

13. Secure the chest tube with a sterile occlusive dressing.

14. Attach the chest tube to a underwater seal drainage system with 10 to 20 cm $H_2O$ suction or per the manufacturer's recommendation. Alternatively, the chest tube may be connected to a Heimlich one-way flutter valve device. Position infant to improve drainage (remember air rises).

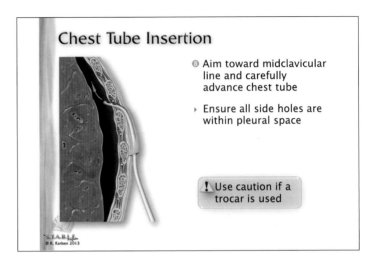

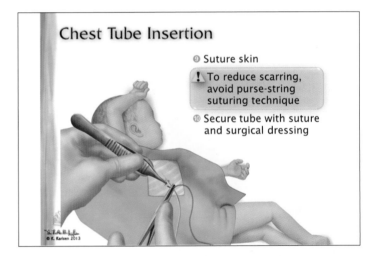

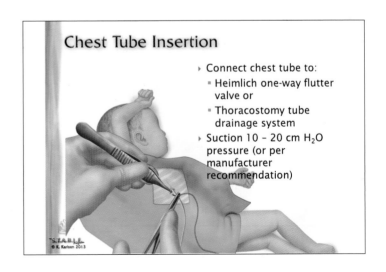

# Pneumothorax Evacuation: Chest Tube Insertion[1-6] (continued)

## Clinical Tip

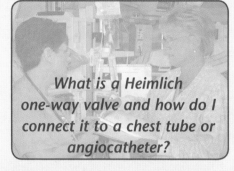

*What is a Heimlich one-way valve and how do I connect it to a chest tube or angiocatheter?*

A Heimlich valve can be connected directly to a chest tube for transport (top photo) or it can be connected to an angiocatheter needle aspiration set-up (bottom photo).

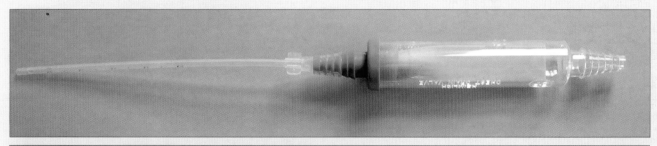

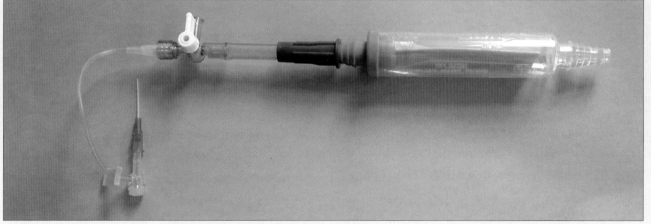

To connect the Heimlich valve to an angiocatheter, take a sterile suction connection tubing and using sterile scissors, cut off the end (as shown). Attach the blue end of the tubing to the Heimlich valve. Attach the trimmed end of the suction tubing to a 3-way stopcock. An IV tubing T-connector is then attached to the stopcock which is attached to the angiocatheter that is in the chest. If the pneumothorax is under enough pressure, it will escape through the Heimlich valve. However, if the patient is unstable, turn the stopcock off to the Heimlich valve and gently aspirate using the 3-way stopcock to evaluate for residual air. If direct aspiration does not help improve the patient's condition, and pneumothorax is suspected as the cause, then the patient may need a chest tube inserted emergently. Chest tube insertion should be performed by personnel with the proper training.

# Pneumothorax Evacuation: Chest Tube Insertion[1-6] (continued)

15. Confirm placement of the chest tube with both an anterior-posterior (AP) and cross table (XT) lateral chest x-ray. This will confirm whether the chest tube is anterior or posterior. For evacuation of air, the chest tube should be placed anteriorly. To drain fluid (pleural effusion or chylothorax), the chest tube should be placed posteriorly.

16. Transilluminate the chest to evaluate baseline appearance of the evacuated pneumothorax. This will enable re-evaluation by transillumination if it is suspected that the pneumothorax has re-accumulated.

17 If air has failed to evacuate following chest tube insertion, try increasing the suction on the drainage device by 5 cm $H_2O$ increments (to max recommended by manufacturer of device), try repositioning the infant to allow air to move towards the chest tube holes, and finally, if these measures are ineffective and the infant's condition is not satisfactory, consider inserting a second chest tube.

**Consult the tertiary center neonatologist if the infant is failing to improve or there are any questions about patient management.**

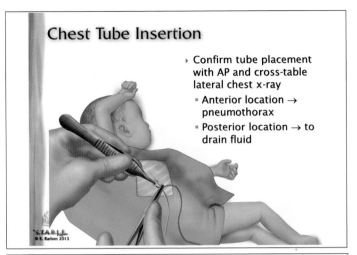

**Chest Tube Insertion**

▸ Confirm tube placement with AP and cross-table lateral chest x-ray
- Anterior location → pneumothorax
- Posterior location → to drain fluid

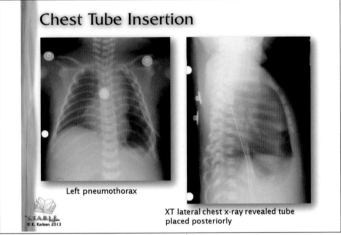

**Chest Tube Insertion**

Left pneumothorax

XT lateral chest x-ray revealed tube placed posteriorly

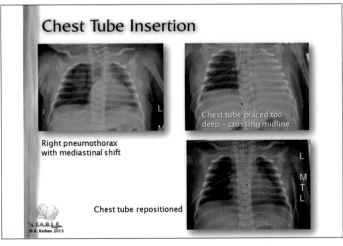

**Chest Tube Insertion**

Right pneumothorax with mediastinal shift

Chest tube placed too deep – crossing midline

Chest tube repositioned

## References
### Needle Aspiration and Chest Tube Insertion

1. Rais-Bahrami K, MacDonald M, G., Eichelberger MR. Thoracostomy tubes. In: MacDonald M, G., Ramasethu J, eds. Atlas of Procedures in Neonatology. 4th ed. Philadelphia: Wolters Kluwer / Lippincott Williams & Wilkins; 2007:261-84.

2. Sigman LJ. Procedures. In: Tschudy MM, Arcara KM, eds. The Harriet Lane Handbook. 19th ed. Philadelphia: Elsevier Mosby; 2012:57-88.

3. Pammi M. Pulmonary Air Leak. In: Cloherty JP, Eichenwald EC, Hansen AR, Stark AR, eds. Manual of Neonatal Care. 7th ed. Philadelphia: Lippincott, Williams & Wilkins; 2012:446-53.

4. Gardner SL, Enzman-Hines M, Dickey LA. Respiratory Diseases. In: Gardner SL, Carter BS, Enzman-Hines M, Hernandez JA, eds. Merenstein & Gardner's Handbook of Neonatal Intensive Care. 7th ed. St. Louis: Mosby Elsevier; 2011:581-677.

5. Abu-Shaweesh JM. Respiratory Disorders in Preterm and Term Infants. In: Martin RJ, Fanaroff AA, Walsh MC, eds. Fanaroff and Martin's Neonatal-Perinatal Medicine: Diseases of the Fetus and Infant. 9th ed. St. Louis: Elsevier Mosby; 2011:1141-70.

6. Bancalari E, Claure N. Principles of Respiratory Monitoring and Therapy. In: Gleason CA, Devaskar SU, eds. Avery's Diseases of the Newborn 9th ed. Philadelphia Elsevier Saunders 2012:612-32.

# Index

# Index

**335**

# Index

Transposition of the great arteries, 107, 108
  blood flow pattern seen with, 107*f*

Tricuspid atresia, 107, 108

Tricyclic antidepressants, risk for neonatal hypoglycemia and, 13*t*

Triponin I, 204

Trisomy 21 (Down syndrome) with duodenal atresia, 47*f*

Truncus arteriosus, 108

Twin-to-twin transfusion syndrome, 199

Type II diabetes, maternal family history of, as risk factor for gestational diabetes mellitus, 18

## U

Umbilical artery catheter (UAC), 35*t*
  abdominal x-ray of term infant showing tip in good position, 42*f*
  actions to take when malpositioned
    high positioned, 44*t*
    low positioned, 44*t*
  chest and abdominal x-ray of preterm infant with, 42*f*
  high, 56
  high versus low positioned
    high line, 41*t*
    low line, 41*t*
  low, 56
  possible complications from, 45
  selection of, 33
  speed in withdrawal of blood from high positioned, 46
Umbilical catheters
  calculating depth using mathematical formulas, 56
  cross table lateral x-ray showing the pathway of, 43*f*
  determining tip location using graph, 57–58
  directions for securing, using sterile transparent semipermeable membrane dressing, 39*f*
  indications for, 33
  safety guidelines for, 38, 40
Umbilical cord accident, 199
Umbilical cord injury, 199
Umbilical vein, 9
Umbilical vein catheter (UVC), 34*t*
  chest and abdominal x-ray of preterm infant with, 42*f*
  chest x-ray of infant showing correct position, 36*f*
  selection of, 33
  tip location and complications related to malposition, 36–37*t*
    central location, 36*t*

complications of malposition in the heart, 37*t*
complications of malposition in the liver or portal venous system, 37*t*
emergency placement, 36*t*
Umbilical venous catheters, 9, 56
  dopamine infusion and, 214
Uncompensated metabolic acidosis, 122
Uncompensated mixed metabolic and respiratory acidosis, 123
Uncompensated respiratory acidosis, 122
Uncompensated shock, 190
  hypotension and, 193
  in premature infants, 191
Uncuffed endotracheal tubes in endotracheal intubation, 135
Universal pulse oximetry screening, 108
Urinary tract infection, as risk factor for neonatal infection, 231*t*
Urine output
  evaluating, 203*t*
  shock and, 193

## V

VACTERL association, 178

Vacuum-assisted delivery, risk factors associated with development of subgaleal hemorrhage, 218, 218*f*

Valvular obstruction, 193

Van't Hoff's law, 69*f*

Vascular integrity, 201

Vascular resistance, increased systemic, 191

Vasoconstriction, 66
  peripheral, 66
  pulmonary, norepinephrine and, 71–72, 71*f*, 72*f*

Venous blood pH, 123, 123*n*

Venous return, decreased volume of, 191

Ventilation, need for adequate respiration and cardiac function in, 113

Ventricular septal defect, 193

Very-low-birth weight infants, bleeding time in, 250

Very-low-birth weight preterm infants, signs of shock in, 191

Viral infection, as cause for cardiogenic shock, 201

Viral organisms, as cause of neonatal infection, 233

Vital signs, evaluating and recording, 97

Vocal cords, swollen, 158

Volume bolus, calculating, 206

## W

Warming mattresses, 76

Washing PRBCs, 207

Well-being, evaluating and recording signs of, 97

Well infants, maintenance of normal body temperature in, 64–65

Wheezing, 102

White blood cells, 239
  types of, 239

Whole blood glucose test, accuracy of, 24